PARADE
Family Health Companion

Jan 97

To Carol and Arnold:

Here's to your

good health!

Love—

Randi

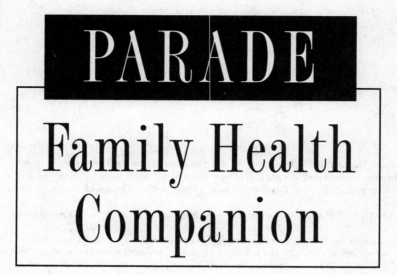

PARADE
Family Health Companion

A REASSURING GUIDE TO DEALING WITH
LIFE'S DAY-TO-DAY HEALTH ISSUES

Earl Ubell

With Randi Londer Gould

PRIMA PUBLISHING

PRIMA PUBLISHING and colophon are registered trademarks of Prima Communications, Inc.

Library of Congress Cataloging-in-Publication Data

Ubell, Earl.
Parade family health companion: a reassuring guide to dealing with life's day-to-day health issues / Earl Ubell, with Randi L. Gould.
p.   cm.
Includes index.
ISBN 0-7615-0307-2
1. Health.   2. Medical care.   3. Medicine, Popular.   I. Gould, Randi L.   II. Title.
RA776.U235 1996

613—dc20   96-42073
CIP

96 97 98 99 AA 10 9 8 7 6 5 4 3 2 1
Printed in the United States of America

HOW TO ORDER:

Single copies may be ordered from Prima Publishing, P.O. Box 1260BK, Rocklin, CA 95677; telephone (916) 632-4400. Quantity discounts are also available. On your letterhead, include information concerning the intended use of the books and the number of books you wish to purchase.

Visit us online at http://www.primapublishing.com

To *Jules Ritholz, Joseph Messina, and Phillip Segall,* who left us all too soon.

—EU

To my *Benjamin,* for his unending love and support; and to *Eileen,* for never letting me forget.

—RLG

CONTENTS

The Brain

The Heart

Diet and Fitness

High-Tech Medicine

Mental Health

Sex

Fertility

Hormones

Immune System

Cancer

Digestive Diseases

Plastic Surgery

Dental Health

Eyes and Ears

Aging

ACKNOWLEDGMENTS

Walter Anderson, the longtime editor of *Parade,* had the confidence in me for this gigantic task of reporting the world of medicine to the world. I have had many editors in my career. Walter is by far the best: a knowledgeable cheerleader who kept me going during hard times and encouraged me to be highly prolific in the good times.

Randi Londer Gould was my researcher for nearly all of this text. In 13 years, I learned to rely on her diligence in digging out the facts and pushing ever forward during many deadlines. These articles are as much her product as they are mine.

To Larry Smith, managing editor, David Currier, executive editor, and Ira Yoffe, design director, of *Parade,* I give special thanks for their patience and support. Similarly, I am thankful to all the people at *Parade* who have been just great, including Gael McCarthy, editor of many pieces, and Anita Goss, who has been indefatigable in rooting out errors and misquotes, saving my life more than once.

My family, in its entirety, also provided support and forbearance. They knew how crazy an author can get around deadline time. I want especially to thank my brother Bob, who found a good publisher for this work. To Steven Martin and Jennifer

xvi Acknowledgments

Basye Sander of Prima Publishing, thanks for their diligence in
bringing this book to fruition. And to my friends Carol C. Flax,
Stuart H. Loory, Carol Berczuk, Gail Levey, Jenifer Woodson,
Colette Le Joncour, and Alvin Moscow—all of whom, each in
his or her own way, contributed to this mighty work.

INTRODUCTION

I wrote these pieces as Health Editor of *Parade* magazine over a period of 13 years and brought them up to date for inclusion in this book. Of course, many things are left as I originally wrote them, mostly the names of the scientists and the patients who people this book. (I haven't counted, but there must be hundreds of them.) It would have been impossible to track them all down prior to the publication date. Besides it isn't necessary to tell you that Dr. X, of Y University, is now working at Z University. Nor will it help your understanding of the subject—medicine and science—to learn that Patient A is now married with six children. You will get to know the cast of characters from the stories I tell about them as they were at the time.

Of this you can be sure: the people quoted are real people, not portraits that I dreamed up to illustrate my story. You will find few John Z's or Helen B's in these pages. My guiding principle was that disease is not a sin, not something to be ashamed of. And those we interviewed largely agreed.

The range of subjects—more than 100 of them—covered in this book is truly awesome, even to me. As you browse, you too will appreciate what has happened in the medical world over the last dozen years. And, at the same time, you will gather much information—information that could save your life, or the life of a loved one. This, then, is a guide to better health for you and your family.

I have tried to arrange the articles using as my guides coherence, logic, and, most important, my own feelings. For example, I put the story of my Parkinson's disease first to let you know who I am and what I, myself, owe to medicine. Besides, the scientific investigation of the brain (which allowed me to live much longer than I had expected) is the leading field of discovery as we move toward the twenty-first century.

In doing this exercise of selection, I found some interesting trends. I have written only four articles on cancer and over a dozen on mental disease. How could that be? The science of cancerology seems to be moving forward extremely rapidly, while mental problems appear to be as dire as they have always been.

I think the answer is as follows: while the biology of cancer has taken long strides in understanding this dreadful disease, the practical applications have not been as forthcoming as we have expected. Yes, when I started science reporting a half-century ago, children with acute leukemia had but a year to live. Today, thanks to chemotherapy, those children will survive long enough and sufficiently disease-free to give birth to their own children. But for most of the cancers, the success rate has been dismal. On the other hand, the discovery and application of chemicals to treat mental disease has been nothing less than astounding, with successful treatment in the range of 40 percent (for schizophrenia) and 80 percent (for anxiety).

Because I zeroed in on medical success, I was more likely to choose current victories than triumphs of the future. I do believe that this will change soon with respect to cancer.

One can say the same about AIDS. Although I frequently refer to AIDS, I did not write a separate story about this terrible disease. Up until 1996, one could not be hopeful about the future of AIDS. What at first seemed like a simple public health problem turned out to be enormously complex. The virus for AIDS (human immunodeficiency virus—HIV) was quickly tracked down in 1984. Everybody, including the secretary of Health, Education, and Welfare, predicted that a vaccine would follow almost immediately. Now, more than twelve years later, scientists are just beginning to test a number of vaccines. And for the first time medical treatments have been developed for the various ills triggered by HIV. Further, laboratories have found chemicals to inactivate, if not destroy, the virus in the patient's body. So, as we enter the twilight of the twentieth century, AIDS patients are living much longer than before. They are finally able to look to the future with hope rather than despair.

In my opinion, the future of medicine and disease prevention has never looked better. Only 50 years have passed since the description of DNA, the basic molecule of heredity. As scientists continue to elucidate the properties of DNA, they will—I am sure—find revolutionary treatments, cures, and preventatives for many of the conditions that now prey on us.

My stepfather lived to the age of 98 (unfortunately, I do not have his genes), thanks to medications, surgery, and his will to see how it all comes out. A couple of months before he died, my brother asked him if he was getting tired of the struggle (he, too, had Parkinson's disease). My stepfather answered in his tiny, disease-ridden voice: "I would not give up one day."

Neither would I.

The Brain

I HAVE PARKINSON'S DISEASE. I'VE SUSPECTED IT ever since I wrote in my diary in 1987: "I am holding my right hand oddly. Parkinson's?"

The thought was reinforced by a telephone call from my bank: "We have a check drawn on your account for $2,000. It doesn't look like your signature." It was illegible, but it was mine.

I also noticed a slight tremble of my right hand. I saw my doctor. He said, not without sadness, "Yes, it's Parkinson's," and turned me over to a bright young neurologist, who confirmed what I had and prescribed my medication.

Because I have been writing about health and science for half a century, I knew very well what future lay before me. I had watched as this "trembling disease" trampled my good friend, Dr. Elliott Osserman. He was 53 and at the peak of his career as a cancer researcher when his symptoms became clear: an odd walk—a kind of stiff shuffle—and a stifled, breathy voice. Nine years later, he was dead.

And I have been watching the ever-so-slow deterioration of my stepfather, who has been treated for Parkinson's for more than 30 years. At 95, he was bedridden—immobile—but with a sharp mind and a tiny voice that still could crack a joke. [He died in 1994 at 98.]

Which way will Parkinson's go for me? At 67, with medicines and exercise, I am striving to hold onto my muscles as they get fewer and fewer signals from a section of my brain that controls movement. Tennis and cycling have kept me fit. Had I not exercised throughout my lifetime, I think I would have lost much more muscle. Now I have stepped up my sessions with a physical therapist. I have the shuffling walk, but I can glide across the floor smoothly when I need to, by remembering to swing my arms.

My medicines are Artane and Deprenyl. Artane all but stops the tremor of my right hand. I take it primarily when I am going to be working among people, so it won't distract them. Deprenyl is supposed to slow the progress of the disease by 2 to 5 years.

With luck, I could still be functioning when I reach my 80s, if in a weakened state. There's always a chance I will die from pneumonia, a heart attack (it runs in my family), or falling down and breaking my neck (Parkinson's throws you off balance). But so could many people without Parkinson's.

1

I am lucky now. I still can hit a tennis ball, climb a staircase, work for long hours, go to the theater, see my friends. For writing, I depend on my computer word processor, although I have slowed down. I also make more typos than I used to, but my computer's spelling checker catches most of them. I expect to do better.

I am lucky that my bosses at *Parade,* where I am the health editor, have encouraged me in every way. I also broadcast daily health and science reports at WCBS-TV News in New York. I have not lost my broadcast ability. My chiefs at the station have recognized that and are very supportive.

I am lucky I escaped the rapidly progressing form of the disease that nearly broke my friend Elliott Osserman's spirit. He worked on his beloved science almost to his last days. I hope to do the same. My medicines bring me as close to normal as I can possibly be.

Parkinson's chemical changes in the brain often throw a cloak of sadness over its victims. So far, I have escaped that depression, which can be more deadly than the inability to move. I know that nobody escapes death. And if dying is like fainting, it's no big deal.

I've had a terrific career in journalism. In 50 years, I've covered nearly every major medical and science development. I have good friends. My children and grandchildren have met with success or are well on their way.

I went to see Dr. Lucien Côté, associate professor of neurology at Columbia-Presbyterian Medical Center in Manhattan. He told me, "You are lucky to have Parkinson's disease. It is one of the few brain diseases for which we have medicines that work. And, as you know, more are coming."

Lucky. I am. And optimistic, too.

Scientists are testing at least three new chemicals that could arrest my deficits as I acquire them. On the horizon: the perfection of brain implants to replace or stimulate the malfunctioning tiny ball of nerves in my brain. A second kind of surgery splits away the sick part of the brain from the healthy region. I am lucky because I don't need them yet and probably won't for many years.

Scientists have hunted down the mechanism that has given so many so much trouble. They know that the nerves in the brain communicate with each other by transmitting chemicals from one to the other. These neurotransmitters set off or block electrical discharges in adjacent nerves. One of these chemicals is called *dopamine*. One organ in the brain stem, a bundle of nerve cells no bigger than a grape, is rich in dopamine. It is called the *substantia nigra*. Ultimately, it feeds dopamine into neighboring clusters of neurons that control your movements: No dopamine, no control.

There are many theories about why the substantia nigra stops producing dopamine. For example, some scientists say an environmental poison could be the cause. Others say your genes may increase sensitivity to everyday materials, such as aluminum. No proof yet.

If the brain doesn't get enough dopamine, you cannot control your movements without concentrating. I can keep my right hand perfectly still by just looking at it. But if I have not taken Artane, and I am watching a movie or just talking to someone, my hand jumps around like a flag in a breeze. When I am broadcasting, I hide my hand. In a conversation, I am often amused by the other fellow's attempts to look and not to look at my shaking hand. So the trick is to get more dopamine to the brain. Oral doses of levodopa often help do this.

In 1994, I started taking levodopa, sometimes called L-dopa, because I was trembling more. L-dopa is converted within the brain to dopamine, which I am growing less able to produce.

Other medicines curb enzymes that break down dopamine, leaving more of the chemical intact in your brain. There also are drugs that behave like dopamine itself. Finally, you can take medicines that hinder the action of other neurotransmitters, chiefly acetylcholine. If not checked by natural dopamine, acetylcholine is the culprit that makes my hand flutter.

My heart leaps with hope when I realize that my doctor can prescribe two or three other drugs that I haven't tried yet and that more medicines are on the way.

Perhaps I'll be lucky enough to hold Parkinson's at bay until the more effective chemicals arrive.

All this drug research was stimulated in 1982, when what was intended to be synthetic heroin was produced in an illegal laboratory. Seven people between the ages of 20 and 40 arrived for treatment in hospital emergency rooms in the west after having injected the illegal substance. It was tainted with impurities, primarily the toxic chemical MPTP, which killed the dopamine cells in their brains. They were affected severely with irreversible immobility, a symptom of Parkinson's later stages. Dr. J. William Langston, now president of the Parkinson's Institute in Sunnyvale, California, saw the first case while working at the Santa Clara Valley Medical Center. He published that discovery in 1983.

From this devastating incident, scientists found a way to create an animal model of Parkinson's on which to test the new surgeries and drugs before trying them on humans. The model works best in monkeys. And progress has been rapid. Once treated with MPTP, the monkeys became Parkinson's patients, and Swedish surgeons implanted them with dopamine-producing cells from the brains of monkey fetuses. Brain surgeons in Sweden, at Yale, and at the University of Colorado later tried human-cell implants with humans. They reported improvements but no cure.

Scientists are developing techniques of changing the patient's own skin cells so that they make dopamine when surgically implanted in the substantia nigra region of the brain. If the implants succeed, the body would not reject its own tissue, and scientists would not have to depend on fetal cells. Success may be 5 or 10 years away.

A dozen or more pharmaceutical companies are testing drugs on monkeys with MPTP-induced Parkinson's. Some scientists have tried electrical stimulation of the brain to control tremors. It may work. In Manhattan, neurologists and neurosurgeons from the New York University Medical Center are working with others at the Hospital for Joint Diseases, rewiring the brain's dopamine circuits by cutting certain nerve pathways. They are optimistic.

I am one of about half a million Americans with Parkinson's. Our ages range from the 20s to the 80s, but the average age at onset is 61. We are all lucky. In the 1960s, patients could anticipate being in a wheelchair 3 to 5 years after the first symptoms and dead 3 to 5 years after that. Now, living 15 functional years is usual. And more help is on the way.

So far, nothing has crippled me. I can still take Parkinson's as a challenge. My job is to keep on going and to get the best out of my future life. If it includes tennis, work, family, and friends—great.

For further information, write to the United Parkinson Foundation, Dept. P, 833 W. Washington Blvd., Chicago, IL 60607.

When Your Head Starts Pounding

HEADACHES COME IN MANY VARIETIES—tension, migraine, and cluster are just three of them—and they merit many adjectives, such as *splitting,* as in, "I have a splitting headache." Also *aching, blinding,* and *terrible.* Few people escape headaches in their lifetimes. In fact, the pain of headaches is so common that we often equate them with troublesome people or situations, which we refer to as "real headaches."

Up until the last century, doctors could offer headache sufferers only mild relief, with such remedies as vapors or poultices of foul-smelling herbs and vinegars. Some of these "treatments" really worked. But, on the whole, if you had a headache, you had to wait it out—let it run its course—in pain.

All that has changed. Now very few headaches cannot be helped in some way, thanks to new discoveries about how headaches arise and new medicines that can ease the headache's pain or even prevent its occurrence.

Practically everyone at one time has suffered a pain in the skull. The ache ranges from a passing pang to a full-blown explosion of agony that some experts say has even caused suicide. Each year, 42 million Americans drop what they are doing and search for relief from their pounding headaches. They visit their doctors 18 million times a year seeking respite.

Headaches occur more often than colds, more often than pain anywhere else in the body. They are the most common sickness signals, passing quickly with or without simple treatment. But if yours are intense and recur, do see your doctor without delay. They might be the first of headache torments to plague you week after week, year after year. Severe headaches interfere with normal work and social activities for perhaps 2 million Americans. Adults lose workdays, and children lose school days because of them.

There is no cure for most obstinately recurring headaches, of which migraines and cluster headaches are the most dreaded, but there is relief. Dr. Seymour Solomon, director of the nation's first headache unit at Montefiore Medical Center in the Bronx, New York, says that doctors cannot eliminate the underlying causes of headaches. "But," he adds, "80 percent of people who come to us with intractable headaches can be helped to lead a normal life. We cannot promise that they will never have another headache, but we can reduce the frequency and severity of the pain."

Here is a headache horror story told by Major Kay Stoops of Franklin Square, New York. Major Stoops, a Salvation Army minister, suffers from migraines.

"Eight years ago," she says, "I started having headaches. In about 3 years, they were lasting 4 to 5 days. I felt someone was grinding a hot knife behind my left eye. I was vomiting so much, I had to go to the hospital emergency room. For a while, this happened every 3 weeks."

Major Stoops saw doctor after doctor for her headaches and tried morphine and the other drugs they prescribed. None helped. "I was beginning to think I'd never get better," she says.

Finally, she found Dr. Richard Lipton of the Montefiore headache unit. He prescribed a form of ergotamine, a drug that constricts the blood vessels. (Expansion of arteries in the brain may be one cause of headaches.) Major Stoops learned how to inject herself with ergotamine. The medicine is expensive—$700 a month—and, because it is experimental, may not be covered by her medical insurance. Still, she values the relief it gives her. As of this writing, Major Stoops says she gets only mild migraines, and they last for just 1 or 2 days. "Now I can exercise and get out of the house," she says. "And I don't vomit anymore."

Major Stoops also sees a psychologist for coaching in relaxation techniques. She is happiest about being able to return to her work—helping prisoners with their Bible studies. "I have really come a long way," she says.

The word *migraine* stems from the Greek and Latin *hemicranium,* for "half a skull," meaning that the pain keeps to one side of the head. Feeling pressure developing on one side of the head is the classic sign of the onset of a migraine headache. Other symptoms include vomiting or nausea, dizziness, and sensitivity to light.

Some migraineurs (the word for migraine sufferers) see spots, lines, or heat waves; some even experience a partial loss of vision before the onset of a headache.

Only 4 percent of reported headaches fall into the migraine category. Two to four times more women than men have migraines. These figures come from a study of 10,000 men and women in their teens and 20s conducted by Dr. Martha Linet and Walter F. Stewart, colleagues at the Johns Hopkins University School of Hygiene and Public Health in Baltimore.

More common are tension headaches. You suffer pains in the neck, shoulders, and the muscles near your skull—you can feel the tension in those muscles with your fingers. One group of scientists says that when these muscles contract in a spasm, you get a tension headache. Others have tried to measure the spasm without success. This kind of headache is relieved nicely by aspirin, acetaminophen, or other over-the-counter drugs called nonsteroidal pain relievers.

A third kind of head pain comes from cluster headaches, which pop up in groups in the course of a day, week, or month. After a period of peace, they return. The pain of cluster headaches is so intense that, in rare cases, it has driven victims to seek relief by banging their skulls against walls.

Blair Hodowal, 35, is a supervisor in the highway department of Centerville City, Indiana. Five years ago, his cluster headaches began with one bad headache. "During the headaches, my eye would tear," he recalls. "My teeth hurt like they had giant cavities. My nose ran. It would incapacitate me for a half hour. The pain is like jamming a knife into your head, and there is nothing that will make it quit. I would scream."

In 1988, Mr. Hodowal found Dr. Ninan Mathew at the Houston Headache Clinic. Dr. Mathew, president of the American Association for the Study of Headache, recommended the use of radio frequency waves to deaden certain nerves.

"They numbed me from the top of my forehead to my upper teeth and to the back of my ear," Mr. Hodowal says. "I can only eat on one side of my mouth. But it was worth it. I can now work and function. After the pain I've been through, this is heaven."

In a test Dr. Mathew and Dr. Wayne Hurt have tried the procedure on 65 patients with chronic cluster headaches. Dr. Mathew reports that 75 percent responded excellently.

Of course, the classification of headaches into three groups is an oversimplification. Some people have both migraine and cluster headaches, or tension headaches alternating with migraines. After years of arguing over how to diagnose headaches, the specialists got together in 1988 and issued a standard manual that covers nearly 100 different kinds of headaches.

"For the first time, we have criteria for diagnosing headaches," says Dr. Lipton of Montefiore. This "headache bible" will allow researchers to know that they are all talking about the same kind of headache.

There are as many theories on the origin of headaches as there are headache specialists. There is agreement that the brain itself isn't hurting, because the brain has no nerves for experiencing pain. However, the arteries in the brain do have pain nerves. If something hurts or inflames them, the arteries transmit pain signals to the conscious center of the brain. That may be why headaches throb. Every time your heart pumps, it sends blood pulsing through the arteries, stretching them. With each stretch, you sense a pain signal if the artery hurts.

But what inflames the arteries? Some evidence suggests that changes in the amounts of various brain chemicals may do it. Dr. Michael Welch, chief neurolo-gist at Henry Ford Hospital in Detroit, has focused high-tech attention and equipment on this problem.

Using an instrument sensitive to magnetism, Dr. Welch follows changes in the brain's magnetic field during a headache. He says he thinks he can see the brain respond to the factors that trigger a headache. Another instrument helped him discover that magnesium drops to low levels in the brain before and during a migraine attack. In a third technique, he follows the ebb and flow of blood in the brain before, during, and after a headache.

Dr. Welch and Dr. Sandra Nagel-Leiby work at putting the pieces together to reveal a picture of headaches—how they vary, who gets them, and why. It turns out that all of us can suffer from a headache. Some of us are more susceptible. Older individuals get more headaches, and so do women (menstruation increases risk of headache). Those who suffer from chronic stress at work or home, or who take oral contraceptives, are prone to headaches.

With a lowered resistance to headaches, other events trigger the actual pain. Chocolate, cheese, wine, and other foods that contain substances, such as tyramine, can touch off a headache. Acute stress—from an auto accident or from taking an important examination, for example—can do the same. Glaring light can spark the pains. So can certain drugs, unfortunate combinations of drugs, or a blow to the head.

However, a serious underlying disease, such as a brain tumor, may cause the headache in patients complaining of skull pains. Here are the warning signs of severe problems, as cited by Dr. Lipton:

- Sudden onset of the worst headache *could* mean you are bleeding in the brain—a stroke. Go immediately to the hospital emergency room.
- Headache with fever and a stiff neck could mean meningitis. The symptoms may signal bleeding into the brain.
- If strong headaches replace weak ones over weeks or months, see your physician.
- Red eyes or blurring vision with a headache point to glaucoma, high pressure in the eye. Untreated, you risk blindness.
- A seizure (a fit) or a new type of headache, at any age but particularly after 55, is a good reason to consult your doctor.

As scientists unravel the causes of various headaches, new treatments are being devised, though exactly why some of them work is often unclear.

Rodney Fritz, news director and morning anchor of WMJX-FM, a radio station in Boston, endured cluster headaches every August for 5 years. "The third year was the worst ever," he says. "It was like someone sticking a hot poker in my eye. I would pace. I wore a path in the rug. Tears were coming from my eye."

Mr. Fritz went to the headache center at Faulkner Hospital in Boston, where they gave him ergotamine and verapamil, a drug that lowers high blood pressure. They also gave him pure oxygen to breathe. The treatments helped ease his pain.

Dr. Egilius L. H. Spierings, director of the headache center at Faulkner, has tested verapamil on 48 cluster-headache patients and says two-thirds improved greatly.

Dr. Lipton categorizes headache drugs this way:

- Abortive—These stop headaches. They include ergotamine and some of the new nonsteroidal antiinflammatory chemicals.
- Prophylactic—These prevent headaches. They include antidepressants, beta-blockers, and calcium channel-blockers. These chemicals act on tiny muscles in the arteries. The last two usually are used to treat high blood pressure. Verapamil is a calcium channel-blocker. Chiefly used for cluster headaches are methysergide, prednisone (a type of cortisone), and lithium, a drug usually prescribed for manic depression.
- Symptomatic—These drugs reduce the pain and other headache symptoms. They include aspirin, codeine, and other painkillers. But sometimes these drugs make the headache worse. Should you get rebound headaches in the morning, your doctor might prescribe Compazine to reduce the nausea of migraine.

At the General Medical Center in Akron, Ohio, Dr. James Dougherty injected patients with Compazine. He says it stopped the cluster headaches without the aid of other painkillers.

Headaches also often respond to nondrug treatments, such as relaxation therapy, meditation, hypnosis, and biofeedback. If chronic stress on the job or at home triggers headaches, it may be important to change your job or adopt a new lifestyle. Psychological counseling may help.

By doing more research on the underlying causes, scientists quite possibly will find new and effective ways to stop, prevent, or ease the pain of headaches.

For referrals to doctors and clinics specializing in headaches, or for additional information, send a self-addressed, stamped business-size envelope to the American Council for Headache Education (ACHE), 875 Kings Highway, Suite 200, Woodbury, NJ 08096; or call (800) 255-ACHE. You can also fax your request to (609) 384-5811.

Finally, Some Answers to Epilepsy

A CONDITION THAT GOES BACK TO CAESAR AND Socrates now is controllable, thanks to new techniques and drugs.

The scene is an ordinary one. Couches. Small tables. Books. John Natale, an appraiser for the federal government, lounges in an easy chair. A movie plays on the TV set.

But take a closer look: There are wires extending downward through the hair at the back of Mr. Natale's head. The wires run from little metal disks glued to his scalp, through a cable ending in a box tied on his belt. And, up in each of the room's four corners near the ceiling, TV cameras follow his every movement.

Mr. Natale is a patient at the Veterans Administration Hospital in the Bronx in New York City. Dr. James Rowan, the chief neurologist, is searching for the cause of his strange seizures. In another room, technicians observe their patient on TV monitors. A slab of white paper moves slowly out of a machine. On its surface, 16 pens write wiggly lines. From the wires the doctors are getting an electrical picture of Mr. Natale's brain. Suddenly, he begins to tremble and shake. He falls to the floor, his body writhing. Later he is shown a videotape of his seizure.

"I was bouncing around, uttering odd sounds, dribbling, mouth all foamy, clamping on my jaw and tongue," Mr. Natale recalled. "My arms got stiff. I was making odd animal noises. I was totally exhausted and went into a sleep."

While this was happening to him, the wiggly lines on the paper went wild. An electrical storm sweeps through his brain whenever Mr. Natale has seizures. Because no doctor had seen his fits before this, the diagnosis of his illness had been in doubt. But because this seizure was monitored by TV and the brain's electrical signals, it was concluded that the cause was neither fever nor emotional upset. It was epilepsy.

Mr. Natale is now one of 2 million Americans diagnosed as having epilepsy. Doctors have prescribed for him Tegretol, one of several antiseizure drugs available. He now suffers a seizure only every 2 months or so and, thanks to his medicine, leads a normal life.

"Sometimes my illness keeps me from work," Mr. Natale says, "but I can function better. I know I will always have seizures, but medication can control them."

More than 500,000 Americans with epilepsy are not so lucky. They have never received a clear diagnosis or definitive treatment. They continue to have seizures; they cannot drive cars; they are often avoided by employers and neighbors. Many become shut-ins.

The Good News

In the 1970s, doctors controlled only 50 percent of their epilepsy cases. Today the Epilepsy Foundation of America puts the number as high as 85 percent, thanks to new diagnostic techniques, drugs, and surgery that removes part of the brain. The modern war against epilepsy has begun.

"Our drug treatment today is far better than in the past," says Dr. Rowan. "Our problem is that many patients fail to get a good diagnosis or they get the wrong dose of a drug or the wrong drug entirely. It's sad, because we now can control nearly every case of epilepsy."

Epilepsy is a Greek word meaning "to seize." In ancient days, people with epilepsy were thought to have divine visitations. But by medieval times, victims were said to be possessed by Satan. Doctors could do nothing, although by 150 A.D. Galen, a Greek physician, knew that the brain was involved in this illness. Napoleon, Julius Caesar, Socrates, Tchaikovsky—all had epileptic seizures, and all went untreated.

Simply put, the electrical storm in the brain occurs because some or all of the brain is damaged or because of a genetic predisposition to the disorder. A blow to the head, some toxic substances, lack of oxygen during birth—all can injure brain cells. So can infections, tumors, strokes, or other circulation problems.

Epilepsy is not a mental disease or an emotional or behavioral problem. But because the seizures can be so debilitating, patients do suffer with emotional and behavioral problems. Long ago, psychiatrists believed it caused criminal or violent behavior. Science has since shown that persons with epilepsy have the same kinds of psychological problems (or lack of them) as persons with other chronic physical diseases. And those with epilepsy are no more or less criminal.

Drug Treatment

Up to the mid-19th century, doctors had no tools to deal with epilepsy. In 1857, a British physician reported success in quelling seizures with compounds of bromine. Sixty years later, phenobarbital also was found to control the spells. Both, however, have unpleasant side effects: drowsiness and coordination difficulties.

Then, in 1938, two American physicians, H. Houston Merritt and Tracy Jackson Putnam, discovered Dilantin, a drug that quieted the spells in most patients without too many side effects. Dilantin freed thousands of patients from mental and epilepsy institutions. Without Dilantin, many would have remained locked up.

Since then, science has created new drugs, and more are on the way. Dilantin controls most seizures. For various types of seizures, doctors also prescribe Zarontin, Klonopin, Depakene, Depakote, Mysoline, Tegretol, and Tranxene.

The drugs do have side effects but less than the old treatments. Dilantin can disrupt coordination, Tegretol can produce blurred vision, and Depakote can cause hair loss. The doctor, ideally, tries to bring the dose to just the point where the side effects and the seizures both disappear.

Marion Clignet of Aspen Hill, Maryland, takes Tegretol to prevent the sei-zures that began when she was 17. The drug controls her condition so well that Ms. Clignet, a cyclist, puts in 300 to 400 miles a week, plus weight lifting and stair climbing.

"I'm not concerned about having a seizure while riding," she says. "At first my family was scared for me, but I proved that I could do it."

Surgery

If the spells persist, doctors consider surgery—cutting out the damaged part of the brain. But first they must map the brain to avoid cutting out parts that control vital functions—speech, hearing, sight, writing, muscular movements.

In the past, doctors kept the patient awake during surgery and mapped the brain during the operation by touching or electrically stimulating various parts. For example, if they put a small electric current through the speech area of the brain, the patient would stop talking. But there's a limit to how long you can keep a patient in the operating room.

Now, doctors map a patient's brain by putting a network of up to 100 electrodes inside the skull and under the dura, the fibrous tissue that covers the brain. The electrodes may stay in for weeks—patients walk around with them. The scientists record the brain's electrical activity to spot damaged regions.

Dr. Ronald Lesser, director of Johns Hopkins Epilepsy Center in Baltimore, is one of the proponents of this method.

"In follow-up after surgery, patients do remarkably well," he says. "You would expect that taking out an area of the brain would create lots of damage afterward, but usually it doesn't."

Mrs. Kathleen Fitts of Oakdale, Connecticut, had surgery twice—in 1970 and again in 1989 at Yale–New Haven Medical Center. "The first time, the doctors went in blind," she says. "They took out tissue they thought was scar tissue. They had left some damaged brain behind." The second surgery identified all the safe and dangerous areas and removed part of Mrs. Fitts's brain. She also takes Mysoline and Tegretol. No more seizures.

As many as 16 different drugs a day could not control the blackouts of Marty Downing of Delmar, Maryland. In January 1988, in a 6½-hour operation, Dr. Sumio Uematsu, a neurosurgeon at Johns Hopkins, took out Mrs. Downing's right temporal lobe—a quarter of her brain. Afterward, her left thumb and index finger were numb and remained so. But the blackouts are gone.

"I am so much different now," she says. "I can teach Sunday school again. I ride my bike. I put on a dress for the first time in 14 years. I had to wear pants all the time before, because I kept falling down stairs."

"It's not simple. It's not like getting your tonsils out," says Dr. Uematsu, "but we do help 75 percent of our patients. The rest are unchanged."

For Beth Usher of Storrs, Connecticut, surgery was the only way to stop her seizures—up to 100 a day. Surgeons at Johns Hopkins cut out the left brain. Miss Usher went into a coma for 5 weeks. After she regained consciousness, the right side of her body was paralyzed, but she learned to walk again with a limp. She has limited use of her right hand. "But there has not been one seizure since the surgery," says her mother, Kathy. "Beth gets stronger every day."

Fewer and fewer people hide having epilepsy now that drugs can control their seizures. Representative Tony Coelho (D.—California) is the first Congressman to announce that he has epilepsy. "When I ran for Congress, my advisers told me not to talk about it," he recalls. "When I got elected, I decided to go public about it. I had my last seizure in 1982. I ride cutting horses. I am a runner. Nothing slows me down."

For further information about epilepsy, write to the Epilepsy Foundation of America, 4351 Garden City Drive, Landover, Maryland 20785.

How to Spot an Epileptic Seizure

If you see someone having a seizure, stay calm and follow these rules:

1. Turn the person gently on his or her side to keep the air passages free of saliva. Do not force a tongue depres-

sor or anything else into the person's mouth—people cannot swallow their tongues. Also, if the person clamps down on a hard object, a tooth or jaw could be broken.

2. Remove potentially harmful objects like dentures.

3. Remove the person's glasses and loosen his or her clothing.

4. Don't try to hold the person down. You cannot stop a seizure, which usually lasts only a few seconds or minutes.

5. Stay nearby. When the person becomes alert, help him or her become reoriented. If you have doubts about the person's well-being, phone a doctor.

Winning Against Stroke

A STROKE HAPPENS SO FAST THAT THE VICTIM often recalls nothing about it. The brain simply does not have enough time to store the event in its memory banks. But the stroke's damage is evident: There may be paralysis on one side of the body. Perhaps there is an inability to speak, indicating brain damage.

A stroke occurs when something shuts off the blood supply to brain cells. Deprived of the blood's essential oxygen and nutrients, the cells die. The blood supply might be stopped when an artery is clogged by a clot, an air bubble, or solid tissue, or when an artery bursts, releasing blood that pools rather than circulates.

William Wylder, 73, a former radio and TV reporter, said his stroke terrified him. The symptoms he described are fairly typical: "In 1973," he recalls, "with no warning symptoms before it happened, I had a stroke while I was doing a radio newscast in Rock Island, Illinois. It was the craziest newscast ever. I could not speak. I could not get anyone's attention. My arms were flailing. I managed to crawl to my car. Somehow, I drove home, and my wife got me to the doctor."

Each year, 500,000 or more Americans experience strokes. Two-thirds survive, many unable to support themselves or live productive lives. Three million U.S. residents have had at least one stroke, and $30 billion is spent for treatment and care each year.

Persons undergoing coronary bypass surgery also are at risk of stroke. A patient's heart is slowed for the surgery. Because of this, there is an increased risk of blood clotting, and 5 to 7 percent of bypass surgery patients suffer strokes from clots that form during surgery.

"Of those patients who undergo bypass, 30 percent are not mentally as good as they were before surgery," says Dr. Denise Barbut, director of the stroke center at New York Hospital in Manhattan. "We are trying to prevent that."

Despite such grim statistics, progress in medication, technology, and research is brightening the picture.

New Advances Can Stop a Stroke

New technology improves diagnosis. Today, doctors sometimes can detect high-risk patients before stroke symptoms even arise.

An important result of all this is a change in attitudes. Physicians once shrugged in defeat at strokes. Now they know that many stroke patients can be rescued, and doctors treat strokes with the same urgency as heart attacks.

The death rate from strokes in the United States has plunged 40 percent in the last 20 years. New treatments cut the risk of stroke by 60 percent in some patients. Many have been helped by the treatment of high blood pressure—a major factor in stroke—through diet or drugs.

"Stroke is one of the most rapidly expanding areas in the brain sciences," says Dr. Michael Walker, who directs the Division of Stroke and Trauma for the National Institute of Neurological Disorders and Stroke (NINDS) in Bethesda, Maryland. Here are some of the important advances in this area.

Physiological Research

It once was accepted that damage from stroke was permanent, because the brain does not replace dead brain cells. But new findings in physical therapy show that, with persistent guidance, the brain can find new pathways, allowing undamaged nerve cells to take over and perform the functions of the dead ones.

Dr. Mark Hallett, a clinical director for NINDS, studies adult stroke survivors who have regained function of a limb after losing partial or total control. Dr. Hallett says he has found that "if you use a body part repetitively, more groups of nerve cells become devoted to it, and this may upgrade its use.

"This suggests," he adds, "that the brain can be trained to use different nerve pathways to control a once-paralyzed hand, for example. We believe that the brain's capacity to reorganize itself will help rehabilitation profoundly."

Chemical/Drug Research

When an artery bursts or is clogged, it can't supply the brain cells with blood, and they die. The injured and dying cells then emit substances that spread the injury to a widening circle of brain cells. Release of these substances allows the entry of excess calcium into the cells, followed by the entry of water, which bloats and destroys the cells. Chemical compounds to reduce the risk to brain cells during stroke are now being tested for human use. They would protect the cells from being flooded with water in this deadly process.

Brain scientists also are testing many chemicals for their ability to dissolve blood clots and stop a stroke in progress. These include streptokinase, an enzyme from bacteria, and TPA, a chemical found in tiny amounts in human blood. Studies show that they destroy clots in the coronary arteries. There is some proof that these chemicals destroy clots in brain arteries.

An experimental anticoagulant called Ancrod comes from the venom of Malaysian pit vipers. It thins the blood, breaks up clots, and has been tested on about 500 persons with some success.

In addition, researchers are focusing on ways to prevent clot formation. Blood clots in the coronary arteries produce heart attacks. Antiplatelet (blood-thinning) drugs, including aspirin and warfarin, are being tested on a large scale to see which ones help prevent stroke. If you have suffered a stroke, the chances are that you will have another. Treatment with blood thinners can extend the life expectancy of stroke patients.

Aspirin therapy—depending on the patient and the dosage—has been found to stop clotting. If you are 50 or older, researchers urge you to consult with your physician about aspirin therapy to help prevent stroke or heart attack.

Warfarin, a prescription drug for humans, is a blood-thinning chemical. It was long known as an ingredient in rat poison. When used to prevent stroke, it requires careful management, including monthly blood tests and adjustments of the dosage, as its effects vary with age.

Technology and Surgery

For stroke victims, diagnosis must be quick and accurate. Within 6 hours, it should be medically determined whether the stroke was due to a hemorrhage (bleeding or burst brain artery) or a clot (blocked brain artery). New imaging methods, including CAT and MRI scans, hasten this discovery, which is crucial to proper treatment. If caused by a brain hemorrhage, surgery usually is considered. For a clot, treatment with an antiplatelet medication, such as aspirin, is considered. In some cases, surgery may be needed.

Felix Ticineto, 79, a self-employed accountant from Flushing, New York, suffered a stroke. "I came home, ate, and started bumping around," he recounts. "I couldn't walk. I had no balance. I went to sleep without telling my wife and woke up with the problem."

Dr. Barbut of New York Hospital used an ultrasound transcranial Doppler to help diagnose Mr. Ticineto. This machine sends out sound waves that bounce off internal organs and produce a colored picture showing the patient's blood flow to the brain. Dr. Barbut says that, with the Doppler, "you can see the clots waft past and even hear them."

Finding that arteries feeding Mr. Ticineto's brain were blocked by plaque, she had them scoured in a surgical procedure called an endarterectomy. "I feel great now," says Mr. Ticineto. "My right hand and arm are a little weakened, but I was very lucky. I work every day."

Recognizing the Symptoms

People seem to recognize the symptoms of a heart attack and react readily to aid the person having one. But a stroke often is mistaken for something else, including drunkenness (there may be slurred speech, clumsy motions), and a physician's care is not sought.

Dr. Stanley Tuhrim, who heads the stroke program at Mount Sinai Medical Center in New York City, says, "We must educate the public and physicians to recognize stroke symptoms and get help. [See the list later for symptoms of stroke.] Heart attack victims get chest pains and call 911. That reaction is needed for stroke."

"We now think that there's a lot we can do in the first few hours after a stroke," adds Dr. Elliot Roth of the Rehabilitation Institute of Chicago, "and that a lot more can be expected and achieved."

Get medical help within an hour if you experience any of these symptoms:

- Weakness or numbness of the face, arm, or leg
- Dimness or loss of vision, particularly in one eye
- Difficulty in speaking or understanding speech
- Severe headache with no known cause
- Unsteadiness, unexplained dizziness, or sudden falls, especially with any of the other signs

You can also take some preventive measures to help avoid such symptoms. See your doctor and get tested for high blood pressure. If you have it, get treatment. If you smoke, stop.

For more information, write to the National Institutes of Health, Neurological Institute, Dept. P, P.O. Box 5801, Bethesda, MD 20854.

Pain

AN HOUR OF PAIN IS AS LONG AS A DAY OF pleasure, says the old proverb. For some, those hours turn into days and years of unremitting pain from torn nerves, a blood-starved heart, cancer. Fortunately, medical science has learned much about pain, its causes, and how to stop it.

That knowledge was a godsend to Arlynn Munro of Fullerton, California, who worked as a secretary at Disneyland. Years ago her sciatic nerve—a nerve exiting the spinal cord—was pinched in an injury, sending waves of burning pain into her leg and back.

"I was in such a state, I couldn't stand myself," says Mrs. Munro. "I limped. I could not sleep. I couldn't hold a steady job."

Mrs. Munro found her way to Dr. Ronald Young, chief neurosurgeon for the University of California at Irvine Medical Center. Dr. Young put fine platinum wires into Mrs. Munro's brain, where the wires deliver tiny electric shocks. The surgeon also implanted a tiny battery-powered shock generator in her chest, with wires leading to her brain's pain-control centers. She can turn the generator on and off with a magnet applied to her skin. When she tried turning it off for a week, the pain came back.

"Shortly after surgery, I had relief," says Mrs. Munro. "I now feel a warm, tingling sensation across my lower back and down the left leg. The pain has stopped. It has changed my life."

Dr. Young, one of a limited number of doctors in the country able to do this operation, admits that nobody yet knows exactly why the method works but says that its effect "can be tremendously dramatic." He adds, "Patients had this pain, and now it's miraculously gone." It works for 7 of 10 patients, he says.

Brain stimulation is for those patients who cannot bear their pain anymore. Doctors and scientists also have developed new techniques to relieve a variety of pains. They have new drugs, new devices, and new ways to use old medicines, all of which can eliminate or reduce pain. Here are some of them:

- Injection of opiates including morphine into the spine to block nerve transmission to the brain
- New painkilling compounds
- Electrical shocks to nerves that shut off the pain patterns
- Hypnosis and behavior therapy
- A system that allows patients to inject themselves with painkillers

Scientists now know which nerves carry the pain signals. They understand how injured tissue releases chemicals that trigger those nerves. They know which nerve channels in the spinal cord carry which pain signals, and they have a general idea of the location of the brain's pain detection center.

Scientists also have unraveled part of the mystery of how aspirin works. First they found that the body reacts to injury by making a chemical called *prostaglandin*. Prostaglandin triggers the nerves that carry pain signals. Aspirin slows prostaglandin's release and thus dulls pain.

Now, in addition to aspirin, there's a whole class of medicines that inhibit prostaglandin. Two of them are sold in over-the-counter drugs: acetaminophen (e.g., Tylenol) and ibuprofen (in both

Nuprin and Advil). Stronger doses of ibuprofen can be obtained by prescription. For more powerful prostaglandin inhibitors, you must ask your physician to consider prescribing them.

Arthritis is a disease marked by pain in the joints, which these drugs lessen. Some of them reduce inflammation of the joints. As a result, patients afflicted with arthritis pain are given aspirin or other prostaglandin inhibitors.

These drugs also work to relieve headache pain. Doctors blame some headaches on inflammation in parts of the brain and prescribe medicines that calm such inflammation to ease those headaches. Because migraine headaches involve blood vessels, doctors may prescribe a drug such as ergotamine to open up or close down the arteries in the head. There is disagreement about how blood vessels in the brain react to cause headaches. And not all drugs work for everyone. (Note: *Never* mix any prescription or over-the-counter drugs with alcohol, diuretics, antacids, antibiotics, anticoagulants, tranquilizers, or other medications without your doctor's approval. Seemingly harmless drugs can, in combination, result in severe—even fatal—health problems.)

Knowledge about the chemicals released when tissue is injured appears to be leading to antibradykinin, a new kind of painkiller. Bradykinin is one of the substances made by injured tissue that triggers pain nerves. Antibradykinin chemicals block the trigger. Its use is still experimental, but studies of the substance indicate it has possibilities of becoming a great painkiller for cuts and bruises.

Dr. John J. Bonica of the University of Washington at Seattle almost single-handedly has spurred on the medical profession to take notice of the patient's pain, particularly in cancer cases. He has long exhorted medical schools to teach their students how to treat the problem of pain. He also has urged scientists to do more pain research. He says doctors today are paying more heed to who's hurting and why.

Dr. Bonica estimates that, world-wide, 40 percent of cancer patients die suffering from pain that could have been relieved. And in advanced cancer cases, 60 to 70 percent needlessly endure pain.

Dr. Kathleen Foley, chief of the pain service at Memorial Sloan-Kettering Cancer Center in Manhattan, agrees that there is no reason that cancer patients must suffer from pain. Narcotics such as morphine, Percodan, methadone, and Dilaudid effectively relieve chronic pain.

"People confuse them with street drugs," Dr. Foley says, "and often doctors fear that patients might abuse them." Patients do become physically (but not psychologically) dependent on narcotics, she concedes, and they suffer symptoms like diarrhea and chills when the drug is stopped. However, says Foley, practically none become dependent on narcotics. They may need increasing amounts, but she asserts that's not addiction. And, she notes, after the drug is stopped, the patients do not seek more of it, as an addict would.

"With these drugs, terminal patients can die relatively pain-free," argues Foley. "It is cruel to deny them."

For a while, there was controversy over the medical superiority of heroin, but studies show that, dose for dose, heroin has proved to be no better or worse than morphine. And now morphine can be taken safely and swallowed painlessly, rather than injected, thanks to new slow-release, 8-hour and 12-hour morphine pills.

For those needing pain relief after major surgery, doctors often allow patients to inject themselves with the right amount of drug, usually morphine, under a procedure called PCA—patient-controlled analgesia (*analgesia* means pain relief). This is done with a device attached to the tube that doctors use to transmit fluid into a vein. When the need for a painkiller arises, the patient just pushes a button, and a pump automatically injects a small regulated amount of the drug into the system.

Joan Glenn, a nurse from Bethel Park, Pennsylvania, had to have a cesarean operation to give birth to her son last May. She got PCA at Magee Women's Hospital in Pittsburgh. "The pump freed me from excess pain," says Mrs. Glenn. "It lets you treat yourself instantly, without waiting for a nurse."

In another important advance, doctors also now inject narcotics—chiefly morphine—directly into the spine rather than into a vein, frequently sidestepping some of morphine's side effects (nausea, itching, and the retention of urine).

And, in really bad cases, surgeons cut the spinal nerves. Pain relief is often instant. However, for some reason still unexplained, the pain returns after 8 months to a year.

There's help, too, for people with moderate pain, as well as for those with acute pain. It's called TENS—transcutaneous (through the skin) electrical nerve stimulation. When it was introduced a decade ago, direct electrical stimulation of the nerves seemed a panacea, but doctors now know that it works for only up to half of such sufferers and that in some cases its effect eventually wears off.

Another pain-relief resource is acupuncture, the Chinese method of sticking needles into various parts of the body. Chinese surgeons long have eliminated patients' pain responses with acupuncture. And many an athlete has had sore tendons and muscles relieved by an acupuncturist's needles.

But, again, acupuncture doesn't work for everybody, and there is no way to predict for whom it will work and how effective it will be.

Somewhat the same is true of hypnosis, one of the oldest methods of dulling pain. Probably you've seen a stage show in which the hypnotist sticks a pin into the palm of a hypnotized person and that person feels no pain. Dr. Martin Orrie, professor of psychiatry at the University of Pennsylvania in Philadelphia, an expert in hypnosis, says, "About 90 percent of the population in pain can benefit from hypnosis, and 10 percent of these can so effectively block pain that they can undergo surgery without anesthesia." Hypnosis has proved especially helpful to those patients with a clearly physical source of pain—like arthritis, shingles, or muscle pain.

Sheryl Johnson, a nurse from Panarama City, California, mastered her arthritic pain by learning self-hypnosis from a qualified doctor. "I have controlled my pain for myself," says Ms. Johnson. "I still feel pain, but I can manage it. I have not taken pain pills for 4 years." Previously, she had been unable to work for 7 months.

Dr. Orne says that if you're in pain, rather than shop for a hypnotist on your own, it's much better to seek out a doctor or pain clinic willing to both deal with your pain and find the best treatment for you. Wilbert Fordyce, a professor of psychology in rehabilitation medicine at the University of Washington School of Medicine in Seattle, runs such a pain service for patients experiencing chronic pain from accidents, surgery, or back trouble. Fordyce says his program is for "those who have healed but still are hurting more than they need to." Using behavioral therapy, he makes patients do physical things that relieve their pain. He pushes them to move, even if it hurts.

Sarah Abbott, of Seattle, injured her lower back in high school. Back surgery relieved her sharp pain, but chronic aches persisted. "I learned in the clinic to get up and bend over and touch the floor whenever I think I must take it easy," she says. "A year ago, I would have sworn this might kill me. I had the thought pattern of a cripple. At one point, suicide had seemed my only option."

Despite the discomfort and difficulties of this approach, Sarah Abbott says it's worth it: "The pain clinic turned me around. It has saved my life."

New Techniques Bring Brighter Future for Those with Brain and Spinal Injuries

YOU DRIFT AWAKE. LIGHTS FILL YOUR EYES. It's hard to see the faces peering down at you. You can't remember exactly what happened a few minutes ago—or was it hours ago? You cannot lift your hands. Your legs don't respond either. You are totally paralyzed. Terror grips your mind.

Slowly, you realize this is no nightmare. This is real. Then they tell you: Two weeks ago . . . auto accident . . . barely made it . . . neck is broken . . . can't tell yet whether you can walk.

And, as the weeks go by, the full reality hits: You will never walk again, never use your arms, hands, or fingers. You can't control your bladder or your bowel.

How would you react? Most people say they would not want to live.

In the past, the victims of injury to the brain or spinal cord lived but briefly. Consigned to back rooms, they soon fell prey to deadly infections, kidney failure, or pneumonia. Today, new medical techniques keep them alive and productive. Thousands live busy, even happy lives.

Leslie Brumagin of Emmaus, Pennsylvania, was paralyzed from the waist down in an automobile accident in 1983. She couldn't think or remember. With treatment, Leslie attended college, drives a car, skis, goes gliding, even plays tennis from her wheelchair.

"I didn't know much about life before the accident," she says. "I just wanted to be popular. Now I am just beginning to live."

Combined, spinal cord injury and brain trauma inflict a stupendous burden on our medical and social systems. According to the National Head Injury Foundation, auto accidents, falls, and flying objects send 500,000 Americans to the hospital each year with injured heads and wounded brains. One in 10 of them dies, and 50,000 more are permanently disabled. More than a million head-injured Americans are struggling with brains that don't work properly.

The National Institute on Disability and Rehabilitation Research estimates that 14,000 Americans suffer spinal cord injuries each year. Forty percent die, most of them almost immediately. But about 8,000 to 10,000 are left paralyzed and in need of care. In this country alone, 300,000 paraplegics and quadriplegics are trying to forge new lives for themselves in wheelchairs.

Estimates of the bill for all this— mostly paid in tax dollars—have been placed as high as $4 billion a year in health care costs and lost productivity.

At the Maryland Institute for Emergency Medical Services Systems in Baltimore, the shock trauma center springs into action on spine or brain injuries four or more times a day.

Dr. Fred Geisler, clinical director of neurotrauma at the institute, says 95 percent of patients treated there survive. He adds, "So far, doctors have done a good job of keeping patients alive, but we haven't been able to help in the long term."

Beyond the emergency phase, medical and psychological advances help patients. The National Institute on Disability and Rehabilitation Research lists 13 model hospitals nationally where the spine-injured get top care. Craig Hospital in Denver is one.

Leslie Brumagin went to Craig Hospital in 1983. "I was convinced that I would walk again," she says. "It took me a while to get it through my head that, actually, I would not get miraculously better."

Says Dr. Dan Larnmertse, medical director at Craig: "The resiliency of the human spirit is incredible. People dig down and come up with inner strength to get through. But some never get over their anger."

In 3 to 4 months, the staff members squeeze every bit of function out of whichever nerves and muscles still work. They teach paraplegics how to get in and out of bed, on and off the toilet, how to dress and bathe. They constantly fight infection, kidney shutdown, and pneumonia. Many quadriplegics cannot breathe without mechanical respirators.

For the brain-injured, the problems are more subtle, more daunting. They must be taught new ways to think—the old thought pathways are blocked forever.

Thomas Kay directs research at the Research and Training Center on Head Injury and Stroke at New York University (NYU) Medical Center in Manhattan. He says that the amount of damage can affect a patient's thinking and emotional changes. A severely injured patient often looks and sounds different, with jerking movements, unclear speech, peculiar gestures, and odd facial expressions.

Yehuda Ben-Yishay directs the head trauma program at NYU's Rusk Institute for Rehabilitation Medicine. He points out that brain trauma cuts across many intellectual functions. The patient's attention may wander. He may not coordinate reasoning with action; even if he finds the solution to a problem, he cannot easily carry it out. He cannot formulate goals either at work or in daily life. He may not even be aware he has memory problems.

Dr. Ben-Yishay's group offers a 20-week program to teach the brain-injured how to think and act. For 5 or more hours a day, the patients solve thinking problems, with both pencil and paper and with computer. Patients also do public speaking—under pressure—so they later can interact with bosses and others without inappropriate behavior. After the training, 63 percent have been able to earn a living.

In 1984, Chris Willner of North Miami Beach, Florida, then an accountant, was driving her car when another hit her broadside. Upon waking up after 2 weeks in a coma, she couldn't speak, write, or remember things. She walked with a limp.

"Dr. Ben-Yishay's program gave me a fresh start," says Mrs. Willner, now working again as a secretary. "I was lost, but they taught me how to remember things and to have more confidence in my abilities. Now I can handle my house, my son. I am pretty darn close to how I was before the accident."

Research points to some inspiring advances. For example, electric stimulation of sperm ejaculation has enabled paralyzed husbands to become fathers. Women whose sex organs are unaffected by their injuries can have babies normally. Karen Silver Karlin of Huntington, New York, had her neck broken in a car crash in 1979. Later she had a trouble-free pregnancy.

Another exciting development is computer-driven electrical stimulation, given directly to leg and thigh muscles. This treatment enables paraplegics to walk. Dr. E. Byron Marsolais of the Veterans Administration Medical Center in Cleveland has developed a system that lets paralyzed patients walk on flat ground and on stairs.

Dr. Marsolais inserts 48 electrodes under the skin and into muscles. A computer controlled by a hand-held device sends electrical signals into the muscles, forcing them to contract in just the right sequences to produce a walking motion.

The system still needs work to make it operate more smoothly, slim its bulk, design an implantable one, and reduce its cost. More than 100 scientists and engineers have worked on it.

Researchers also stimulate the diaphragm, the large muscle in the abdomen that pumps air in and out of the lungs. They help patients breathe by activating the paralyzed diaphragm to contract. The Food and Drug Administration has approved a device for this function.

Engineers are also working on an electrical stimulator to help patients empty paralyzed bladders.

Biologists are still testing transplants of animal fetal tissue to reestablish the broken nerve connections. Fetal tissue grows rapidly and could help injured nerves before they die.

At the Medical College of Pennsylvania in Philadelphia, scientists partially have healed spinal cord injuries in rats by transplanting nerve tissues from rat fetuses into the spinal cord.

Across the nation, scientists are hard at work trying to make paralyzed bodies respond and to lift the victims from their wheelchairs.

Should Infants Have Surgery Without Anesthesia?

HE LOOKS SO HELPLESS, STRAPPED TO THE TINY operating table. Premature, newborn, weighing less than 2 pounds, the infant has a severe heart malformation. Surrounding him, hunched over, masked doctors and nurses strive desperately to repair what nature forgot to do.

The surgeon's scalpel cuts through skin and muscle and nerve. The infant emits a muffled cry. He has been given a muscle relaxant but no painkilling drug, no anesthetic. Why?

First, doctors have long argued that premature infants could not feel pain because their nervous systems had not fully formed. Second, confronted with a tiny, sick baby barely clinging to life, surgeons and anesthetists often fear that a painkilling drug might endanger an already weak breathing system or stop a heart hardly able to beat.

Dr. David Swedlow, assistant professor of anesthesia at Children's Hospital of Philadelphia, says, "The judgment call is whether you think this child can survive the anesthetic, balanced against whether the child will survive the pain."

Concerned doctors and nurses estimate that physicians withhold anesthesia in half of all major surgery for prematurely born infants. Every year in this country, 200,000 preemies spend the first weeks, sometimes months, of their lives hospitalized in intensive care units.

But protests were mounting as parents like Jill Lawson of Silver Spring, Maryland, discovered that doctors have kept painkillers from their babies. Mrs. Lawson's son, Jeffrey, was born in February 1985, 14 weeks premature and weighing less than 2 pounds, suffering from heart and lung problems. He underwent surgery.

"Jeffrey had holes cut on both sides of his neck," Mrs. Lawson says. "Another hole was cut in his right chest, an incision was made from his breastbone around to his backbone, his ribs were pried apart, and an artery near his heart was tied off. He was totally conscious throughout $1\frac{1}{2}$ hours of surgery." Jeffrey died 5 weeks later.

When Mrs. Lawson learned that no anesthesia had numbed her child to the pain, she first felt agony, then fury, and, in the end, vowed to change this practice. She wrote letters to medical organizations and government agencies and finally "went public" in a newspaper story.

Doctors have struggled with the problem for years. It was discussed at a 1970 conference of anesthesiologists held in Palm Springs, California. There a doctor stated that preemies did not need anesthesia, just some adhesive tape to hold them down.

Dr. Richard J. Ward, then of the University of Washington School of Medicine in Seattle, was in the audience. He countered that comment angrily, saying, "May I just mention that in no animal laboratory in the world could you get away with anesthetizing a puppy with adhesive tape. Some of us feel that perhaps an infant is worth at least the same amount of care as a puppy."

Parade has learned that Mrs. Lawson's efforts and Dr. Ward's biting comments have not gone unheeded. Through interviews, we found that many, but not all, anesthesiologists now make every effort to ease an infant's agony.

Dr. Fritz Berry specializes in pediatric anesthesiology at the Children's Medical Center at the University of Virginia in Charlottesville.

"With new techniques," says Dr. Berry, "we can anesthetize preemies as we do any patient with an unstable circulatory system. But there are doctors who do not feel secure about giving anesthesia to very sick preemies. Some fear that as soon as they do, these children will die."

But the opposite may be true: Killing their pain may help these babies live. Dr. K. J. S. Anand, a researcher in the anesthesia department at Children's Hospital in Boston, studied preemies who needed surgery to repair an artery near the heart.

Doctors gave one group of babies the muscle relaxant curare plus nitrous oxide (laughing gas), a mild anesthetic. The others received fentanyl, which puts the patient to sleep. Dr. Anand found that, following surgery, those given fentanyl had fewer problems with breathing and heart stability. His measurements of blood hormones showed clearly that, without full anesthesia, the babies experienced great stress and pain.

"I assume these babies feel pain," says Dr. Swedlow, "and we try to give them an anesthetic—as much as we feel they can tolerate. We really have no way of knowing just how much is really safe and effective. It is better to survive and perhaps feel discomfort than die and not feel any discomfort."

All of this leaves parents in a quandary. Debra Scharg of Oakland, California, an obstetric nurse, gave birth 3 months prematurely to Jacob Eli. He weighed 1½ pounds and had a severe bowel infection. The Schargs say they gave permission to operate on the 18th day of Jacob's life, on the condition that he be anesthetized. Jacob did not survive the surgery. The Schargs say they later found that medical records showed no evidence of Jacob having received painkillers.

"As it turned out," Mrs. Scharg says, "our son was much too sick to go through the operation. We wished that the doctors had just let us hold Jacob to say good-bye to him. Instead, he died on the operating table in pain."

Jill Lawson, determined to help other babies avoid Jeffrey's fate, urges that parents discuss the issue with their pediatrician and the anesthesiologist, not the surgeon or assistant surgeon. It's the anesthesiologist who makes the decision to give painkillers.

As of now, no laws compel a doctor to follow the wishes of an infant's parents. If the doctor feels that anesthesia might impose too great a risk, he can order the drugs withheld. "Doctors need to spend more time talking to the parents," says Dr. Berry. "We, too, are extremely concerned about the child."

The Heart

YOU COULD HAVE HIGH BLOOD PRESSURE AT THIS moment and not know it. Usually, there are no symptoms of this sneaky disease that slowly and secretly undermines your organs.

Then, one day, a blood vessel bursts in your head, and a stroke paralyzes you. Or a blood clot forms in one of the coronary arteries, which feed blood to your heart. A clot prevents blood (and, therefore, oxygen) from getting to the heart muscle. Starved for oxygen, a chunk of the heart dies.

Or your body fills up with water—your heart and kidneys cannot get rid of fluid.

Still, there is hope for the 70 million Americans with elevated blood pressure that warrants some type of therapy or regular monitoring. In more than half the cases of high blood pressure, or hypertension, doctors can control the disease with drugs. And many don't even need drugs; doctors simply prescribe losing weight, lowering the intake of salt and alcohol, exercising, and learning to relax.

The lowering of salt in food is somewhat controversial. Not all types of high blood pressure respond negatively when you eat too much salt. The pressure in these types of hypertension does not increase with salt intake. But only a doctor can tell you whether your high blood pressure is salt sensitive.

"Thanks to the progress made in treating high blood pressure over the last 30 years, largely with new drugs and greater patient awareness of a healthy diet and lifestyle, tens of thousands of lives have been saved," says Dr. Ray Gifford. He works at the Cleveland Clinic Foundation and is one of the nation's leading experts on high blood pressure. Since 1973, deaths from stroke have dropped by more than 50 percent, and deaths from heart attack have fallen 35 percent.

"Better hypertension control has contributed to the remarkable decline in deaths," says Ed Roccella of the National Heart, Lung, and Blood Institute. "The precise contribution is still not clear, but evidence from clinical studies has clearly demonstrated the effects of lowering blood pressure on reducing stroke deaths. The effects of reduced blood pressure on heart attack are less clear but still apparent."

Three of four individuals with high blood pressure are being treated today—

that's twice the number of patients who were under treatment in 1972, adds Dr. Roccella.

Normally, as your heart contracts, it pushes blood out into that giant web of arteries and veins. Arteries carry blood away from the heart; veins carry blood back to the heart and lungs to refresh the blood with oxygen.

With the heart pumping, the blood, which, of course, is liquid, pushes against the walls of the blood vessels. That's the pressure that doctors talk about. The pressure rises to a peak when the lower half of the heart muscle squirts blood into the arterial tree. That's called *systolic pressure.*

When the heart relaxes, the pressure drops but the blood continues to flow. That's called *diastolic pressure.*

In the United States, 28 million hypertensive adults have systolic pressures greater than 160 or diastolic pressures greater than 95. An additional 20 million Americans have less severe but still serious readings: systolic pressures between 140 and 160, and diastolic pressures between 90 and 95.

Many people are unaware of the health risks imposed by even so-called "mild" blood pressures, such as 140/90, and often discontinue their therapy. An 18-year study in Framingham, Massachusetts, shows clearly that, at all adult ages, men and women with elevated blood pressures run an increased risk of heart disease. For example, the risk for a 50-year-old man with "mild" hypertension is 40 percent higher than for one

with a "healthy" pressure. Of course, at higher pressures (such as 160 systolic), that 50-year-old's risk of heart disease runs even higher—75 percent greater than for a man with a healthy pressure.

Figures collected by the National Center for Health Statistics in Hyattsville, Maryland, show that one white adult in four has high blood pressure; among blacks, it is one adult in three. Regardless of race, women adhere to treatment better than men and, therefore, control their hypertension better.

Blood that courses through your arteries under high pressure takes a heavy toll on your other organs. Bit by bit, the high pressure of circulating blood serves to pile more and more cholesterol, calcium, and scar tissue into the linings of your blood vessels. Soon, their tubelike openings are blocked, closing down the flow. The high pressure can damage the wall of the aorta, the giant artery that carries blood from the heart to the rest of your body. After years of being subjected to high pressure, the heart muscle thins and then can balloon out and burst. Albert Einstein died of this condition.

The pressure also hurts your tiny blood vessels, making it tougher for the heart to push blood through the body's billions of narrowed channels. In a vicious cycle, your heart pumps harder, raising your blood pressure still higher and causing more injury.

As the blood pressure increases, the left side of your heart works harder and harder to push the blood through. Like any hard-working muscle, the heart gets bigger, but, overworked, it eventually can't keep up with the demands placed on it. The volume of blood pumped by the heart drops. As a result, you go into congestive heart failure. Once this happens, water piles up in your tissues because, under the reduced blood flow, your kidneys cannot eliminate it. Eventually, you "drown" in your own fluids.

What Causes High Blood Pressure?

Many things contribute: heredity, overweight, high emotional stress, no exercise, and too much alcohol. For some patients too much salt in the diet makes the pressure rise.

Salt is composed of two chemicals: chlorine and sodium. However, each element can play a role when attached to other chemicals or other elements. Sodium in any situation triggers increased blood pressure in those patients sensitive to it. Some experts say sodium results in hypertension in only 20 percent of the population; so if your pressure isn't going up, you need not change your salt-eating habits. But if it is rising, cut back to 2 grams a day by shunning the salt shaker and avoiding processed foods high in salt or sodium.

Contrary to what you may have heard, your blood pressure need not increase with age. Dr. Lot Page of the National Institute on Aging in Bethesda, Maryland, studied the natives of the Solomon Islands in the South Pacific. He found no increase in either their body weight or their blood pressure as they grew older. Scientists have made similar findings in studies of other primitive peoples. The lifesaving lesson for survival: exercise—and don't gain weight.

In the last 20 years, scientists have learned that blood pressure is controlled by many different systems in the body. For example, your kidneys release chemicals that either increase or decrease blood pressure. So do your adrenal glands, found atop each kidney. Doctors have also discovered a hormone produced by the heart called atrial natriuretic factor (ANF). As blood pressure rises in the heart, ANF is released, causing a reduction in pressure.

Drug Therapy

From their research into the body's own blood-pressure control mechanisms, scientists have developed several classes of drugs:

- Diuretics (water pills). These chemicals stimulate the kidneys to remove water and salt from the blood system, reducing blood pressure.
- Beta-blockers. These medicines block the action of epinephrine (also known as adrenaline) and norepinephrine, thereby decreasing the heartbeat rate and the vigor of each contraction.
- Calcium channel blockers. They prevent calcium from entering the tiny

artery muscles and causing them to constrict, which raises blood pressure.

• ACE inhibitors. ACE stands for angiotensin converting enzyme. Angiotensin II, a hormone originating in the kidneys, raises blood pressure by constricting the artery muscles. The new drugs inhibit or halt production of angiotensin II. Without angiotensin II, the arteries relax and blood pressure drops.

• Vasodilators. These drugs work directly on the artery muscles, relaxing them.

• Central agents. These chemicals work primarily in the lower part of the brain, where they prevent nerves from sending out signals to release the hormones that, in turn, raise blood pressure.

Several studies, involving more than 10,000 patients, clearly show that these drugs not only lower pressure but also reduce the incidence of strokes and other cardiovascular problems, thereby lowering death rates.

Tests of the newest classes of drugs—calcium channel blockers and ACE inhibitors—show that they do lower blood pressure, but proof that they save lives is lacking. Doctors are increasingly prescribing them because they have fewer side effects than the old medications. The chief drawback is that they are expensive ($1,000 or more a year for treatment).

Katherine Echols of Atlanta discovered that her blood pressure was 162/113, placing her at risk of a stroke or heart attack. Doctors prescribed diuretics, which reduced the pressure. She also lost weight, cut her salt intake, and began a walking program for exercise. Her pressure came down. Then she tried one of the new drugs, and her last reading stood at 119/85—definitely within the healthy range.

"Once you get high blood pressure, it's a lifetime thing," says Ms. Echols, "It's not a cure, but you can be helped."

How Science Is Saving Your Heart

WHEN A HEART ATTACK COMES, YOU FEEL AS though a lightning bolt had struck the ground beside you. Sharp pain crashes through your chest. It can also sizzle up your arm, your back, your neck. And the pain doesn't let up.

Over 1.5 million Americans will suffer a heart attack each year. And 550,000 of them will die. But advances in surgical techniques and drugs in the last decade now give you the best chances in 50 years of surviving an attack. This means that people who have had heart attacks are living longer and without pain. Increasingly, they are winning the war against heart disease.

Leslie Schield, 56, is a heart attack victim who became a victor.

"I woke up with pressure in the center of my breastbone," says Mr. Schield, a plumbing superintendent in Houston. "And I had a pain in my right shoulder. I thought it was heartburn."

Four hours later, Mr. Schield lay on an operating table at Herman Hospital of the University of Texas Medical School. X rays showed that a blood clot was blocking a coronary artery. This blood vessel, no thicker than a soda straw, carries blood and oxygen to the heart. Without enough oxygen, Mr. Schield's heart screamed in pain.

The medical team had to act fast. Drs. Richard Smalling and Lance Gould and their associates slipped a long hollow tube—called a catheter—through an artery in Mr. Schield's groin up to his heart. Guided by X-ray pictures of the patient's heart that were projected onto a television screen, the doctors jiggled the catheter so that it rested at the face of the blood clot. Then they squirted the clot with a drug called streptokinase and actually watched the drug dissolve the blockage. Within an hour, the artery channel was clear. Life-sustaining blood flowed freely once more.

"I saw the whole thing on television while it was happening," says Mr. Schield, "and except for a hot flash when the drug went in, I got relief right away."

New drugs can save lives after a heart attack, but doctors must act fast. In the 1970s, Mr. Schield (and any other patient with a similar condition) would have either died or been crippled for life by a weak and painful heart.

Streptokinase is only one answer, though an important one, to heart disease. Doctors also can insert small but powerful pumps into the heart's main artery, the aorta. The pump can help a weakened heart muscle circulate blood. Surgeons also open up clogged coronary arteries or bypass them with sophisticated plumbing jobs.

A drug that fights organ rejection has made heart transplants viable for far more patients. Other drugs calm irritable hearts and reduce high blood pressure, one of the heart's most powerful enemies. And researchers are seeking and finding new clues to help you prevent heart attack.

Patients with irregular, irritable hearts that could stop at any moment are candidates for pacemakers. This year, surgeons will implant these tiny (each is smaller than the powder puff in a woman's compact) battery-powered boxes into the chests of 200,000 Americans. Via electric wires, the pacemakers deliver weak shocks to the heart to keep it beating in rhythm.

Another heart saver, one of the most successful in use today, was invented in

1966 by Dr. Adrian Kantrowitz, now of Sinai Hospital in Detroit. He devised the balloon pump, a highly effective aid for a weakened and dying heart. It squeezes blood through the arteries.

Stanley Burkoff, a Detroit advertising executive, lay dying from a heart attack. His blood pressure dropped dramatically, sending him into coronary shock. No medicine could raise his pressure. Such patients, Dr. Kantrowitz knew, have only one chance in a hundred of surviving.

Mr. Burkoff vividly remembers how it felt. "I was driving the car over a cliff. I was going into shock."

In a procedure similar to the one that the Texas doctors used to squirt streptokinase at Mr. Schield's blood clot, Dr. Kantrowitz opened an artery in Mr. Burkoff's groin and slipped a catheter up into the aorta near the heart. But at the end of the catheter, Dr. Kantrowitz had placed a 10-inch-long, sausage-shaped balloon.

Within 15 minutes, helium gas, which was driven by a pump outside the body, pulsed in and out of the balloon, blowing it up and collapsing it. With each cycle, that little pump moved an ounce of blood through Mr. Burkoff's heart, brain, and body. This kept him alive throughout the day and the next night until Dr. Kantrowitz could bypass the clogged artery. Then the pump was removed.

After his balloon-pump experience, Mr. Burkoff retired to writing, happy that Dr. Kantrowitz's invention was there to help him.

Approximately 30,000 balloon pumps have been temporarily inserted each year into arteries where they pump blood for anywhere from a few days to 6 months. They save a third of the heart attack victims in shock. Dr. Kantrowitz has developed a permanent balloon pump, which is now under test.

In essence, the balloon pump can be considered the grandfather of the artificial heart that kept Barney Clark alive for 112 days until he died of multiple organ failure at the University of Utah Medical Center on March 23, 1983. It was the balloon pump that first proved you could put a mechanical device inside the body to pump blood and keep the heart going for weeks and months.

In 1972, Dr. Kantrowitz sent Haskell Shanks home with a permanent balloon pump sewn into his aorta wall. But that experiment raised some disturbing doubts.

Three months after surgery, Mr. Shanks died from infection. Germs had apparently crawled along the tube that brought gas from the outside. Although there has been no official report, the same kind of infection may have killed Barney Clark.

In fact, infection may bar permanent installation of a total artificial heart regardless of how well the pump operates. But Dr. Kantrowitz's team believes it has the answer: a plastic skin plug that creates a biological home for skin cells. The cells grow into the plastic, making the seal between skin and plastic so tight that germs cannot pass through.

Many doctors, however, insist that the artificial heart is too complicated and too expensive ($250,000 per patient) to be practical, except for a few patients. So research teams, including Dr. Kantrowitz's and others at the Cleveland Clinic, at Stanford and Harvard Universities, and in Hershey, Pennsylvania, are racing to complete cheaper and simpler pumps that will give the heart partial assistance. Several of these devices already have been implanted in patients with otherwise poor chances of survival. About a third of them have survived.

The hottest development is called the L-Vad—Left Ventricular Assist Device. It replaces the left side of the heart—which does most of the pumping—with a mechanical pump. A couple of hundred have been installed to help the patients in the waiting period to get a human heart transplant. The FDA has approved a model that can be installed permanently. If the partial heart is as effective as the total mechanical heart, treating bad heart damage will be relatively inexpensive and safe.

While artificial hearts still seem the stuff of science fiction, heart transplants have become frequent lifesavers. For more than a decade now, surgeons have been replacing sick hearts with healthy ones. Dr. Norman Shumway of Stanford University has had the greatest success—more than 50 percent of his heart transplant recipients survive. And a drug called cyclosporine, which prevents rejection of the foreign heart, has increased Dr. Shumway's success rate to 85 percent.

But donor hearts are scarce, because they must come from healthy people who died of brain injuries. Unless scientists can find a way to transfer hearts from other species, transplants may never become widespread. Each year only 2,000 hearts become available for transplant. Experts say that heart surgeons could use 10,000.

However, doctors have developed ways to open or bypass clogged coronary arteries. Such arteries are the result of atherosclerosis, a disease in which fatty deposits coat and narrow the channels of the coronary vessels leading to heart pain and often to heart attack.

The most common method, coronary bypass surgery, became the chic surgery of the 1980s. In 1964, Drs. Michael De Bakey and Edward Garrett of Houston did the first such coronary artery plumbing job on a human being. They removed a length of vein from a patient's leg and used it to bypass the clogged section of artery. It promptly relieved the patient's heart pain, and he survived 9 years.

Today, 250,000 persons a year undergo coronary bypass surgery. The patients include two former secretaries of state: Henry Kissinger and Alexander Haig. For a while, doctors argued over whether bypass surgery prolonged patients' lives, although most agreed that it relieved heart pain.

"About 80 to 85 percent survived 10 years after their surgery," he told me, "and half of the people under 65 years of age are working full-time." Physicians can also stretch partially clogged arteries with a procedure called balloon angioplasty. Again, they use the long catheter with a tiny balloon at the end. They work the catheter into the artery, blow up the balloon, and stretch the opening of the artery.

Other new drugs can prevent heart attacks, heart pain, or both. One chemical, called a beta-blocker, opens up the coronary arteries and reduces the heart's need for oxygen. Studies show that patients treated with beta-blockers suffer less pain, have fewer heart attacks, and survive longer.

Even newer are the calcium channel blockers. They also open up arteries and reduce the heart's oxygen use. But their life extension properties are not yet proved. Both types of drug dramatically drop blood pressure; this, by itself, can prevent heart attacks.

Finally, you may be able to prevent or reduce your risk of heart disease if you stop smoking, increase exercise, and cut down your blood cholesterol level by eating less animal fat.

While medical science cannot yet give you a foolproof prescription to prevent heart attack, it has shown you ways to increase your chances of doing so by changing your lifestyle. And the magnificent progress in coronary medicine and surgery has given you a better chance of surviving heart disease—pain-free.

The Truth about Cholesterol

IF YOU HAVEN'T HEARD OR SEEN THE WORD cholesterol in the past month, you've probably been stranded on a desert island.

Because everybody's talking about it—often with confusion—*Parade* has surveyed the latest scientific research and consulted the major experts about cholesterol. We now can tell you what it does, how it gets into your body, how it could clog up your arteries, and how to get it out of your body.

But is all that information going to make any difference to your health?

Yes, says Dr. John C. LaRosa, of the American Heart Association. He says, "In the last decade, we have had a really substantial increase in certainty that there is a cause-and-effect relationship between cholesterol levels in the blood and heart disease. We are also certain—beyond reasonable doubt—that we can reduce heart disease."

Data from the National Center for Health Statistics show that from 1971 to 1996, deaths from heart disease dropped nearly 50 percent. People are taking action: exercising, limiting the fat and cholesterol in their diet, and reducing other risks by quitting smoking and lowering high blood pressure.

You may have heard that cholesterol is a fatty substance. In a way it is, sort of. But cholesterol is not fat. In large amounts, fat is yellowish-white and oily; cholesterol is white and waxy.

Your body needs fat, which is a source of energy, and cholesterol, which goes into the making of hormones, digestive bile, and the "skin" of your cells. Your body can create fat and cholesterol. The foods you eat contain both, but only animal foods (including butter, cream, ice cream, cheese, meat, eggs) have cholesterol. Your body stores *pounds* of fat as lumps everywhere, but it stores only *ounces* of cholesterol, which are distributed to every organ of the body.

The kind and amount of fat you eat is linked to how much cholesterol your body makes and how much cholesterol runs in your blood. This link is the key to the cause of heart disease. If you eat too much fat from animal sources, the cholesterol in your blood rises. Each day, a little sticks to the walls of your arteries. In a few years, sacs of cholesterol pile up on the arterial walls. These sacs have been found in men as young as 19.

In a few decades, enough cholesterol can collect on the arteries' walls to slow or block the flow of blood through them. Often this narrows the coronary arteries, which feed blood to the heart muscle. With flow slowed or blocked, heart pain (angina) signals that the heart muscle itself lacks enough blood to give it oxygen and enough energy to keep it pumping. Result: a heart attack.

If a blocked artery leads to hemorrhage or to a lack of blood in part of the brain, a stroke—with paralysis, loss of speech, or other mental functions—could result. In the legs, cholesterol-clogged arteries can so block circulation as to cause severe muscle cramps and sometimes gangrene.

Neither fat nor cholesterol dissolves in water. And both float. So, how do they get through the watery bloodstream to the organs and cells that need them?

The body ingeniously produces a microscopic waterproof boat of fat, cholesterol, and protein, called lipoprotein (*lipo* means fat). The protein forms a skin around the fat and the cholesterol, creating a watertight lipoprotein bundle. The bundle then rides easily in the water of the blood.

The body also creates different types of lipoprotein. You've heard of two of them—HDL, the "good cholesterol," and LDL, the "bad cholesterol." HDL stands for high (to help you separate the bad from the good, let *H* stand for *healthful*) density lipoprotein, which means the bundle is small and tightly packed with cholesterol and fat. The bad stuff, LDL (let *L* stand for *lethal*), is low density lipoprotein. Its bundle is large and lightly packed.

LDL, the "bad cholesterol," transports cholesterol to the cells of all organs. If you have too much LDL in your blood, the lipoprotein bundles dump the excess cholesterol onto your artery walls. HDL, the "good cholesterol," hauls cholesterol away from the walls. Studies show that if you can depress the LDL levels in blood and raise the HDL levels, your body actually can clean cholesterol out of the artery walls.

A test for cholesterol levels usually reveals not only your total blood cholesterol level but also how much and what kinds of cholesterol are in your blood. Even 15 years ago, the tests were not so detailed.

Most people are puzzled about what the test scores mean, because doctors give cholesterol amounts in metric units rather than in ounces or pints. They use milligrams—a milligram is $1/1{,}000$th of a gram, or $1/28{,}000$th of an ounce. They also use deciliters—a deciliter is $1/10$th of a liter or $2/10$ths of a pint, a bit more than 3 ounces.

Many studies have shown that you're safest if your total blood cholesterol stays below 200 milligrams for each deciliter of blood or, as a doctor would write it, 200 mg/dl. At 240 mg/dl, your risk of heart attack doubles that of a person with less than 200 mg/dl. And at 300 mg/dl, the danger is undeniable.

To prevent the rise of cholesterol in your blood, you must, quite logically, eat less cholesterol and saturated fat. Most red meats, animal and dairy products, and commercial baked goods contain goodly amounts of both. Cut back on saturated fats. These stimulate the liver to make more cholesterol than you need. Most vegetables contain little saturated fat. Read your food labels, even when you see the words *no cholesterol* or *low cholesterol*. Check and avoid products high in saturated fats such as coconut, palm, and palm-kernel oils; whole-milk solids; whole-egg solids; chocolate; coconut; suet; lard (pig fat); and butter fat.

Dr. Jeremiah Stamler, for many years a leading cholesterol researcher at Northwestern University Medical School in Chicago, says to be wary of the cholesterol you eat, too. "Cholesterol in the diet raises LDL," Dr. Stamler says, "even though not as strongly as saturated fat."

Clearly, we must cut down on saturated fat. The American Heart Association says that no more than 30 percent of our calories should come from fat of any kind. Today the average American's calories total 37 percent fat. That's down from 45 percent just 20 years ago, and many scientists say that's why heart disease is decreasing. In the same period, our average blood cholesterol level dropped from 240 mg/dl to 220 mg/dl.

Here are some general guidelines:

Substitute fish, seafood, skinless chicken, and turkey for red meats, and choose lean cuts (beef flank or round steak, pork tenderloin) when you do eat meat. Limit meat and fish portions to 6 ounces a day, and limit eggs to three or four a week. Use egg substitutes freely, and, suggests dietitian and writer Gail Levey, for baking, try using two egg whites instead of one whole egg. Also, she mixes 3 tablespoons of cocoa and one tablespoon of oil to substitute for one square of baking chocolate. Instead of ice cream, Ms. Levey says to try low- and no-fat yogurts, regular or frozen. Plain popcorn also makes a healthful treat, she advises.

Replace the calories lost by the elimination of animal foods with complex carbohydrates—starches like bread (preferably whole-grain), cereal, pasta, rice, dried peas, and beans. Let half or more of your calories come from starches.

Eat more vegetables and fruits to raise the amount of vitamins and fiber in your diet. You also will get fiber from breads and other starches. Fiber, especially the water-soluble kind found in oat bran, helps lower your blood cholesterol.

Use vegetable oils—such as corn, safflower, and olive. They contain unsaturated fats that lower cholesterol. Says Dr. James Cleeman, head of the National Cholesterol Education Program in Bethesda, Maryland, "Exercise is very important in lowering cholesterol. Vigorous exercise may raise levels of good cholesterol."

The Education Program, comprised of panels of experts, was convened by the National Heart, Lung, and Blood Institute. It helps spread the word about cholesterol, and the number of patients going to doctors has increased by nearly five times since the program began in 1985.

First, one panel suggested that all adults be tested for total blood cholesterol. Levels below 200 mg/dl need only sensible dieting.

Borderline scores between 200 and 239 mg/dl may require action, depending on other risks you may have, such as heart disease, smoking, high blood pressure, a family history of early heart disease, diabetes, or severe obesity (more than 30 percent overweight). Being male also raises your risk.

If you have heart disease or two of the other risks, you're in the high-risk group. If you have none of these, you're in the low-risk category.

If your cholesterol level is borderline, doctors will urge you to keep your diet below 30 percent fat. Have your level checked yearly. If you're at high risk with the middling score, your doctor will warn you to lower your cholesterol.

The first thing to be checked is your level of LDL, the bad cholesterol. If you have less than 130 mg/dl in your blood, your diet should be kept healthful. If your LDL is between 130 and 159, barring other risks, you may not have to do anything more than watch your diet and moderate your intake of saturated fats. If your LDL level puts you in the high-risk group, you're certainly going to have to enlist in a strong diet program.

Your goal is to push your blood LDL down to under 130 if you have heart disease, or under 160 if you do not. If you don't succeed in 6 months, your doctor may consider prescribing drugs.

Fortunately, there are many, including nicotinic acid, Questran, or Colestid. The last two are resins that trap bile in the digestive tract and carry it out of the body. Normally, your intestines reabsorb unused bile and reprocess the cholesterol it contains. When the resins remove the bile, they remove its cholesterol, too. Because it needs cholesterol to make more bile, the liver will remove new cholesterol (especially LDL) from the blood.

Doctors prescribe resins because, although they cause occasional constipation and heartburn, they are known to be safe and can lower the LDL count quickly. With a resin drug, my cholesterol level fell from 270 to 180, my LDL dropping along with it. And it definitely cut my risk of heart disease.

In large amounts, nicotinic acid stops the liver from making certain lipoproteins that give rise to LDL. Result: the body slows production of the "bad cholesterol." Nicotinic acid's side effects include your face and body possibly becoming very flushed, and nausea may occur. If you can get through the first 3 or 4 weeks, the side effects vanish. Nicotinic acid also cuts the risk of heart disease.

Three other drugs—gemfibrozil, lovastatin, and probucol—slow the making of LDL to varying degrees and help lower cholesterol in the process. In a study done in Helsinki, Finland, gemfibrozil was shown also to cut the risk of heart disease.

If your total cholesterol count exceeds 240 mg/dl, your doctor will order the LDL tests for you. If you're at high risk, or if your LDL level soars above 160 mg/dl, you will be told to follow a stringent diet program and, depending on the doctor, a regular exercise regimen too. If this fails to lower your cholesterol, drugs probably will be prescribed.

Some people maintain that if you have a high HDL level, regardless of how high your total cholesterol is, you have nothing to worry about. Still, the experts also caution that if the LDL level is high, there is cause for concern.

Dr. DeWitt Goodman, a professor at Columbia-Presbyterian Medical Center in New York who headed a panel of experts for the National Heart, Lung, and Blood Institute, says data show that lowering LDL lowers the risk of heart disease. "The vast majority of people," he says, "can reduce their risk of heart disease by lowering total cholesterol."

If you get your total blood cholesterol below 200 mg/dl, you have optimized your chances of escaping a heart attack.

Will programs to lower cholesterol result in a higher risk of cancer, as some people have said? All the experts we consulted denied that it was a proven risk. In fact, Dr. Goodman says, by eating a lowered-fat diet, you may reduce your chances of colon cancer a well as several other kinds of cancer.

Dr. LaRosa of the American Heart Association says, "It is most important for one with high cholesterol levels and other risk factors to reduce those levels."

Dr. Jeremiah Stamler says you can add up to 8 years to your life expectancy,

---

Like Father Not Like Son

Forty-eight years ago, I saw my father, at the age of 44, succumb to two of the human heart's greatest enemies— fatty diet and smoking. Not until 10 years after his funeral did I learn that there was a connection between his death of a massive heart attack and his lifestyle. A short man, at least 40 percent overweight, my father smoked two packs of cigarettes a day. Based on his diet, as I remember it (he ate lots of beef, butter, and other animal fats), I would guess that he had a very high blood cholesterol level.

A decade after my father's death, I met the late Dr. Norman Jolliffe, then head of the Bureau of Nutrition of New York City's Health Department. He invented the Prudent Diet—low in fat, low in cholesterol—because the scientific evidence (even as early as the 1950s) began to show that heart disease and diet were interrelated.

At that time, I weighed 190 pounds—35 pounds more than was healthy. Dr. Jolliffe put me on his Prudent Diet. Eventually, I went down to my normal healthy weight of 160. In the 1960s, I had my blood cholesterol level measured. It rang the alarm bell at 300 mg/dl. My risk of heart attack stood four times higher than that of a man with 170 mg/dl.

I had inherited my father's chemistry. I did not want to inherit his heart disease.

I changed my eating habits even more: no beef, butter, or eggs; more fish, more complex carbohydrates, more vegetable oils. Finally, I knocked my cholesterol down to 240 mg/dl. And it stuck.

In the 1980s, a massive study proved that the medication Questran was safe and effective for lowering cholesterol. I took it. My cholesterol dropped to 170 mg/dl of blood. Later, I took lovastatin, which cut my cholesterol further. I never smoked. I exercise vigorously four or five times a week. I have outlived my father by 34 years. I wish both he and I had known all this when he was alive.

and even more under some conditions. He compares two men: One smokes and has a high cholesterol level; the other doesn't smoke and has a low cholesterol level. The chances are that the low-risk man will live up to 10 years longer than the other man.

Some critics assert that lowering cholesterol would yield only small increases in life expectancy, from a few months to a year. Dr. Goodman counters that if the cholesterol treatment delays the onset of a heart attack, that alone makes it all worthwhile.

When Is Heart Surgery Really Called For?

EACH YEAR IN THE UNITED STATES, DOCTORS invade the chests of more than 750,000 patients to repair their hearts and clear their coronary arteries. Heart surgery once meant almost certain death for patients. Today, some say it has risen to the level of mass production. The annual surgical scorecard for the United States reads as follows:

- 400,000 bypass procedures, in which unclogged veins from legs and arms, and unblocked arteries from chests, are used to bypass clogged ones
- 300,000 angioplasty operations, in which doctors snake tubes from the leg artery to the narrowed blood vessel, where they insert a balloon to push aside cholesterol blockage
- 58,000 repairs to damaged heart valves
- 2,000 transplants of healthy hearts into patients whose own hearts cannot be repaired

The cost of these operations is roughly $50 billion a year, or 6 percent of the nation's annual $900 billion medical bill. But is this money well spent? Can patients be helped with far less risk and at considerably reduced expense? Experts are now asking, How necessary is heart surgery?

If you're slated for heart surgery, heed the saga of my good friend, Mimi Cole of Wayne, New Jersey.

Years ago, Mimi danced with the Martha Graham Company. On stage, she was a luminous young woman—a pleasure to watch as she swept across the floor. She is now 70 and still teaches dance occasionally. Mimi thought she was in good condition. But, in 1992, trouble arose.

"My chest felt funny," she recalls. "I could not easily walk up a hill. I had a pain in my shoulder. My cardiologist in

New Jersey sent me to a surgeon who examined me, found my arteries were blocked, and recommended surgery. I was terrified."

Blood could not pass through the plugged blood vessels to feed oxygen to Mimi's heart muscle. Her doctor's plan was to allow the blood to bypass the obstruction by taking unblocked veins from her legs and grafting them onto the heart arteries. But there was no way to accomplish this: the appropriate veins, which had become varicose, had been surgically stripped from her legs years ago.

The alternative, her doctor said, was to use arteries from her abdomen or chest. He recommended a specialist at the Cleveland Clinic in Ohio. Mimi did not want to go so far from home. Instead, she found her way to Dr. Eric Rose, chief of cardiothoracic surgery at Columbia-Presbyterian Medical Center in Manhattan. Dr. Rose told Mimi he could work with her arteries, but first he wanted her to be examined by Dr. Michael Cohen, a heart specialist at Columbia. She agreed.

Two days before the scheduled surgery, Drs. Rose and Cohen called Mimi in and announced that they preferred to treat her condition first with medication rather than surgery. It proved a good decision. They prescribed beta-blockers, which controlled the rhythm and power of her heart, eliminating her pain and shortness of breath. Mimi resumed play-

ing tennis. In her case, the surgery remained unnecessary.

Mimi Cole's experience forces us to wonder how many other heart patients could have survived with an affordably priced pill instead of a costly and painful operation.

This problem of unnecessary surgery has been the subject of study for nearly a decade by the Rand Corporation, a policy research center in Santa Monica, California. In the early 1980s, Rand researchers checked the records of patients in one western state who'd had coronary bypass surgery. They found that, of 386 coronary surgeries performed there, 14 percent were unnecessary.

Given estimated average costs of $20,000 per heart-related operation, it seems safe to project that Americans paid $1 billion in taxes and insurance premiums just to cover those costs.

In the early 1990s, however, the Rand Corporation studied bypass surgery in New York State. The scene appears to have changed dramatically: It was found that among 1,500 operations, only 2.4 percent were unneeded. And, reports the New York State Department of Health Cardiac Survey, the death rate also dropped on the operating table—from 3.53 percent in 1990 to 2.51 percent in 1992.

The indications are that doctors keep acquiring skills and that the newer drugs and technology are gaining in their power to heal without injury. Some states keep track of cardiac surgeries. Through New York State Health Department data, in fact, you can discover a heart surgeon's batting average—how many surgeries he or she performed and their outcomes.

At Columbia-Presbyterian Medical Center, where Mimi Cole's Drs. Rose and Cohen work, physicians have opened a new Heart Failure Center. Here, the doctors turn first to drugs to heal damaged hearts and reduce the battered heart's workload. Dr. Milton Packer, the center's chief, says that this approach has:

- taken 40 percent of heart failure patients off the transplant waiting list,
- improved the conditions of 70 percent of people with heart failure, and
- cut the mortality rate by 25 percent.

"Drugs are not as exciting as transplants or mechanical hearts," Dr. Packer says, "but we have got to give drugs a chance to work."

A growing number of patients seem to be opting for the drug-treatment-first approach.

One of them is Howard Mills, 48, a British citizen living in Redondo Beach, California. In November 1992, a viral infection had attacked his heart muscle, leaving it weak and flabby. Mr. Mills opted for medication over surgery. He became a patient at the UCLA Cardiomyopathy Center.

"I was taking a lot of different drugs," says Mr. Mills, recalling the start of his treatment. "I could barely walk. But my heart and body came back. Now I can walk 4 miles an hour, I can swim, and I can ride a bike. I'm glad I escaped the transplant."

Open-heart surgery wasn't part of our medical landscape until the mid-1970s. A brief history lesson reminds us that there are records of such surgery dating to Greece in 400 B.C. The first successful heart operation on a human being didn't occur until 1896, when a doctor in Frankfurt sutured a heart wound for a young German soldier and saved his life. In World War II, shrapnel was removed from the hearts of American soldiers. In 1945, the first repairs of congenital abnormalities of the heart were made.

Surgeons in the early 1900s had the techniques to operate but were unable to do so on a still-beating heart, a problem that wasn't resolved until the mid-1950s and early 1960s.

Scientists had found early on that they could stop and restart the heart, but they had less than 3 minutes to avoid irreparable brain damage to the patient. Dr. John Gibbon of Philadelphia developed a machine that took over blood circulation. His machine was tested on animals in 1931. But it was 1953 before Dr. Gibbon performed a successful operation on a human patient using total cardiopulmonary bypass. It was not until the mid-1970s that machines were widely available. Now, by-pass (heart/lung) machines can maintain a patient's complex circulatory system during surgery for hours without serious side effects.

The other innovation allowing heart surgery for extended periods was the introduction of extreme cold to preserve a heart that has been stopped.

The red-letter day for heart surgery was December 3, 1967, when Dr. Christiaan Barnard performed the first hu- man heart transplant in Capetown, South Africa. And the first angioplasty was performed in Zurich in 1977; the first in the United States was done in 1988. An angioplasty is a surgical procedure in which the physician snakes a fine tube to the mouth of a clogged heart blood vessel. From there the catheter enters the artery itself. When the doctor encounters a blockage, he inflates the balloon at the end of the catheter. That opens a channel through the blocked artery so that blood carrying oxygen can once more invigorate the heart muscle.

The angioplasty is less invasive yet apparently as effective as heart bypass surgery and better for patients at special risk. The artery often becomes clogged again within a year, however, and the Washington (D.C.) Hospital Center estimates that roughly 30 percent of all angioplasties are repeated.

Dr. Spencer King III heads the department of interventional cardiology at Emory University in Atlanta. He led a 3-year study that compared the results of angioplasty and bypass.

Selected patients—392—were allotted either of the surgeries at random: half had angioplasty, half bypass. "Either way," Dr. King reports, "they came out the same in terms of death, heart attack, or the decreased blood flow to the heart.

"Initially," he continues, "the costs for bypass surgery were much higher." But, because repeated angioplasties were required, in 3 years' time the comparable costs were equal. Twenty percent of angioplasty patients later require a bypass operation.

Those who choose a bypass should know that, according to the American Heart Association, 20 to 28 percent of bypass surgeries need to be repeated, for reasons that vary among patients. And, although life improves for 90 percent of bypass patients, reclogging recurs in about 10 years for approximately 40 percent of them, reports the *Mayo Clinic Heart Book*.

The surgical choice, then, is between a bypass, if you want to avoid frequently repeated procedures, or an angioplasty, if you'd prefer to avoid major surgery.

Meanwhile, researchers are working hard to find ways of preventing the collapse of angioplasty patients' blood vessels. Two are currently in use. First, a surgeon can place a tiny metal cylinder in the patient's artery to support it. Second, the doctor and patient may treat arteries with medication and a healthful lifestyle.

The patient-controlled treatment prescribed for clogged arteries includes regular checkups, a low-fat diet, exercise, relaxation, and no smoking. Success depends on the patients' willingness and determination to trade in their harmful old habits for healthful new ones that will enable them to enjoy longer lives. The heart transplant—the most dramatic surgery of all—probably pays off best in the number of years of life gained.

A transplant replaces the failed heart that, weakened by heart attack or infection, produces a blood flow that has declined to a trickle. While anywhere from 11,000 to 20,000 patients are eligible for heart transplants, on average, only about 2,000 hearts are available yearly in the United States. It becomes a waiting game.

To maximize the survival chances of those who wait for a heart transplant, these choices are offered:

• The use of new mechanical hearts to sustain the patient waiting for a donor heart. These machines, intended for temporary use, are working increasingly well and may prove equal to or better than transplants, which have a 5-year survival rate of 50 percent.

• The use of animal hearts with medications to prevent rejection. This technique has been tried four times, but the recipients rejected the organs and died.

• Heart-strengthening medications to help transplant candidates' survive while on the waiting list for a new heart

But a crisis is emerging.

"If we continue to list so many [noncritical] patients for transplantation as we now do," says Dr. Stevenson, "in 4 years' time we will reach a point where none of the unhospitalized patients will have a chance for a transplant. People have to wait too long. They deteriorate, making their chance for survival poor."

One heart transplant recipient, Brenda Butler Hamlett, then 48, of Jamaica Plain, Massachusetts, says, "Before my transplant, I was too tired to blink." Now, Mrs. Hamlett reports, she happily exercises, watches her diet, and keeps track of her blood pressure.

Dr. Adrian Kantrowitz, professor of surgery at Wayne State University College of Medicine in Detroit, was the first to implant a human heart in the United States, at Maimonides Hospital in Brooklyn, New York, 3 days after the world's first human heart transplant by Dr. Barnard in 1967. Dr. Kantrowitz cites good results from heart surgeries for infants, too.

"We repair congenital defects extremely well," says Dr. Kantrowitz, "and we successfully operate on infants born with impaired connections between the heart arteries." He places the mortality rate for that surgery at less than a tenth of 1 percent. For valve replacement surgery, when using plastic or stainless-steel devices or valves taken from pigs, the rate is 2 percent, he says.

The final verdict on the effectiveness of these procedures is not yet in, but all heart disease must be treated—by you as well as your doctor.

Artificial Hearts That Work

DR. ERIC ROSE, THE CHIEF HEART TRANSPLANT surgeon of Columbia Presbyterian Medical Center in New York City, knew that because her tissue type was so very unusual, his new patient, Janet Harris, then 36, would have a perilously long wait for a heart transplant. She would get no help until someone who had her same rare tissue type died—without a heart injury.

But Mrs. Harris had little time left: her heart was growing weaker. She was in danger of death at any moment. Dr. Rose was convinced that her only other chance lay in an experimental, mechanical heart that could keep her going until the right donor came along.

Acting quickly, he performed the surgery at 2 o'clock in the morning, August 31, 1990. Dr. Rose implanted a HeartMate, a mechanical device no bigger than two adult males' fists. It features a high-tech pump designed to take over temporarily the function of a weakened left side of the patient's heart. HeartMate was designed by Victor Poirier, president of Thermo Cardiosystems of Woburn, Massachusetts, working with Harvard University.

Mrs. Harris's own heart stayed in her chest, pumping as much as it could. Unlike the Jarvik-7, the totally artificial heart with which surgeons replaced Barney Clark's heart in 1982, the HeartMate was built to assist an ailing heart and to be removed when surgeons replaced the patient's heart by implanting a heart from a donor. Scientists call the HeartMate machine an LVAD, for left ventricular assist device. The lower left chamber of the heart, called a ventricle, does most of the pumping.

Almost immediately, Mrs. Harris said she felt stronger as the water retained by her sluggish circulation flowed out of her tired body. In just days, she was on her feet. She used a wheeled table to move around with the electronic controls that kept her pump operating. Compressed air entered her body via a plastic tube to drive the artificial blood pump inside her. Mrs. Harris learned how to maintain the equipment throughout her daily activities. She took no medication except vitamins and an aspirin daily.

"I knew then I was going to make it," Mrs. Harris told me, when I visited her 3 months after the surgery. "Before the operation, they said I had only 24 hours to live."

Mrs. Harris remained attached to portable controls for 11 months before a suitable heart transplant was found. Her case shows that mechanical pumps probably can take over for the heart for a long time, perhaps for many years. Six months after her heart transplant, Janet Harris was dead. Her body had rejected her heart.

What a contrast to Barney Clark: Blood clots formed in his brain, and infections assailed his body. He lived only 112 days, connected to a 400-pound air-electronic system.

Michael Templeton, 34, a gas and oil pipeline technician from Humble, Texas, was HeartMate's user of longest duration. For Mr. Templeton, like Mrs. Harris, a viral infection led to a failing heart. With no suitable heart donor in sight, surgeons at the Texas Heart Institute in Houston implanted the machine in him.

Mr. Templeton was not hooked up to a console. His life support was powered and controlled by an electric wire that ran from a backpack containing batteries to the pump implanted in him.

"I'm in pretty good shape now," Mr. Templeton said. "Sometimes my back hurts from carrying the batteries. Having to stay overnight [at St. Luke's Episcopal Hospital in Houston] was the hardest part." In September 1991, the Food and Drug Administration (FDA) okayed daily visits home including overnight stays but said he still needed to spend 8 hours a day at the hospital.

Surprisingly, Dr. Howard Frazier, Mr. Templeton's surgeon, said the right and left ventricles of his heart improved notably. "If we cut back on the pump function," Dr. Frazier reported, "his own heart can work again. He can go home. Mike is in better shape than I am." After the pump, Mr. Templeton may not have needed a transplant after all; however, he died before he could get his donor heart.

Doctors say his death was unrelated to the LVAD.

The stories of Michael Templeton and Janet Harris lead some scientists to say that the ventricle aids could make total heart replacements unnecessary. Hundreds of patients who otherwise might have died have survived on them for varying periods.

Today, at least 65,000 Americans are desperately sick with failing hearts. These are patients who can barely move and must lie in bed all day. They need heart transplants to stay alive. But only about 2,000 human hearts are available for transplant each year. As a result, many of these patients won't last 6 months, unless they get an artificial pump. More than 40,000 will die each year for lack of that pump.

At this writing, however, the FDA, which oversees medical machines, has yet to approve a left ventricular assist device for sale. But it has allowed surgeons to implant them for testing as a temporary bridge to transplants. At least four manufacturers, all with their own designs, are racing to get FDA approval to sell the devices as transplant stopgaps. Approval could be speeded up, thanks to the devices' improvements regarding the infection, clotting, and the destruction of blood that had plagued the Jarvik-7.

Novacor is an implantable device from the Novacor Division of Baxter Healthcare, in Oakland, California, first tested at Stanford University, later at the

University of Pittsburgh. Novacor has been tested on 130 patients. Novacor and HeartMate are the only two LVADs that are implantable with only an electric wire emerging from the patient's body.

One of the earliest of pump implants, the Thoratec ventricular assist device, was conceived at the Penn State University Milton S. Hershey Medical Center in Hershey, Pennsylvania. Worldwide, the Thoratec device was tested in nearly 200 patients, until they got their transplants. A 57-year-old man is its longest-surviving patient. He was implanted with the Thoratec device on December 19, 1990. It was removed when his donor heart was transplanted 225 days later, on August 2, 1991, at the University of Pittsburgh Medical Center.

A fourth machine is the BVS 5000 Bi-Ventricular Support System, made by Abiomed Cardiovascular of Danvers, Massachusetts. Generally for bedridden patients, it uses a tube to connect the atrium—the upper chambers of the patient's heart—with a compressed air–driven pump stationed at the bedside.

More artificial mechanical heart assistance is given by a pencil-size device, the Hemopump. It rotates about 25,000 times a minute to take blood from the left ventricle and pump it down the aorta. Intended for only a week or so of use, it has been tested on 200 patients. Taken over for further refinement by Johnson & Johnson of New Brunswick, New Jersey, the Hemopump was developed by Nimbus, a company headquartered in Rancho Cordova, California.

All the data on individuals who have benefited from such machines lead surgeons like Dr. Rose and Dr. Frazier to call Novacor and HeartMate good enough *now* for permanent use by many who otherwise might die without them.

Says Dr. Rose, "We propose that desperately ill patients who have a horrible prognosis without a new heart be offered the HeartMate as an alternative to waiting and risking that a transplant might not occur before it is too late. Patients with HeartMate could leave the hospital. Janet Harris took care of her heart-pump equipment for 11 months.

"There are 40,000 deaths per year from congestive heart failure; that is three times the mortality rate of AIDS," Dr. Rose continues. "It is frustrating to see this device puttering along so slowly in the regulatory system." Dr. Robert Jarvik, developer of Jarvik-7, agrees.

Janet Harris told me she felt good with her donor heart. She added that she is required to take a lot of expensive drugs to prevent her body from rejecting her human transplant. "I don't like to take medication," she said, "but I have to."

Sadly, Mrs. Harris's heart transplant developed an immune reaction and stopped beating. She died just a few months after her transplant operation after living a healthy life for 11 months with her LVAD.

"It may be," says Dr. Frazier, "that some patients actually are better off with the pump than the transplant, particularly younger patients. After heart transplants, 85 percent do well. But the survival rate drops to 60 percent after 5 years."

If the artificial, blood-pumping device could function for at least 5 years, would a patient be better off with a pump than with a transplant? That's asking a lot of a piece of machinery.

"The reliability level of these machines has to be higher than a manned spaceship going to the moon and back," says Dr. John T. Watson, head of the artificial heart section of the National Heart, Lung, and Blood Institute in Bethesda, Maryland, since 1976. The institute has backed the four leading machines.

The human heart beats 40 million times in a year. Generally, if it is injured, the body can repair it. If a mechanical heart breaks down, however, it cannot be repaired. If it stops, blood stops flowing, then clots in a huge lump.

Dr. Adrian Kantrowitz, senior heart surgeon at Sinai Hospital in Detroit, is testing the Cardiovad, a frankfurter-shaped pump that sidesteps this clotting problem. The pump is inserted in the wall of the aorta. Electronically controlled to expand under air pressure when the natural heart's valve closes at the aorta's entry, the pump can do up to 50 percent of the left ventricle's work. When the heart contracts, the pump relaxes; when the left ventricle empties, the pump expands, pushing the blood along with extra force. This device might help hundreds of patients needing temporary but long-term assistance while their hearts heal or as surgeons repair damage to heart muscle or arteries. Because the balloon is outside the stream of blood, you can turn it on and off without fear of blood clots. Dr. Kantrowitz says he hopes the Cardiovad one day will eliminate the need for heart transplants.

Dr. Claude J. M. Lenfant, director of the National Heart, Lung, and Blood Institute, says, "I am absolutely convinced that the mechanical and clinical aspects of these devices will be resolved by the end of the century."

To criticism from heart scientists that his institute, budgeted at $1.2 billion, is not giving enough money to the development of the devices treating heart disease, Dr. Lenfant replies, "We also must put some of our research money into the *detection* and *prevention* of heart disease. In the last decade, such research has contributed to a dramatic drop in the rate of death from heart disease."

Other projects are under way to develop a completely implantable total-heart replacement like the Jarvik-7, but with no wires or other protrusions. Experts say the controversy surrounding the Jarvik-7 obscured its scientific contribution. A Jarvik-7 sustained William Schroeder for 620 days. The FDA had granted permission for its use while the patient waited for a transplant but withdrew it because of poor manufacturing quality. Dr. Jarvik, pursuing research privately, reminds critics that the Jarvik-7 did work. "It could have been made portable," he adds.

Another possibility for very sick heart patients could be the use of a transplant from another species. A baboon's heart has been transplanted into a human child. The patient died.

Dr. Thomas Starzl, director of the University of Pittsburgh Transplantation Institute, says animal hearts may be transplanted successfully to humans. Because the baboon heart is too small for human adults, surgeons will turn to cows or pigs.

"Most important is to control the antibodies present that reject other species," he adds. This has not proved a problem for patients using the artificial pumps because there is no immune reaction to the plastic and metal of the artificial hearts.

As the various devices become more plentiful and surgeons become more skilled with them, patients will spend less time in costly intensive care. Best of all, they might even get these heart savers when they need them.

Protect Your Heart

PAIN IN THE CHEST: ANGINA. THIS DREADED signal of clogged arteries and a possible heart attack is a frightening warning indeed.

Heart attacks kill or incapacitate more Americans than any other condition, but science has the death rate dropping.

Millions of people, young and old, have atherosclerosis, in which plaque—a lumpy, fatty material—builds up inside artery walls by attracting to itself clumps of excess cholesterol in the blood. The plaque can build up until it fills the arteries, lessening or blocking the flow of blood and oxygen to the heart. Lacking oxygen, the heart muscle cramps in pain; eventually, some heart muscle dies. The resulting wound can kill or weaken the heart so that it pumps inefficiently.

New uses of chemicals, surgery, and gadgets today can clear the plaque or bypass an artery blockage with transplanted vessels from the leg or chest through which blood flows freely. But, in 30 percent of these cases, if the plaque buildup and clogging isn't slowed or stopped, the artery closes after 5 to 7 years.

Dr. Eugene Passamani directs the Division of Heart and Vascular Diseases at the National Heart, Lung, and Blood Institute in Bethesda, Maryland. "Since 1963, there has been a 50 percent drop in coronary death rates in this country," he says. "We have better prevention, better use of high-tech approaches."

Still, repairs do fail—some right on the operating table, some years later. But progress continues in both known and new methods.

Coronary Bypass Surgery

The coronary arteries sit like a crown of branches on your heart. (*Coronary* is from *corona,* Latin for crown.) Only the three main coronary arteries, none thicker than a soda straw, bring fresh, oxygen-filled blood into your heart muscle, which needs oxygen to pump your blood.

In 1967, surgeons first opened the chest of a patient, stopped the heart, and put the patient on a heart-lung machine. They then grafted a vein from the lower leg onto the artery at points before and after the blockage, to bypass the clogged area and keep the blood flowing freely to the heart muscle. A substance called plaque, composed in part of cholesterol, builds up on the walls of the arteries and eventually clogs them. General medical estimates are that, from 1967 to the end of 1990, a total of 3.5 million bypass operations were done in the United States.

"I never thought I'd feel this good again," says Hay Brown, 63, a retired tobacco company executive in Durham, North Carolina. He had three blocked arteries bypassed in 1987. He adds, "I like to go golfing, hiking, jogging—anything that gets me outside."

How long will it last? Bodies producing enough plaque to clog the arteries *before* surgery will keep doing so—and clog the arteries again. Diet, exercise, and lifestyle adjustments can control this tendency.

Dr. Passamani says his reviews of 10- and 12-year follow-up studies of bypass patients show that, in 10 years, a third of the average vein grafts close, a third have atherosclerosis, and a third are open. The bypass lengthens life by a few years in the patient whose major (left) coronary artery is diseased, he adds, and it relieves angina pain, but it does not greatly prolong the patient's life. "We have no data that surgery will help more than medication," Dr. Passamani says.

No one knows why *newly* grafted arteries close. But, in 4 to 6 months, up to 25 percent of all bypasses shut down, probably because the artery's damaged inner walls grow out toward the center, as if to heal the wound. Hoping to avoid this, doctors take arteries from inside the chest rather than veins from the leg.

Arteries or veins reclogged by plaque often do shut down years later, and it's generally agreed that the early bypass patients got little guidance on how to control this. But Hay Brown is learning. At the Center for Living at Duke University in Durham, North Carolina, he attends a program on how to follow a low-fat diet, exercise regularly, and stop smoking to help lower cholesterol levels and prevent or curb new plaque buildup.

Medically Cleaning the Arteries

Doctors have proved that by lowering their patients' cholesterol levels to about 150, the patients could—and did—reverse the process. They actually removed plaque from their artery walls by taking a prescribed combination of the drugs cholestyramine and lovastatin.

Cholestyramine removes bile from the digestive tract so that it cannot be used to make cholesterol. Lovastatin stops the manufacture of excess cholesterol in the liver. This combination works for me. For more than 20 years, I struggled to lower my blood cholesterol. Finally, with a low-fat diet, I went from the extremely dangerous high of 300 to 240. A few years ago, I added cholestyramine, and my cholesterol level dropped to 170. In November 1990, I added lovastatin; my cholesterol level dropped to 150. It is as yet unproved that this method can completely clean arteries.

Ballooning the Arteries

In Switzerland in 1977, a decade after the first bypass surgery, the late Dr. Andreas Gruentzig performed a balloon angioplasty and opened a blocked artery. (In Greek, *angio-* means vessel, as in blood vessel; *-plasty* means to change.) Since then, probably a million such procedures have been done in the United States. The physician opens an artery in the inner thigh. He or she snakes a thin wire up to the main artery, the aorta. From there the physician finds the mouth of the troubled coronary vessel and watches the progress of the wire on X-ray motion pictures. This is a guide wire.

With the thin strand of metal in place, the doctor runs a catheter—a thin plastic tube—up the wire. At the end of the catheter is a plastic balloon. Once the plastic balloon presses against the plaque, the doctor inflates it, flattening the plaque against the artery wall. That opens the channel allowing blood to flow where the blockage was. The procedure takes less than 2 hours, costs about $8,000, and requires only 2 days in the hospital. A coronary bypass costs $20,000 and requires a week or more in the hospital. If the artery closes during the angioplasty, doctors may perform an emergency bypass.

Frederick Swan, 63, of Bridgewater, New Jersey, a hardware wholesaler, had an angioplasty in 1987. But by late 1990, he says, "I could not walk without chest pain." X rays showed blockage in another artery.

Lasers—Hot and Not

Lasers are machines that emit hot beams of light. Some can burn through steel in 10 seconds.

Dr. J. Richard Spears, of Wayne State University in Detroit, uses a laser that heats to 212 degrees Fahrenheit, water's boiling point. He conducts it through the balloon to the artery's blockage. Pressing the balloon against the heat-softened plaque, he molds it against the artery wall. Its success rate in 3 years, he says, is "nearly 100 percent." Other physicians continue to evaluate the plaque-removing system.

About 10 years ago, heart specialists began to remove plaque with another laser whose tip heats to 750 degrees Fahrenheit and that most experts now say damages the artery lining, causing it to close down in spasm. Dr. Robert Ginsburg, of Stanford Medical Center, calls this hot-tip laser "a disaster."

A newer laser, called the excimer laser, issues a very intense beam of ultraviolet light that vaporizes plaque yet leaves surrounding tissue cool. "This is my laser of choice," says Dr. Thomas Linnemeier, of St. Vincent Hospital in Indianapolis. "Of 130 cases, 120 were successful." He says he does not know whether it will prevent the closing of newly channeled arteries.

But Frederick Swan knows that it unclogs arteries. He was treated with the excimer laser in December. "I felt no pain, no burning," Mr. Swan says. "It was like someone tapping fingers on my bones. I'm back to working, walking— my regular activities."

Rotary Blades and Chemicals

Dr. John Simpson, of Sequoia University in Redwood, California, developed a catheter with a motorized steel blade that rotates 2,000 times a minute to shave off plaque from a patient's coronary artery. X-ray motion pictures show blood flowing through the newly opened channel.

To stop the overgrowth of cells in a bypassed artery, Dr. Harvey Wolinsky, of Mount Sinai Medical Center in New York, invented a perforated balloon catheter. Into it he sends the chemical heparin to leak through the balloon and slow or stop the cells' growth in animals. He soon may try it on human patients.

The New Powers of Aspirin

SCIENTISTS RANK ASPIRIN HIGH ON THEIR research priority lists now, even though this fascinating drug is over 100 years old. In recent years, they've found it does wonders—and not just for headaches.

Doctors have prescribed large doses of aspirin to cool inflamed and painful joints, quell a fever, and ease pain anywhere in the body. Now scientists have new evidence of aspirin's potential to:

- lessen the risk of a fatal attack of high blood pressure during pregnancy;
- head off migraine headaches;
- retard cataracts, the clouding of the lenses of the eyes;
- quiet gum disease; and
- increase immunity to infection.

Most important, they have proved that aspirin prevents (and maybe heals) some heart attacks and strokes. Many doctors now prescribe doses of regular aspirin (325 milligrams) daily or every other day. Experiments show that daily doses of one baby aspirin (81 milligrams) also protect you. The right dose for you? Ask your doctor.

In 1987, Ed Koch, then mayor of New York City, suffered a minor stroke—a blockage of a capillary in his brain. He said then that the left side of his face felt funny and his speech was slurred.

"I was very worried," Mr. Koch says. "I knew strokes could leave you paralyzed and speechless." He left the hospital 4 days later with only this prescription: Lose weight. (He ultimately lost 40 pounds.) Exercise more. (He exercises daily.) Take an aspirin every day. (He does.) Now a busy lawyer, newspaper columnist, author, and radio commentator, Mr. Koch says he feels fine.

Low doses of aspirin thin the blood, making it less likely to form an oxygen-blocking clot. A stroke can occur when a clot forms in an artery that feeds blood to the brain. A heart attack can occur when a clot forms in a coronary artery—an artery that feeds blood to the heart muscle. Without the oxygen carried by the blood, a section dies in the brain (stroke) or heart muscle (heart attack).

Studies of more than 100,000 patients taking half an aspirin daily were analyzed at Oxford University in England. Among the most startling findings was that in men with a history of cardiovascular problems, aspirin can slash the clotting of a coronary artery by one-half to two-thirds and reduce the risk of heart attack.

More findings on low aspirin doses:

- Giving patients aspirin immediately after a heart attack reduces by 23 percent their risk of further heart attacks.
- Aspirin taken every other day lowers the likelihood of stroke by 25 percent in people with heart problems.

That's quite impressive for a drug dating to ancient Greece. A chemist at Bayer, a German chemical company, developed the first aspirin in 1894; it went on sale in Germany in 1899 and has been in demand ever since. Even now, an estimated 80 million tablets are consumed daily in the United States alone. And its many wonders are still unfolding.

For example, the Physicians' Health Study, headed by Dr. Charles H. Hennekens, a professor of medicine at Harvard Medical School, was begun at Harvard in 1982 and is scheduled to last through the 1990s. Its focus is on 22,071 volunteers, healthy male doctors between the ages of 40 and 84.

One segment of the study focused on the effects of taking aspirin every other day. Half the volunteers were given regular aspirin, half placebos (dummy tablets). Five years into the study, it was found that the aspirin takers had developed 44 percent fewer cases of heart disease than the placebo takers. So, the monitoring board decided to terminate the aspirin study and share its findings quickly, possibly saving millions from experiencing a heart attack. The study also tested beta-carotene against cancer and heart disease. It had no effect at all.

Dr. Hennekens was among the volunteers given placebos. "I found that out on January 25, 1988—the date the aspirin segment of the study ended," he says. "I was 47 years old, had low cholesterol, low blood pressure, was active physically—I was then the number-one squash player in the country in my age group—and I'd never smoked cigarettes." But then, Dr. Hennekens adds, a friend with a similar lifestyle had a heart attack. Both men also had fathers who had suffered early heart attacks. "My doctor and I decided that I would start aspirin," he says.

Dr. Hennekens advises, "Use aspirin as an adjunct to, but never a substitute for, the proper management of other risk factors, including lowering cholesterol to below 200 by diet and/or drugs, treating even moderately high blood pressure, losing weight, exercising, and stopping smoking."

Aspirin hinders blood from clotting by acting on tiny blood cells known as platelets. Platelets have only an 8-day life span. Aspirin permanently stops the platelets from clumping, but it must be taken every other day to be effective on new platelets. That's why you have to take the aspirin for life: it has to act on ever-new platelets.

Most of the research on heart attacks and stroke have been done on males because men have more heart attacks and strokes than women. So when research on men is done, the scientists can more quickly come to a conclusion than among fewer women. The saving in time reflects itself in saving of lives because the therapy will be in place for a longer time. The time saving also means that the research is cheaper when done with men.

However, women have protested being left out as subjects of research projects. Male scientists have often made the point that what works for the gander works for the goose; that is, women can expect the same benefits as men.

In the discussion of male/female research, women often point out that they have different hormones, give birth, and retain more fat, any or all of which could result in a different response to drugs and other therapies.

It appears that the male scientific community has heeded the complaints. A study of women nurses over 50 is in progress at Harvard. Other female-oriented research shows that aspirin helps women avoid second heart attacks and second strokes. In that respect, then, women resemble men.

Aspirin does have drawbacks:

• Because it thins the blood, inordinate bleeding can occur. Doctors advise not to take aspirin within 7 days before having surgery or dental work.

• Aspirin may aggravate a stroke that is caused by a bleeding artery, rather than by a blocked artery. And, says Dr. Hennekens, findings in the Harvard study hint that aspirin might slightly increase the risk of brain hemorrhage.

• Aspirin can cause gastric (stomach) bleeding or irritation and intestinal discomfort. Many doctors suggest that long-term users of aspirin with stomach problems, including those prone to ulcers, take aspirin tablets with a chemical coating that prevents their breakup in the stomach. Some brands are coated to neutralize the aspirin's acidity in the stomach. Still others are coated to ease swallowing, and some have ingredients to help neutralize stomach acids. Coatings can slow the aspirin's effect, which makes some brands better for headaches, others better for joint pain, so read the labels and ask your doctor to find the right one.

• Relatively rare but potentially fatal, Reye's syndrome can afflict children and teenagers treated with aspirin for fever during flu or chicken pox. The reason is not yet known.

Still, aspirin's pluses predominate. For instance, research shows that low doses of aspirin reduce by 20 percent the frequency of migraines in men. (A women's study is being considered.) And researchers are tantalized by aspirin's as yet unproved potential in the following ways:

• Slow the development of cataracts. Dr. Edward Cotlier, an ophthalmologist in Manhattan, noticed fewer cataracts among arthritis patients taking high aspirin doses (sometimes more than four a day) for joint pain and inflammation. He showed that aspirin blocks cataracts in lab animals, especially those with diabetes.

• Strengthen the immune system. Dr. Judith Hsia, an assistant professor of medicine at George Washington University Medical Center in Washington, D.C., found that, in healthy volunteers, low doses of aspirin increased the white blood cells' effectiveness. (They attack invading viruses and bacteria.) She also found that, in adult lab mice, aspirin enhanced the white cells' ability to make antibodies in response to flu vaccine. This, says Dr. Hsia, may lead to work that helps the elderly respond well to flu shots. Research finds that the immune system in elderly persons is often too weak to respond to the flu vaccine to prime the body's white cells to recognize an invading flu virus.

• Prevent preeclampsia. Scientists also are studying the use of one baby aspirin a day to prevent this lethal complication of pregnancy that sends the expectant mother's blood pressure skyrocketing. If not treated properly, it can end with a brain hemorrhage, kidney shutdown, or heart failure.

All that from aspirin, a chemical found in willow bark a century ago.

A Quiz That Can Save Your Life

FOR THE FIRST TIME IN DECADES, HEART specialists are tremendously optimistic about the number one health problem in the United States—cardiovascular disease. Each year, 550,000 Americans die of heart attacks and 200,000 from strokes. Now doctors see ways to cut down those gruesome death rates as well as $60 billion in annual medical costs.

Listen to Dr. Claude Lenfant, director of the National Heart, Lung, and Blood Institute: "Only in the last 15 years have we had effective medical treatments; only in the last 20 have we discovered ways in which people can lower their danger."

So, in 10 to 20 years, we will see a 25 to 50 percent reduction in the death toll from heart disease, predicts Dr. Lenfant. "We will give people more years of useful life," he says.

To help you understand the giant steps that have been taken to control heart disease and strokes, here is an adaptation of the heart-health IQ test developed at the heart institute. If you score high— that is, if you get many of the answers right—you can apply your knowledge, and you may live longer. If you score low, go over your answers and compare them with the correct ones. Then apply your new knowledge to lead a healthier life.

1. True or false: The three most potentially dangerous conditions that you can do something about are high blood pressure, high cholesterol in your blood, and smoking.

True. If you have all three of these risk factors, you run eight times the risk of heart disease as someone with none of them. But you can reduce blood pressure and cholesterol and quit smoking. Other risk factors, such as age and a family history of heart attacks, cannot be changed. And if you are overweight, do no exercise, and live a high-stress life, you are at greater risk, too.

2. True or false: A heart attack or stroke is often the first symptom of high blood pressure or cholesterol or both.

True. If you have high blood pressure or high cholesterol, you may feel fine and look great. But both conditions work silently until, without warning, a heart attack or stroke hits.

3. True or false: People with high blood pressure are generally nervous, tense people.

False. Calm people also have high blood pressure. High blood pressure means that the blood flowing in your arteries is pressing too hard against the blood vessel walls. It does not mean that you are too tense.

4. True or false: A blood pressure reading of 140/90 or more is generally considered to be too high.

True. The higher your blood pressure, the greater your risk of heart disease or stroke. The number 140 is the pressure in your arteries when your heart contracts; 90 is the pressure when your heart relaxes. A better pressure would be 120/80. To reduce blood pressure, (a) bring your weight down to normal; (b) decrease your sodium intake, not only table salt but that in snacks and processed foods; (c) take prescribed medicine regularly. Many doctors also prescribe exercise and relaxation training to lower blood pressure.

There is some controversy over the dietary input of salt. Most experts suggest lowering the salt content of your food. Salt, indeed, can aggravate your high blood pressure if your high blood pressure is sensitive to salt. If you do not have this specific type of high blood pressure, salt will not do you harm. However, only a proper test can determine your blood pressure type. If you're not sure, see a blood pressure expert.

5. True or false: It is only a scientific theory that elevated blood cholesterol is related to heart disease.

False. If you have too much cholesterol in your blood, scientific studies show, it will stick to and clog the inside of your arteries. If your cholesterol level is over 265 milligrams per deciliter of blood (mg/dl), your risk of a heart attack is four times that of a person with 190 mg/dl. Reducing cholesterol either by diet or medication can reduce the risk to your heart.

6. True or false: The most effective dietary way to lower blood cholesterol levels is by eating less cholesterol.

False. You do get cholesterol in your blood by eating foods containing the chemical, but your liver also makes cholesterol. When you eat saturated fat (fat that is usually solid at room temperature), you trigger your liver to make more cholesterol. If you substitute polyunsaturated fat (liquid at room temperature), you reduce your blood cholesterol. So avoid cholesterol-rich foods—eggs, red meats, fried foods, and such dairy products as whole milk, cream, ice cream, cheese, and butter—as well as foods high in saturated fat. Choose instead lean meats, skinless chicken and turkey, fish, and low-fat or no-fat dairy products.

7. True or false: A food product labeled "no cholesterol" is safe for people with elevated cholesterol.

False. It may contain large amounts of saturated fats, including coconut and palm oils or a heavily hydrogenated vegetable oil. Look for oils high in polyunsaturated fat, such as safflower, corn, and soybean.

8. True or false: Smoking increases your risk of heart attack.

True. The heart disease rate among smokers is 70 percent higher than among nonsmokers. If you also have a high blood cholesterol level, your chances of a heart attack jump dramatically. In addition, you put yourself at higher risk for cancer and emphysema, a deadly lung disease that makes it difficult to breathe.

9. True or false: Heart disease is the number two killer of women.

False. Heart disease is the number one killer of women in the United States. Of the 750,000 Americans who die each year of heart disease, 350,000 are women. And almost 100,000 women die each year from strokes. This means women have to follow the same heart-healthy rules as men. No smoking. Eat a diet low in saturated fat. Cut your calorie intake if you are overweight. Increase your dietary intake of fiber.

10. True or false: Physical inactivity is related to heart disease.

True. People who are inactive tend to have more heart disease than people who are physically active. Regular, brisk, and sustained exercise often can reduce blood pressure and help you lose weight and may even help you stop smoking.

Get some regular (three times a week or more) exercise that leaves you puffing. If you are sedentary, increase your exercise slowly. If you are over 40, check with your doctor before you begin your regime.

Diet and Fitness

Are We Choosing the Right Foods?

THE RICHEST PEOPLE ON EARTH—AMERICANS—do not eat a healthy diet. It's not because we haven't the money but because we simply do not know better, or we ignore the facts. Two of three Americans eat high-fat, high-sugar foods that may increase their risk of cancer, heart and liver disease, obesity, diabetes, stroke, and high blood pressure.

But large numbers of Americans, perhaps as much as a third of the population, are improving their eating habits, responding to the guidelines laid down by government agencies and health organizations.

These health-conscious eaters are consuming fewer calories but more fruits, vegetables, grains, beans and low-fat dairy products. They are cutting down on fats, limiting sugar and salt, and switching from beef, lamb, and pork to chicken, turkey, and fish.

The American Way

There is no longer a typical American eating pattern, according to the Community Nutrition Institute in Washington, D.C. Five distinct eating styles emerge, some healthy, some unhealthy. The good news,

says Dr. Rodney Leonard, executive director of the nonprofit institute, is that "people are moving away from the traditional American meat-eater pattern." Dr. Leonard analyzed Department of Agriculture data and reports that beef eating dropped 20 percent since 1975, with an equal shift toward poultry.

Betty Peterkin, an associate administrator at the U.S. Department of Agriculture Human Nutrition Information Service, points out, however, that "we need red meat for zinc because it is one of the better food sources of zinc." She adds, "Without red meat, it is difficult to get a diet that has all the vitamins and minerals."

The Fat Issue

Without question, one of the major culprits in the American diet is fat. Up to 43 percent of the calories we eat every day comes from fat—almost half of our total daily intake of food energy. These figures come from Drs. Helen Guthrie of Pennsylvania State University and Annemarie Crocetti of the New York College of Medicine. They examined data from the Department of Agriculture on the eating patterns of 21,579 adults. Three of four people ate more than 35 percent of their calories in fat.

Many studies show that a high fat intake goes with higher rates of heart disease and probably of cancer. Guidelines issued jointly by the Department of Agriculture and the Department of Health and Human Services—and adopted by such major health agencies as the American Heart Association and the American Cancer Society—recommend that daily fat intake be below 30 percent of total calories.

Vitamins and Minerals

More than half of Americans take in less than the recommended level of at least one of the vitamins and minerals they need for good health, say Drs. Guthrie and Crocetti. Mostly, they fall short in vitamins A, B_6, and C and the minerals calcium, iron, and magnesium.

One way to ensure that you get the right amount of these micronutrients (so called because we need them in such tiny amounts) to eat a balanced diet every day from the following four food groups. Scientists suggest you emphasize grains, vegetables, and fruits and reduce fat and animal proteins. This cuts your risk of heart disease and some cancers.

- Milk and milk products: This group includes liquid milk (preferably skim), low-fat cheese, yogurt, and ice cream.
- Meat, chicken, turkey, and fish: Avoid fatty meats.

- Fruits and vegetables: The modern view emphasizes six or more portions a day.
- Grains: Cereals, bread, potato, rice, and pasta comprise this group.

Drs. Guthrie and Crocetti found that 86 percent of Basic Four eaters got enough micronutrients; and the more that people departed from the diet, the more they fell short nutritionally.

However, sticking to the Basic Four does not guarantee a healthy fat intake. Experts now urge Basic Four eaters to choose low-fat foods, such as lean meats and skim dairy products.

Only 3 percent of the nation follows the Basic Four scheme for three consecutive days. Still, almost half of us seem to get enough vitamins and minerals from the foods we eat.

Sugar

Huge increases in the amount of sugar that modern people eat have stirred many nutritionists to issue warnings against excess sugar. The Department of Agriculture reports that annual consumption of sugar rose from 87.5 pounds a person in 1909 to 142 pounds a person by 1983. (Most of this sugar is hidden in processed foods.) Since then sugar consumption has leveled off, but the use of noncaloric sweeteners has skyrocketed.

Sugar does not actually lead to disease, except for tooth decay. It provokes symptoms in diabetes; it does not cause diabetes. But sugar contains only empty calories—it provides no vitamins, protein, or fiber, all essential to a healthy diet. And if you eat a lot of sugar, you are taking in calories that could be better divided among foods with important nutrients.

Fiber

Americans need to eat more complex carbohydrates—starches such as potatoes, rice, and pasta—and fiber. Fiber is the indigestible (but not inedible!) part of all plant foods. It's what your mother called "roughage." Scientists now say that a diet rich in fiber and complex starches may protect against cancer, bowel disease, diabetes, and other ailments. The average American gets about 10 to 20 grams of fiber a day—less than an ounce. Many experts recommend between 30 and 40 grams. You get fiber from fruits, vegetables, whole grains, dried beans, peas, lentils, nuts, and seeds.

Convenience Foods

We Americans depend more on processed foods today than ever before. Almost half the calories we eat comes in foods that have been prepared fully or partially outside the home, reports a team of food scientists from Virginia Polytechnic Institute. Food experts call these "convenience foods" and break them down into three types:

1. Basic convenience (17 percent of all calories consumed by Americans today) foods include processed cheeses, powdered milk, quick-cooking cereals, peanut butter, as well as canned and frozen fruits, vegetables, and juices.

2. Complex convenience (27 percent of our total calories) foods are salad dressings, frozen desserts, baking mixes, hot dogs and luncheon meats, and ready-to-eat canned and frozen meals.

3. Manufactured convenience (12 percent of our total calories) foods are those with no home-prepared counterpart, such as ready-to-eat cereals, sodas, breakfast toaster pastries, and soy-based infant formula.

Snacks

No scientific evidence indicates that snacking leads to obesity or any other unhealthy condition. Some nutritionists, in fact, advocate several small meals during the day to reduce appetite.

Betty Peterkin of the Department of Agriculture says that, as a nation, our snacking habits changed very little between the 1960s and the 1970s. On average, people eat three to five times a day and get 20 percent of their calories from snacks. Children and teenagers snack the most.

Dr. Karen Morgan, of the University of Missouri at Columbia, has studied snacking extensively. "Where and when foods were consumed had very limited impact on their nutritional status," she says.

A Perfect Day

Can you really get all the protein, carbo-hydrates, fats, fiber, vitamins, and miner-als you need every day? *Parade* asked Gail A. Levey, a registered dietitian, to plan a day's menus that include every-thing the experts say you need in perfect proportion. The total number of calories is about 2,700, enough for the average man. A similar diet for a woman, with smaller portions, provides about 2,000 calories.

Breakfast
1 1/2 cups oatmeal, topped with cinna-mon, a sliced banana, and 2 tablespoons of walnuts

1 cup skim milk

Lunch
Italian tuna, bean, and pasta salad (1/2 cup water-packed tuna, 1/2 cup cooked beans, 1 cup cooked pasta seasoned with 2 table-spoons mayonnaise, 1 teaspoon mustard, 1 tablespoon cider vinegar, curry powder to taste)

1 sliced tomato topped with 1 tablespoon oil and vinegar, dash of oregano

Steamed broccoli, 1 cup

Whole-wheat bread, 2 slices

1 apple

Club soda, with a lemon slice

Afternoon Snack
1 cup vanilla low-fat yogurt

Dinner
Roast chicken (no skin), 5 ounces

1 baked sweet potato

Summer squash, 1 cup sautéed in 1 table-spoon oil and fresh garlic

Cranberry juice, 1 cup

Chocolate pudding (made with skim milk), 1/2 cup

1 orange

Evening Snack
Popcorn, 4 cups, unbuttered and unsalted

How the Experts Want Us to Eat

The guidelines below are endorsed by the Department of Agriculture, the Depart-ment of Health and Human Services, the American Heart Association, the Senate Select Committee on Nutrition, the Food and Nutrition Board of the National Academy of Sciences, and the American Cancer Society.

Variety
Every day, you need at least two servings of low-fat milk products: two servings of protein-rich foods like meats, fish, poul-try, eggs, and legumes; four servings of fruits and vegetables; four servings of grains, including whole-grain breads and cereals. Keep these additional points in mind, too:

• Ideal weight. Take in only as much food energy as you burn up. You may need to eat less or exercise regularly.

• Total fat. Reduce overall fat intake to 30 percent of calories or less. Trim fat off beef, pork, lamb. Remove skin from poultry. Eat more fish, lentils, dried beans, peas, whole grains, low-fat dairy products, fruits, and vegetables. Saturated fats stimulate production of cholesterol, which clogs up your arteries. So limit beef, pork, lamb, solid shortenings, and palm and coconut oils.

• Cholesterol. Try to keep your daily ration of cholesterol down to less than 300 milligrams, the amount of cholesterol in one egg yolk. Organ meats, beef, pork, lamb, veal, and butter also contain goodly amounts of cholesterol.

• Starch/fiber. Eat more fiber-rich dried beans, peas, lentils, whole grains, fruits, and vegetables. Starchy foods, rich in vitamins and minerals, are low in fat and free of cholesterol.

• The sugar trap. Sugary foods squeeze high-nutrient foods off your menu. So cut back on sugared soft drinks, candy, ice cream, frozen desserts, cakes, cookies, and pies.

• The salt connection. Controversy rages over the role of salt in the human diet. Many people have thought that salt triggers high blood pressure. Evidence is building that excess sodium may worsen high blood pressure in certain individuals, but it doesn't cause the disease. Healthy individuals need not worry about salt.

However, because we don't know who has or will get this salt-sensitive hypertension, the best strategy is to keep your daily salt load between 1/2 and 1 1/2 teaspoons.

• Alcohol. Limit daily intake to one or two drinks. Alcohol has no important nutrient; like sugar, it pushes other foods off the menu. Pregnant women are advised to avoid alcohol altogether.

What's Your Eating Style?

Nationwide, there are at least five styles of eating, according to a 1982 study by the Marketing Science Institute in Cambridge, Massachusetts, and the Community Nutrition Institute in Washington, D.C.

1. The meat eaters. They are the last of the meat-and-potato Americans. They take meat—mostly beef—for breakfast, lunch, and dinner. They also eat plenty of eggs, sausage, TV dinners, and hot dogs. Hence, they have the highest consumption of fat and cholesterol.

2. People on the go. They eat away from home more than any other group. They consume lots of dairy products, especially yogurt, cheese, and butter. They also eat whole grains, but few sweets and below-average amounts of vegetables, fruits, beans, and nuts.

3. All mixed up. They skip the most meals, but when they do eat, they eat away from home. They go for convenience foods—TV dinners, frozen pot pies, cake mixes, presweetened cereals, donuts, cookies, candy, bacon, potato

chips, soft drinks. They have the poorest diet of any group.

4. Conscientious eaters. They eat what most experts consider a healthy diet—more than average amounts of beans, nuts, whole grains, and low levels of cholesterol, red meats, salt, and processed foods. They eat most of their meals at home.

5. Healthy eaters. They eat the most vegetables, fruits, and whole grains. Like Conscientious Eaters, they reduce cholesterol, sweets, total fat, and red meats. Instead, they eat lots of chicken, turkey, and tuna. They love bananas, cantaloupe, whole-wheat bread, broccoli, carrots, and cucumbers, but they do not eat a lot of beans.

How People Really Diet

DIETING IS ONE OF AMERICA'S FAVORITE INDOOR sports. Half of the people in the United States have dieted at least once in the last 5 years. For a substantial group of people, dieting has become a compulsion, even though almost every dieter has lost weight and then failed miserably to keep the pounds off. The compulsive dieter thinks, "I know what went wrong last time; I can fix it this time." It almost never succeeds.

Parade randomly telephoned 1,000 men and women nationwide to ask them how they dieted. They told us things about themselves that identified what it takes to be a successful dieter—one who can take off weight and keep it off for at least 6 months.

Based on the results of that survey, we created a questionnaire to show how successful you can expect to be on your next diet. The quiz follows this special diet report.

Important Findings from Parade's *First National Diet Survey*

- The average dieter loses 16 pounds when dieting.
- Men lose a little bit more than women.
- But there are lots of heavy dieters: one of three took off 20 pounds or more.
- One person in 20 dropped 50 pounds.
- The most popular way to diet is just to eat less of the usual foods.
- Half the people lost their weight this way.
- But one in five opted for a special diet to take off weight. Equally popular was fasting or eating very little. (Men dieted this way more than women.) About 7 percent took a liquid formula diet, women favoring this two to one.
- Half the dieters in America get no vigorous exercise at all. That means that

when they diet, they do not benefit by cutting appetite with exercise. Almost as many women as men exercise. It is the people over 65 who hardly get any exercise. But large numbers of people exercise three or more times a week.

- Women diet 50 percent more often than men. Even so, one man in three diets to lose weight. And one person in four hits the diet trail five times or more in 5 years.

- A lot of people—about a third—found dieting tough because somebody made it tough for them.

- Married people complained most frequently about their spouses. Dieting men got less help from their wives than dieting women got from their husbands. Children and coworkers didn't make it easy either.

- Many dieters have trouble because they continue to eat even though they are no longer hungry. Women are just as troubled by this habit as men, but those who have the most difficulty with it are young people aged 18 to 24.

Although many people diet for aesthetic reasons—they want to look better—many more say they diet for health motives. Almost everybody knows that being overweight certainly does no good. The statistics show unequivocally that overweight people have a higher risk of death and disease.

Researchers now tell us that overweight may have many causes, including genetic makeup. Surely some of us have inherited our tendency to overweight. Others eat their way there.

Now researchers have identified four hereditary factors—genes—that determine whether a person will be thin, chubby, seriously overweight, or pathologically obese. The scientific game plan is to find out which of your body's chemicals are controlled by which genes. Then the chemists can design a molecule that blocks or enhances the obesity genes as needed.

Personally, I believe that such an approach is the only hope for seriously or pathologically overweight people. Every study of every method ends the same way. The dieters lose weight, often 50 pounds or more. At the end of 3 years, most patients regain almost all the weight they lost; some—a small minority—keep some of the poundage off, and some gain back more fat than they originally jettisoned.

Many overweight people do no exercise, so they don't burn up the calories they take in. Some of us eat to soothe our nerves.

But some universals ring true for most dieters.

Losing pounds and keeping them off means a change in the way you live and eat.

Keeping company with other dieters increases your chance of success.

Radically and rapidly changing the way you eat decreases your chance of success. In other words, crash diets don't work in the long run.

Losing a lot of weight gradually means you'll probably shut off the regaining mechanism. The most successful dieters in the *Parade* survey were those who lost a lot of weight over a long period of time. For example, people who lost 20 pounds kept a greater proportion of the weight off longer than those who lost only 10 pounds.

Vigorous, sweaty exercise helps you lose weight and keep the extra pounds off. In our survey, half the people did no exercise at all.

Eating less of your usual mix of foods may work best, but for many heavy eaters that is hard to do.

Every Diet Works for Somebody

I cannot recommend a particular diet. After all, no single diet scheme works for every overweight person. But every diet works for somebody—even this former fatty. So, if you seriously want to lose weight, find a diet plan that fits your personality and problem.

That's how I did it. Up to 20 years ago, I weighed 185 pounds. By standard weight tables, I was at least 30 pounds overweight. So I started to count calories. I changed what I ate, how much I ate, where I ate, when I ate. It took a long time—at least 2 years—to get used to eating the new way, but nothing has changed since. My scale fluctuates between 154 and 158—never more, never less.

Now you can turn to the other reports in this section to find the kind of diet program that might work for you. And if it succeeds, you'll end up looking better, feeling better, and, perhaps, living longer.

Getting Help from Others

Theodore B. Van Itallie, of St. Luke's–Roosevelt Hospital Center in New York, says, "Anybody can diet for 2 weeks with any diet. It's losing all the overweight and keeping it off that counts. And that's hard."

Without anybody around to support you, it's harder still. And if somebody actively interferes, losing weight may be impossible. A quarter of all the dieters surveyed by *Parade* said that a family member or friend made it difficult for them to succeed.

One dieter in seven blamed a spouse. (Wives were blamed more often than husbands.) Coworkers were no help, either. And while few dieters indicted their offspring, the presence of children in the household deterred dieting.

It's no wonder that so many overweight people turn to peers for help. Each week, 500,000 Americans attend classes at Weight Watchers. Probably an equal number end up at TOPS, Overeaters Anonymous, the Diet Workshop, and dozens of other groups where they lose weight and keep it off.

Dr. Richard B. Stuart, of the University of Utah, found that, 15 months after reaching goal weights, more than half of Weight Watchers' clients stayed close to their goals.

Weight Watchers started out by dispensing low-calorie diets to its members. Under Dr. Stuart's influence, Weight Watchers has added behavior modification and an optional exercise plan.

Fasting with Care

What's the allure of "protein-sparing fasts"? These low-calorie diets offer liquid protein formulas or small amounts of chicken, fish, and beef. They motivate you because you lose pounds quickly. One person in five polled by *Parade* fasted on his or her last diet. Men seemed to fast more than women.

Protein fasts are risky, particularly over a long period. Total fasting, in which dieters eat nothing at all, is especially dangerous because it uses up the body's stores of protein, such as the muscles (including the heart muscle). It also depletes your potassium level, which could send your heart into a paroxysm. Some years ago, several people on a liquid protein diet died. At best, liquid formulas claim 50 percent success.

Doctors who use protein fasts to treat the grossly obese (people who are 80 or more pounds overweight) prescribe 400- to 600-calorie daily diets of either a special liquid egg formula or tight portion control of protein foods and no carbohydrates.

Dr. George Blackburn, of Harvard Medical School, says that 25 percent of those he treats with controlled portions of protein foods achieve normal weight and stay there. But his program stresses exercise and behavior modification to teach people to eat normally after they've lost weight; the diet is supplemental.

Parade's survey found that people who drank liquid formula diets were more successful in keeping weight off 6 months or longer than those who followed other methods. But if you try these protein fasts on your own, the chances are that you'll eventually gain the weight back and possibly endanger your health.

Exercise Pounds Away

The dieting equation is simple: food = energy. And the energy you don't use, your body puts away as fat.

Our survey shows that only half the population exercises vigorously at least once a week for 20 minutes.

Dr. Bernard Gutin, of New York's Teacher's College, calls exercise the key to lifelong weight control. "People who take up vigorous exercise," he says, "lose weight without even trying to control their food intake." Exercise not only burns up calories, it also cuts your appetite, changes your self-image from a fat to a thin person, improves the condition of your heart and lungs, and changes the way your body burns food.

Unfortunately, when you cut down your food intake, your body burns calories more slowly, as if to hoard the fat that is already stored. That's why dieters find it hard to diet for long periods. Since the body uses less energy during a diet, the dieters have to eat less and less to lose the same amount as they did earlier in their weight loss program.

Exercise speeds up your body's chemistry and counteracts the slowdown. So even though jogging for 10 minutes uses up fewer calories than those in a slice of bread, its impact on the way your body handles calories is greater.

Most obese people shy away from exercise. They drop out of exercise programs faster than thin people. Half of the overweight people who exercise stop within a year. *Parade*'s survey found exercisers among only a quarter of the people over 65, the nation's most overweight group.

If you are so inclined:

- Pick an exercise that's fun.
- Exercise with other people. Use the buddy system; it's harder to disappoint a friend than to get outside on a gray morning. (I rarely miss a tennis date, but it was easy to stay in bed longer when I was not pledged to play.)
- Start slowly, and *never* exercise to the point of pain.

When All Else Fails: Surgery

There are some people who are 100 or more pounds overweight. They are in imminent danger of death from heart attack, kidney problems, diabetes, or stroke. Many of them have tried every diet program known, and they have failed every one. For them, there may be only one solution: surgery.

The most promising methods narrow the stomach so that only a small amount of food can pass through. The surgeon employs a special stapling gun to shut off two thirds of the stomach. These procedures are risky. About one person in 100 dies from the operation, but the health risks of being so obese are probably greater.

Obese patients usually slim down by about 100 pounds because, after stomach-altering surgery, they can eat only tiny meals of ordinary foods. If they wolf down too much food, they have an instant feeling of fullness and loss of appetite.

But this drastic stomach stapling can be defeated. After surgery, one man I knew began to drink milk shakes by the gallon. The liquid easily went down the opening, and he gained back all his weight.

In another operation, the surgeon bypasses a part of the small intestine so that food is not absorbed. This, too, produces permanent weight loss. But the complications are serious: kidney stones, diarrhea, liver disease, arthritis, and infection. Few surgeons now use this method.

Other surgical methods either don't work as well or carry greater risks. Wiring the jaw shut so that the patient can ingest only small amounts of liquid food causes massive weight loss, but the pounds come back once the wires are removed.

Diets to Make You Wary

Here are some diet programs that doctors say to shy away from:

- Single-food diets. These diets (e.g., all-fruit) don't retrain your eating habits and can be dangerous because they are nutritionally unbalanced.
- Highly restrictive diets. The weight you lose from these (e.g., low-carbohydrate plans) is mostly water, which you will gain back when you stop the diet—as, eventually, you must.
- Diet pills without a doctor's prescription. Again, pills don't correct your bad habits, and some appetite killers can be addictive.
- High-fat diets. Most medical experts say these can increase cholesterol levels and the risk of heart attack. They also are hard to stick with. Unfortunately, *Parade*'s survey could not determine the success of high-fat diets.

Act Thin to Be Thin

To lose weight successfully, you have to change your eating behavior.

Psychologists have discovered how to do that with behavior modification. In essence, you reward yourself for appropriate eating behavior and punish yourself for bad eating habits.

Unfortunately, eating is its own reward: The taste gives us pleasure; food assuages our hunger and, for some people, calms nerves. Because eating is so pleasurable, why aren't we all as big as mountains? Our body punishes us with uncomfortable feelings of fullness. We don't overeat.

But some people continue to eat even when they are not hungry. In *Parade*'s survey, one person in five said he or she eats when not hungry. That leads to diet failure.

Behavior modification works by making you aware of your eating—to counter the pleasure of food that overrides your sense of fullness. To begin, write down when you eat, what you eat, where you eat, and how you feel when you eat.

If you find that you nibble all day, restrict your eating to mealtimes. If you munch all over the house, eat only at the table. Stop eating when you read or watch television.

And if you eat to calm your nerves, find alternatives to food, like phoning a friend or, better, exercising.

Dr. Albert J. Stunkard, of the University of Pennsylvania, says that, although the amount of weight lost is modest, behavior modification works better than almost anything in maintaining weight loss over the long run.

Will You Succeed on Your Diet?

Here are seven questions that we asked the 1,000 men and women in *Parade*'s first national diet survey. To test yourself against their results—and to determine how successful you can expect to be on your next diet—check the box beside the answer that fits you best. After you have answered the questions, you will find explanations for each. Checking your answers against the prescriptions will give you an insight to your own behavior and motives. That insight may make you more successful in your next diet.

The Seven Questions of Dieting

1. How many times have you tried to lose weight in the last five years?
   ____ 0
   ____ 2–3
   ____ 4–5
   ____ More than 5

2. Which one of the following methods did you follow most the last time you went on a diet?
   ____ Ate less of my usual mix of foods
   ____ Ate a special diet for weight loss
   ____ Ate very little or nothing at all
   ____ Ate a liquid formula diet

3. How often do you continue to eat even after you realize that you are no longer hungry?
   ____ Often
   ____ Sometimes
   ____ Rarely
   ____ Never

4. How many times a week do you exercise vigorously for 20 minutes or more?
   ____ 0
   ____ 1–2
   ____ 3–5
   ____ More than 5

5. How many pounds did you lose last time you went on a diet? ____

6. How often do you feel emotionally upset?
   ____ Often
   ____ Sometimes
   ____ Rarely
   ____ Never

7. When you were on a diet, was there anyone around who made it difficult for you to stay on the diet?
   ____ No
   ____ Yes

Now, some helpful background for each question in *Parade*'s diet survey (check these notes against your answers):

1. The more often you try to lose weight, the less successful you are likely to be. And men fail more frequently than women.

2. It is difficult to lose weight by eating less of your usual foods, because success depends on your ability to resist eating what you like most. Special diets are especially difficult for women, and, along with eating very little or nothing at all, special diets seldom bring lasting results. People on strict liquid formula plans do better than other dieters because they are allowed very little choice and, therefore, can resist impulse eating.

3. Obviously, if you can't stop eating, even after you are full, dieting is going to be difficult. Pay attention to what your body is telling you.

4. Dieters who regularly exercise are more likely to lose pounds and keep them off. Exercise is one of the best ways to control weight and appetite.

5. According to our survey, the more weight you lose, the better your chances are of keeping it off.

6. Surprisingly, in *Parade*'s survey, it was the men who called themselves "emotionally upset" who reported the most success in dieting. Perhaps they sought help for problems, which, in turn, positively influenced their eating habits. Emotionally upset women, on the other hand, were less affected. Remember, however, emotional distress is no excuse for overeating.

7. Spouses, friends, and fellow workers can make it hard to stick to a new eating regimen. Children are a special dieting deterrent because they can make it hard to limit the kinds and amounts of foods available in the home.

What lessons can be learned from all this? Dieting is hard, very hard—and the outcome is uncertain. But, if you're determined, you can succeed. Good luck!

Eat Wiser, Live Longer

YOUR BODY CHANGES EACH DECADE—SO FAST in your early years that you wonder where "the old you" went, so gradually in your later years that you scarcely notice becoming another person.

Whether slow or quick, your life's shifts require that you eat the kinds of foods that will keep pace with an altered body and body chemistry. If you eat right, you can escape many of the tolls of aging.

Parade has surveyed the science of nutrition and come up with a plan for seven stages of eating for the seven periods of your life when you have to adjust what you eat to the biological person you become.

First, we found general rules of healthful eating for almost everyone of any age. Follow them, and you'll give yourself the best possible odds for a long, healthy life.

Calorie Control

Take in neither more nor less food than you need for growth and energy consumption. If you eat more calories than you burn up (calories are units of heat, or energy), you will get fat. And fat people, in general, sicken and die earlier than lean people.

Fat Control

By keeping your fat intake down, you can easily control your calories. Laboratory mice who've been given all they want of a high-fat diet of items taken off supermarket shelves—cakes, cheeses, candies—become obese. Their fellow mice who've been offered only low-fat, high-carbohydrate foods stay slim, sleek, and sound.

The American Heart Association suggests that healthy people over the age of 2 keep fat down to 30 percent of each day's total calories. However, the American Academy of Pediatrics says that children aged 2 to 12 can take 30 to 40 percent of their calories in fat.

Lower your intake of animal fats from whole milk and cream products, beef, veal, lamb, pork, and some vegetable fat, particularly oils of coconut, palm, and palm kernel. Such fats stimulate your liver to create excess cholesterol.

A Varied Diet

Except for infants, who obtain all they need for the first months from human breast milk or formulas, we all benefit from eating *many different kinds of food.* A diverse diet provides all the vitamins

and minerals we need—without pills. Choose daily from the Basic Four food groups.

The Basic Four

1: Breads, Cereals, Pasta, and Rice Eat at least four servings a day. This group supplies most of our carbohydrates—the energy source burned most readily by the body. Such starches don't necessarily add pounds if you don't fatten them up with butter, gravies, sauces, and creams.

Just as important, be sure you take in fiber, the undigestible portion of plant foods. Fiber is important in relieving several digestive diseases and helps keep weight down. It also aids in controlling cholesterol and blood sugar and may protect against some cancers. Good fiber choices: whole-grain breads and cereals and brown rice.

2: Fruits and Vegetables Eat a total of four or more servings a day. These foods are rich in vitamins A and C and fiber. Deep green and yellow/orange vegetables like broccoli and carrots are especially rich in vitamin A. Citrus fruits, tomatoes, and strawberries are high in vitamin C.

3: Fish, Fowl, Meats, and Beans Eat two servings a day, emphasizing dried beans and lentils, skinless chicken, turkey, fish, and seafood. Go easy on beef, veal, lamb, and pork. Select low-fat cuts. Limit egg yolks to two per week.

4: Milk Products For adults, two servings per day; for children, three; for teenagers, four. Milk is a calcium-rich food but fatty. Best picks are skim milk, low-fat yogurt, low-fat cheeses, and ice milk. Instead of butter, use soft margarines made with oils from corn, safflower, sunflower, or other seeds. Avoid processed cheeses and (alas) ice cream.

Seven Ages of Man

Let's take a look at the seven ages of man—and woman—to see what we all need to keep healthy and fit.

Stage 1: Infancy (under age 2)

Breast-feeding supplies needed nutrients in just the right amounts. Bottle-feeding with formulas often turns out heavier babies, which can lead to obesity in later life.

At 4 to 6 months, introduce solid foods one at a time and 3 to 4 days apart to check for food allergies.

Don't allow a baby to use a juice- or milk-filled bottle as a pacifier at any time. It can destroy your child's teeth. If you must, use water—at least it won't destroy baby's teeth.

Don't limit fats: Infants need them for their rapid development now.

Stage 2: Childhood (2 to 12 years)

At this stage, we develop lifelong habits of eating and exercise. A parent who pushes food at a child sows seeds of future weight problems. Obesity is controlled largely by our genes—that is, our heredity—but a high-fat diet can ensure increased poundage.

Limit TV watching; promote lots of physical activity instead: cycling, skating, swimming, climbing. Serve low-fat, high-carbohydrate, good protein foods.

Stage 3: Teen Years

In their preteen and teen years, children shoot through a growth phase. Boys especially require protein for muscle.

Teenagers' bones grow rapidly, and girls in particular need to build up thick bones now to avoid osteoporosis—brittle bones caused by the thinning of bone mass later in life. Four or more glasses of skim milk a day will do the trick.

Menstruating girls need to replace the iron lost each month in menstrual blood. Lean cuts of beef and liver, once a month, are good sources of iron. Beans, whole-grain breads and cereals, baked potatoes (when you eat the skins, too), and dried fruits also are rich in iron.

Stage 4: Young Adulthood

If you build a foundation of good eating habits in your childhood and teen years, you probably can coast on it up to age 40. For those of you who once played active sports and who now take your sports via TV, flab begins to replace muscle. This may be your last chance to control weight easily by adopting eating and exercise patterns for a lifetime.

In young adult women, pregnancy and nursing increase their bodies' need for protein and all vitamins and minerals. Most of these new demands can be met by dairy products and foods from the meat/fish/ beans group. Doctors often prescribe vitamin supplements, including iron and folic acid to prevent spinal malformation in babies.

Stage 5: The Middle Years

For most of us, our body weight creeps up between ages 40 and 60, initiating "middle-aged spread." Our metabolism—the process by which our bodies burn energy—slows down now, so our bodies are burning fewer calories. Much of that extra weight—and danger—also comes from less activity and taking in more high-fat foods and alcohol.

Stage 6: Senior Years

After age 60 and before 80, food problems multiply. For many older people, a

---

Here's to Your Good Health

You are what you eat, say scientists, who are discovering more and more health power in food. Here are some guidelines based on the latest research:

• Be beware of diet fads that wear the mask of science. They suffer from the "popcorn effect," in which a kernel of truth becomes so inflated with hot air that it can mislead and possibly harm. If some food or nutrient is good, more is not always better. Too much of one vitamin or mineral could block the body's ability to absorb another.

• Eat oats, dried beans, peas, and lentils. These foods harbor fibers that trap sugar in the digestive tract, slowing its entry into the bloodstream (a boon to weight-watchers and diabetics). And colon bacteria feed on these fibers, producing chemicals that sup-

press the liver's cholesterol output and protect you from heart disease.

• Eat fish several times a week. Scientists still are unsure whether it's the fish or its oils that help in heart disease, breast cancer, rheumatoid arthritis, psoriasis, and migraines. Use low-fat cooking methods, such as broiling, poaching, or baking—detailed in the cookbook *Seafood*, by Janis Harsila and Evie Hansen, $16.95 from National Seafood Educators, P.O. Box 6006, Richmond Beach, WA 98160 (800-348-0010).

• Add olive oil to your "OK fats" list. Monounsaturated fat, the kind of fat in olive oil, can lower blood cholesterol, as do polyunsaturates. Other foods with monounsaturated oils are almonds and avocados. Reminder: To keep your heart and waistline happy, limit intake. Fat packs a lot of calories.

loss of taste produces a decline in food variety, with a loss of vitamins and minerals. Nutritionists recommend adding herbs and spices, in place of salt. Too much sodium can aggravate high blood pressure.

As we age, our stomach acid production drops, interfering not only with our digestion but also with our absorption of calcium, which can lead to osteoporosis. More than half of us in the 60 to 80 age group often can't easily digest lactose (milk sugar), and milk is a prime source of calcium.

Stage 7: The Over-80 Years

Even minor changes in our diet can lead to substantial improvements. Upping our intake of high-fiber foods can clear up much digestive discomfort, including constipation. Iron supplements can help relieve anemia.

With small changes for each stage, each of us can design a diet to enrich the times of our lives. It's simple: We should vary our choices daily from the Basic Four food groups, lessen our intake of animal fats, and keep up our intake of carbohydrates.

A Powerful Medicine

FOOD IS POWERFUL MEDICINE. IT CAN PROTECT against a score of diseases, including heart attack and stroke. You may even live longer—if you eat right.

You can say the same about exercise. Regular, heart-pounding, lung-heaving movement also can cut your risk of heart attack. It, too, might help you live longer—if you do it right.

As with all powerful medicines, food and exercise have to be taken in the right doses, at the right time, and be of the right type for you. Too much food sends your weight shooting up. The wrong kind shifts your blood cholesterol up. Too much exercise can hurt your joints. The wrong kind does no good at all. *Parade* surveyed the experts and scientific reports and came up with some guidelines for eating and exercising at any age. First, review three general life-enhancing rules before you choose the exercise and eating patterns that suit you.

• General Rule 1: Less is more. Try to keep your weight to the poundage printed in the healthy weight tables. Common sense tells us that if we eat too much food, we gain weight. If we are overweight, we tend to run greater risks of high blood pressure, diabetes, even cancer. And, usually, we do not live as long as people of ideal weight.

• General Rule 2: Make aerobic exercise a three-times-a-week habit. Most

Americans are couch potatoes—their main form of exercise is walking from the TV set to the dinner table and back. Studies show that this is true for adults and children.

Yet aerobic exercise—the kind that makes you breathe hard—can lengthen your life, reduce fatigue, and keep your weight down. Many experts agree that if you do 25 to 40 minutes of aerobic exercise three times a week, your heart and lungs will benefit substantially.

• General Rule 3: Most people should keep their fat consumption down to 30 percent or less of their daily total of calories. For infants up to the age of 2, fat intake need not be limited. For children between the ages of 2 and 12, fat can comprise between 30 and 40 percent of their daily calorie intake. On average, adult Americans consume 37 percent of their calories from fat. This may explain why 25 percent of us are overweight.

Per ounce, fat contains twice as many calories as carbohydrates or protein. Worse, we get most of our fat from animal sources. And this kind of fat increases the damaging type of cholesterol in our blood, which, in turn, increases our risk of heart attack.

To lower animal-fat intake, cut back on whole-milk products. Eat less beef, veal, lamb, pork, and oils of coconut, palm, and palm kernel. Switch to other vegetable oils, fish, and poultry. You can get all the nutrition you need without pills by adopting the following Basic Four foods plan:

1. Breads, cereals, pasta, rice. Eat at least four servings a day. You won't gain weight—unless you swamp them with fats. For extra fiber, choose whole-grain breads, cereals, and brown rice.

2. Fruits and vegetables. Eat four or more servings a day. This group gives you vitamins A and C and fiber. For vitamin A, choose the deep green and yellow/orange vegetables. Get vitamin C from citrus fruits, tomatoes, and strawberries.

3. Fish, fowl, meats, and beans. Eat two servings a day. You get your protein here. Beans also provide fiber. Some seafoods provide special heart-saving oils. Limit beef, veal, pork, and lamb; make it lean. No more than three egg yolks a week.

4. Milk products. Servings per day: adults, two; children, three; teenagers, four. Look for skim milk or low-fat products; these are your best sources of calcium. Watch out for cheeses—they're high in saturated fat, with the exception of cottage, pot, and farmer cheeses.

Now let's see how eating works with exercise at each stage of your life.

Diet and Exercise for Every Age

1. Infancy (under age 2). The latest fad is exercise for infants. The experts say it can't hurt, but it probably does no more good than the usual infant play. As for food, just follow the pediatrician's advice. Breast-feeding is best, with solid foods added at 4 to 6 months.

2. Childhood (2 to 10 years). A diet high in fat—whole milk, ice cream, cake, candy—can promote obesity. Try more outdoor games and activities, more high-carbohydrates but low-fat foods.

3. The teens. Like their younger brothers and sisters, inactive teenagers can pile on pounds. And a diet of hamburgers, ice cream, and soda adds to their avoirdupois. Acquire an exercise habit that will last a lifetime—tennis or some other racket sport, cycling, swimming, jogging, skiing. On the diet end, stick to the Basic Four with extra emphasis on skim milk.

4. Young adulthood. If as a teen you've developed healthy eating and exercise habits, in young adulthood you will cash in on the results—good health and strength. Young adult women will need to change their diet for pregnancy.

5. The middle years. Danger signs pop up. We slow down. We gain weight. Our bodies burn less energy. We may have to redouble our diet discipline by restricting fats and calories still more and by increasing exercise to retain fitness.

6. The senior years. Between 60 and 80, we face the major results of poor food and exercise patterns. A loss of the sense of taste, common as we age, often leads to a loss of interest in eating and to too little food intake.

But it's never too late to catch up. Adding spices to foods spikes their flavor. A medically supervised aerobic program can recapture half of the heart's capacity, and flexibility exercises will reduce the pain of arthritis.

7. The over-80 years. We may need supplemental pills of iron and calcium to compensate for an outflow of these nutrients. Studies show that even modest leg movements lead to reduced calcium loss and improved lung function.

Summing Up

Keep to the Basic Four. Change what has to be changed with each decade. Build an eating-and-exercise habit for life. If you do, the payoff comes in the form of life's best bonuses: good health and added vigorous years.

A Tragic Disease Called Bulimia: When Staying Thin Is a Sickness

SHE COULD BE YOUR CLOSEST FRIEND. EVEN YOUR wife or your sister. And you wouldn't know that a terrible disease had gripped both her mind and body, threatening her very life.

But she would know.

Gayle Cappelluti, an elementary schoolteacher in Brooklyn, knew that something was terribly wrong each time she shut herself into her room to eat.

"I'd have a whole pizza—one of the big ones. And a couple of pounds of candy and more cookies," she recalls. "Then I'd telephone a Chinese take-out restaurant and order $30 worth of food.

"It was like being in a dream. I didn't think of anything. I'd just eat all night long."

Yet Ms. Cappelluti never gained much weight. At 5 feet, 4½ inches, she weighed 109 pounds. And that was the second part of her guilty secret: she vomited all of the food she ate.

"I'd do it many times a day," she says. "I'd try not to think about what I was doing. But when I did, I hated myself. 'Ugh,' I'd think, 'how could you do a thing like this?'"

Until recently, few doctors considered in an illness when people like Ms. Cappelluti would binge on food and then throw it up or take laxatives. Today, the affliction is called bulimia (from the Greek word meaning "ox hunger") or, simply, binge-purge disease.

Physicians and psychologists rank bulimia as a major physical and mental health problem. But figures are hard to come by. Previous studies suggested that the ailment strikes 5 to 20 percent of female students, ages 13 to 23. Dr. Harrison G. Pope, Jr., of McLean Hospital in Belmont, Massachusetts, says estimates show that 1 man in 20 is bulimic but as many as 7 million women, aged 10 to 52, are trapped some time in their lives in the binge-purge syndrome. Jane Fonda says she was bulimic as a teenager.

You may be bulimic and hide it from yourself. Here are some of the signs:

1. Eating huge amounts of food
2. Vomiting or using laxatives to purge
3. Hiding your binges from others
4. Trying to control your weight by binging and purging
5. Feeling out of control once you start eating

Bulimics may maintain normal body weight and look healthy, but they are prone to such ailments as swollen salivary glands, an inflamed pancreas, and gallbladder problems. Constant vomiting harms the stomach and food pipe, or esophagus. Stomach acid coming up into the mouth erodes tooth enamel. I saw a bulimic with so much enamel gone, only tiny stubs of teeth remained.

At its worst, bulimia can kill. Purging empties the body of potassium; this makes the heart irritable and prone to stop. The estimated death rate for severe bulimics is 1 to 10 percent.

Some bulimics spend up to $300 on food. They isolate themselves at work and at home, even from their spouses. Sometimes they cannot work and lose their jobs.

Bulimia is related to anorexia nervosa, a condition in which patients refuse to eat anything at all and waste away.

Dr. C. Philip Wilson, Columbia University's College of Physicians and Surgeons in New York City, calls anorexia nervosa and bulimia two sides of the same coin because both are rooted in the fear of becoming fat. Every bulimic I spoke to confessed that fear. "Even at 100 pounds, I felt fat," Gayle Cappelluti said. She weighs 120 now.

Nobody knows why the binge-purge syndrome snares mostly women. Dr. Pope and Dr. James I. Hudson, also of McLean Hospital, call bulimia a form of a major depressive disorder. Says Dr. Pope, "Among our bulimic patients, 80 percent suffer from major depression or manic depressive illness."

Dr. B. Timothy Walsh, of Columbia University's College of Physicians and Surgeons, reports success with antidepressant drugs. "Bulimics not only stop binging and purging," he says. "For the first time, they feel better."

One of Dr. Pope's patients, Sheri Swanson, bulimic since she was 18, says she hid the problem from everyone: "It's so shameful." All treatments failed until Dr. Pope prescribed an antidepressant drug, desipramine. Sheri noticed a difference right away. She says, "This oppressive cloud was lifted. Within a matter of weeks, the binging was gone. It was astonishing."

Studies also show that bulimic women have other psychological disturbances. Up to a third have attempted suicide. Bulimics tend to abuse alcohol and street drugs. "We think a third of our patient have kleptomania too," says Dr. Pope. "Imagine a middle-class woman who can buy anything she wants yet steals a bottle of perfume."

Treatment for bulimia varies. Daniel Baker, Ph.D., director of the eating disorder program at University Hospital of the University of Nebraska Medical Center, Omaha, trains bulimics to turn away from food and build self-esteem.

Associates for Bulimia and Related Disorders, a group of psychologists in New York City, teaches clients to turn to other people rather than to food. Says Ellen Schor, Ph.D., a codirector, "We tell them, 'You have a food addiction. Food has been your secret lover, your confidant, and worst enemy. If you go on like this, you will never get close to people.'" In groups, patients are taught the facts about bulimia, urged to keep diaries and to make contracts with themselves to change. Codirector Judith Brisman, Ph.D., reports that after a year, a third of the group no longer binged and another third cut their gorging by half.

When all else fails, Dr. Katherine Halmi, of Cornell University Medical College in White Plains, New York, takes a drastic step. She hospitalizes her patients for an average of 3 months. Hospitalization keeps the bulimic away from food; in serious cases, it can save the person's life. Step by step, patients are taught to eat normally. At $370 a day, the cost for 3 months would come to about $33,000.

Aided by group meetings at the American Anorexia/Bulimia Association in Teaneck, New Jersey, Gayle Cappelluti is a recovered bulimic.

For information on bulimia and related disorders, write to the American Anorexia/ Bulimia Association, 293 Central Park West, Suite 1R, New York, NY 10024.

Will a Diet Help You?

IF YOU'VE NEVER HAD TO DIET TO SLIM DOWN, you really are exceptional. Medical surveys show that more than half of all Americans have tried dieting at least once to drop poundage. Many have succeeded, too—only to regain the weight. At this moment, spurred on by the millions of newspapers, magazines, and books that constantly promote diets, 40 percent of the nation's women and 20 percent of its men are struggling to lose weight and keep it off. Keeping it off is the issue.

There are all sorts of diets. They range from simply counting calories to very low-calorie liquid diets to heat-and-eat, portion-controlled, low-fat meals. And with them, almost everyone can take off weight—for a while.

For example: In 1983, at the University of Pennsylvania, three effective weight loss methods—a very low-calorie liquid diet, behavior therapy, and a combination of the two—were tested by Dr. Albert Stunkard and Dr. Thomas Wadden. Subjects using either method alone lost large amounts of weight. Those who combined

methods lost even more. But, within 3 years, each regained all the weight lost, and then some.

For most people trying permanently to shed at least 30 pounds, dieting is probably futile. Conceding this has led many overweight persons to join a growing "nondiet" movement and raise the cry, "No more diets! Accept me as I am." Some have joined the National Association to Advance Fat Acceptance. The group's chief, Sally E. Smith, says of its goals, "We're trying to end discrimination and to help fat people demand and make use of their rights."

Jill Fuller, 40, of Denver, says that, having tried them all, she won't follow diet programs anymore. She is 5 feet 10 and "thinks" she weighs 300 pounds (she avoids the scales). For more than 20 years, hers was the "yo-yo" diet/weight syndrome typical of most obese men and women: If she was dieting, her weight dropped down; if not, it bounced up.

"Yo-yo dieting had destroyed my metabolism," she says. "My body didn't know if I was fasting or feasting."

Now, with a new lifestyle, Ms. Fuller is slowly losing weight. She eats foods low in fat—30 grams or less daily. She does not count calories and eats as much as she wants. She walks her dogs at least a mile a day and says she opts for stairs over elevators.

"A couple of years ago, when I weighed 350 pounds," she says, "I decided to stop dieting. Since then, I've been eating low-fat foods. I think I've lost 40 pounds—I don't know. I probably will level out at 240 pounds. I feel really good."

By not aiming for the weight that insurance tables term "ideal" for her, Ms. Fuller may be on the mark. Some suspect that the "yo-yo" pattern might lead to diabetes, arthritis, heart problems, even cancer.

O. Wayne Wooley, as codirector of the eating disorders clinic at the University of Cincinnati, knows uncontrolled eaters intimately. He says erratic dieting is unhealthier than excess poundage and adds, "After a failure, it takes twice as long to lose the same amount of weight, but only half as long to regain it." Our bodies, he says, were designed to hang onto fat to survive as cave dwellers.

Dr. Stunkard points out that, prehistorically, humans burned calories while hunting and foraging for food. Now, we sit and devour unneeded food, our bodies store unused calories, and we gain weight. Then we diet to lose it. This works at first. But eventually, after prolonged dieting, the body burns fat slowly

(to avoid starvation), and losing weight gets increasingly harder.

So, is dieting all for naught?

"No," says Dr. George Blackburn. "There's a lot of hope. Dieting may not take off 50 to 100 pounds, but it certainly will take off 10 to 20 pounds."

Dr. Blackburn heads a center for the study of nutrition and medicine at Deaconess Hospital in Boston. He says that, all by itself, too much weight can affect health gravely. He contends that losses of 5 or 10 pounds in even the very obese can improve high blood pressure and diabetes.

He calls overweight a national problem. Indeed, the Centers for Disease Control in Atlanta estimate that 25 percent of all Americans are overweight. Dr. Blackburn says, "We must bring our weight down. Just a 10-pound loss per overweight person in the U.S. would reduce the national health bill by $100 billion." He bases this prediction on a 1992 National Institutes of Health report.

People endanger their health, Dr. Blackburn warns, even when they weigh only 15 percent more than their medically established ideal weight. If, for example, your ideal weight is 120 pounds and you weigh 138, you are 15 percent overweight and at risk. If you are 100 pounds overweight, you are pathologically obese and face the highest health risk of all.

Medical ideas are changing. The realization that dieting won't result in permanent major weight loss has become the central focus for treating obesity, Dr. Stunkard says, which has led to other alternatives that focus on treatment and prevention.

About 5 years ago, Dr. Michael Weintraub, associate professor of community and preventive medicine at the University of Rochester (New York) School of Medicine, found that the drugs phentermine and fenfluramine suppress appetite, but each works differently on the brain and has different side effects.

He combined the drugs to curb hunger in doses so low as to produce few side effects. A 3 1/2-year study ensued. In some cases, drugs were given periodically and then withheld. Subjects lost weight, but most regained all or much of it when the drugs were discontinued.

Pat Kania, 55, who teaches practical nursing in Rochester, was a subject in the study. She says she lost weight with the drugs, regained it without them. But, Dr. Weintraub notes, "The study's prime importance is to lead doctors to reexamine feelings about weight control medications." Maybe, like diabetes, fighting fat requires lifelong medication. The safety of that concept must be studied carefully.

Dr. Rudolph Leibel, a researcher at Rockefeller University in New York City in search of genes that trigger obesity, says, "I am confident that in the next decade, as we better understand the biological basis for the control of body weight, we'll develop more and more powerful drugs for weight loss and, even more important, for the comfortable maintenance of body weight."

One Lump or Two?

TO HEAR SOME FOLKS TALK, YOU'D THINK THAT refined sugar caused or contributed to nearly every known disease. The actual list includes cancer, diabetes, low blood sugar, heart disease, high blood pressure, hyperactivity in children, rotten teeth, gallstones, obesity, and hypercholesterol. From scientists both in and out of government, the verdict: In the amount currently consumed, sugar is safe for almost everybody. It triggers no major disease, makes few if any people fat, and it doesn't make kids climb walls. It does contribute to tooth decay, but no more than other foods.

The worst you can say about sugar is that it is pure calories, devoid of any other nutritive value—"empty funcalories," nutritionists call them, meaning that if you eat too much sugar, you cut down on nutritious food and leave yourself undernourished by an unbalanced diet.

"Most people will use sugar reasonably in amounts that don't drive out good food," says Dr. Walter H. Glinsmann, who headed a special Sugars Task

Force for the Food and Drug Administration. His group wiped out almost all of the indictments against sugar.

Still, nutrition experts worry about teenagers, who may consume up to eight sugar-sweetened soft drinks a day, or 1,200 calories out of the 2,500 an active young person will eat. That doesn't leave much room for vegetables, fruits, cereals, beans, meats, and dairy products—all essential to a well-balanced diet.

The American Dietetic Association (ADA), which speaks for most nutritionists, says it's OK to eat sugar in a well-balanced diet. Too much sugar, the ADA agrees, does interfere with getting the good foods.

How much is the right amount? It varies from person to person, but the ADA suggests that you're safe from an unbalanced diet if you eat no more than 15 percent of your calories in sugar. If you consume 2,500 calories a day, take only 375 calories in sugar—about the amount in two soft drinks. But keep in mind that you'll get added sugar in other foods you eat, such as breakfast cereals, breads, canned goods, frozen dinners, and desserts. Now food manufacturers often tell you clearly how much sugar there is inside.

The bad effect of sugar on the teeth is real. The bacteria in your mouth turn the sugar into acid, which dissolves the dental enamel. However, the latest research blames the number of times you eat rather than specifically what you eat. "If you eat cookies, bread, potato chips,

raisins, apples, bananas, milk, soda—it's all the same," says Dr. Stephen Moss, chairman of the department of pediatric dentistry at New York University College of Dentistry. "Every snack starts the bacteria working again. Limit kids to snacking only two or three times a day."

Scientists have had a hard time killing the myth that sugar turns calm children into fidgety, talky, aggressive terrors. But a number of careful tests have failed to find sugar-triggered hyperactivity. Dr. Markus Kruesi, a child psychiatrist at the National Institute of Mental Health in Bethesda, Maryland, checked 29 children for hyperactivity after sugary meals. Parents of some of the children had reported that sugar turned the kids into jittery robots. "We just did not find it," says Dr. Kruesi. "Not a single child."

People with diabetes need to control the amount of sugar they eat because their bodies lack insulin to burn up sugar. And the high blood-glucose levels can lead to serious problems. But in no way does sugar cause diabetes. Another myth states that if you take in a lot of sugar at a meal, your body rapidly burns up or stores that sugar, and you are left with too little in the blood. That's called hypoglycemia. In the 1970s, it was blamed for everything from the tyranny of bosses to Monday-morning blues to cancer. But, except for people with diabetes, a rare few suffer from hypoglycemia.

Nor can you especially blame sugar for putting on pounds. In fact, it turns out that most of the calories in sweet foods come from fat. Sugar plays a part by making the fatty foods—cake, candy, pie, ice cream—tasty.

The Sugars Task Force systematically reviewed all the diseases with alleged sugar causes. High blood pressure? No. Atherosclerosis and heart disease? No. Cancer? No. Gallstones? No. Blocks vitamin and mineral absorption? No.

Some consumer groups contend, however, that many children's cereals have much more sugar than fiber and that Americans in general eat far more sugar than the task force reports, killing their appetite for the good foods and rotting their teeth. But that's all just supposition, the task force says.

In short, there are no major bad effects from the amount of sugar that most Americans eat today.

How Doctors Can Treat Deadly Obesity

YOU'VE SEEN THEM ON THE STREETS: HUGE human beings, rolls of fat enclosed in oversized clothing. They weigh 250 pounds, 300 pounds, even 400 pounds. Sometimes they elicit hurtful smirks from others.

Lourie Greenblatt, 57, of Manhattan, weighed 267 pounds. "People in restaurants stare at me in the rudest possible way," she says. "It makes me feel just horrible."

Our national obsession with weight is such that a hoaxer easily fooled several reporters for radio and TV stations, newspapers, and wire services when he said he'd formed a "fat squad" whose agents purportedly were hired to trail dieters and keep them honest.

Doctors define as "morbidly obese" individuals whose weight reaches 100 pounds more than the average listed by insurance tables for their size and age. Morbidly obese people fall prey to sudden death from heart attack, to stroke, and to high blood pressure, diabetes, arthritis, kidney disease, swollen ankles, infection, and sleep apnea, a condition in which they stop breathing during sleep. Sleep apnea can trigger heart arrest or leave victims so tired they can't stay awake during the day.

But more than the physical risk, the morbidly obese often become social cripples. Some employers won't hire them. They find travel difficult because seats are too small. They don't visit friends and relatives, fearing they'll sit on furniture and break it.

Almost all of these too-fat people have tried to diet to lose those killer pounds, but few have succeeded. About 95 percent of those who lose large amounts of weight regain it.

But doctors are making progress against gross, deadly obesity. They have developed surgical procedures to stifle appetite—risky but successful in two of three morbidly obese patients, depending on the surgery. They also prescribe diets very low in calories—about 400 to 800 a day. Patients on the regimen enjoy a success rate similar to that of the surgery, but this approach also is risky, and the relapse rate is higher.

Doctors have other new drugs and techniques now under intensive study:

• Balloon treatment. The patient swallows a balloon to keep the stomach feeling full. As the balloon inflates and as the patient eats, very little room is left in the stomach to accommodate more food. Although this creative approach seemed promising at first, most doctors who tried it did not seem to achieve the same weight reduction as the inventors of the balloon did.

• Drugs that suppress appetite. Promising medicines are on the horizon but not yet for sale. Some of these drugs may be addicting.

• Drugs that help burn energy

• Drugs that hinder fat absorption. Again, the safety and efficacy of this treatment need to be established.

• Psychological methods that help overcome the desire to eat. A psychologist can teach a person to control eating habits. For example, Dr. Thomas A. Wadden, assistant professor of psychology at the University of Pennsylvania School of Medicine in Philadelphia, has helped the morbidly obese lose weight with behavior modification alone. One patient, Joan Wozniak 58, of Stratford, New Jersey, lost 50 pounds by keeping a food diary, exercising, and following Dr. Wadden's psychological tips. Powerful as such methods are, the chances for long-term success are low for the hugely overweight.

Most experts contend that the tendency to be fat is inherited. But, says Dr. Theodore Van Itallie, codirector of the Obesity Research Center of St. Luke's/Roosevelt Hospital Center in Manhattan, "Obesity results from a combination of genetics and environment. You have to eat a lot to get fat."

The obese body contains more fat cells—living sacs that make up the fatty flesh—than does the never-obese body. A 400-pound person may have four times more fat cells than does a normal-weight person. And the fat cells are bigger.

If you lose weight with any method, the fat cells block winning. It seems to work this way: As the obese person gains weight, the number of fat cells increases. That occurs because the specialized fat cells increase with the excess calories that the fat person consumes. When the fat cell reaches a certain diameter, the cell divides. Now the fat person not only has more pounds, he or she also has more cells.

When the morbidly fat person tries to lose weight, the fat cells become starved for more nutrition. When they shrink to a particular size, they do not die. Instead, they send chemical signals to the appetite centers in the brain. Those chemical semaphores tell the brain, "Eat! Eat! Eat!" And the weight-gaining process starts all over again. Scientists are avidly searching for chemicals that will block the "eat" signals.

The Last Resort: The Knife

Carla DeKok, 29, of Fort Morgan, Colorado, tipped the scales at 248 pounds on April 29, 1982. On that day, she went under the surgeon's knife in a last-ditch effort to take off those pounds. At 5 feet, 5 1/2 inches, she was almost twice her ideal weight.

Like most obese persons, Ms. DeKok had failed in all weight-loss attempts. Finally, fearing that his wife's weight could kill her, Dennis DeKok told her on their wedding anniversary, "You know what you can give me for our anniversary? Fifty more years. Have the surgery."

In the months following the operation, Ms. DeKok achieved a weight of 149, down 99 pounds. Her coat size went from 26 1/2 to 14. Infertile before surgery, she has since had two babies. Her stomach capacity shrank from quart size to the size of a couple of tablespoons. It cannot

hold big meals. If she tries to overeat, she immediately feels stuffed.

The operation she had is called a vertical-banded gastroplasty. It was developed by Dr. Edward E. Mason, professor of general surgery at the University of Iowa College of Medicine in Iowa City. Dr. Mason creates a small pouch at the opening of the stomach. At the bottom of the pouch, he places a plastic ring so that the exit cannot grow larger.

Dr. Mason estimates that 30,000 persons a year undergo surgery for obesity, most of them having their stomachs "pouched." There is some risk. About one person in 200 dies from the surgery or its complications. Some patients require surgery later to correct problems that result from the pouch.

There is no proof that patients live longer because of such surgery, but they do lose pounds as well as their symptoms of diabetes and high blood pressure. And their arthritis symptoms are relieved, even if their ideal weight is not reached. Overall, most experts consider this surgery only as the last resort.

Testing New Antifat Pills

All fat persons dream of taking a pill that will magically cause pounds to melt away. A dozen pharmaceutical companies are working hard to turn that dream into reality—and cash.

"We are trying to design molecules that intervene in the body's regulation of fat storage and food consumption," says

Ann C. Sullivan, director of pharmacology and chemotherapy for Hoffmann-La Roche Inc., in Nutley, New Jersey. The pharmaceutical companies are now testing some of these molecules in human beings. Preliminary results indicate that they might work. The experiments are in their infancy but promising. The drugs being tested could help you lose weight in three ways:

1. Appetite suppression. One stomach hormone, released while eating, has been found to mildly suppress the appetite. But so far, an increased supply can be given by injection only.

Another group of drugs acts on a brain chemical called serotonin. Preliminary tests on obese patients resulted in weight loss.

Naloxone, a drug used to treat heroin users, blocks the brain's reaction to opium products. Tests show it also has some effect in suppressing the appetite of persons who do not use such narcotics.

2. Fat and carbohydrate absorption. Fat forms if the digestive system sends an excess of fats and sugars into the blood. Several drugs block either fat or carbohydrate absorption.

3. Stepping up energy expenditure. Since the obese person's body burns energy very efficiently, it simply uses fewer calories to maintain itself during weight loss. And as the body's fuel-burning system burns less and less energy, weight loss becomes harder and harder. (It also results in the obese person feeling cold while dieting.) To counter this, three drug companies are testing compounds that might increase body energy use. If successful, they can step up the number of calories burned.

So far, none of the drugs being tested is available. Until they're proved safe and marketed, you'll have to lose weight without the aid of antifat pills.

Starving Yourself Thin

In a sense, it is easy to lose weight by fasting because, after about 5 days, you no longer have an appetite. There's only one problem: Fasting can kill you. Fasting kills by thinning the muscle of the heart or by upsetting the mineral balance in the blood. No one can predict whether the lethal effects will strike you. Eating a small amount of high-protein food plus mineral supplements spares the heart and keeps the blood well supplied with minerals.

Rick Pisauro, 36, a photographer in Columbus, Ohio, dropped 160 pounds (from 410) in 7 months by eating 420 calories a day of Optifast, a high-protein and high-glucose liquid made primarily of eggs and milk with vitamins and minerals. After switching to regular food, he began a running regimen, lost 55 pounds more, and currently weighs 195. "Life is more exciting now," says Mr. Pisauro.

Drs. Victor Vertes and Saul Genuth, professors of medicine at Case Western Reserve Medical School in Cleveland, developed Optifast. Their 26-week-long program costs between $1,500 and

$3,000 for the liquid plus doctors' fees. Nationwide, more than 750,000 patients have tried the Optifast program, which includes exercise training, instruction for transferring to regular food, nutrition education, medical monitoring, and behavior modification to form new eating habits. Patients must be at least 30 percent above their ideal weight to enter the program.

Dr. Vertes reports that 80 percent of all patients stick with the program. After a year, about a third regain most of their weight, a third gain back half of what they lost, and a third stay within 10 pounds of their lowest weight.

For the gigantically overweight person, the turn in research may be the dark before the dawn. Researchers seem to be closing in on the causes of uncontrolled obesity, and from that understanding they may be able to find ways of preventing or curing this peculiar plague.

Are You an Apple or a Pear?

"WHAT GOES PAST MY LIPS SETTLES ON MY hips" is an oft-repeated lament that is literally true for many women and some men. When these "hippy" types become obese, their excess body fat clings to their thighs and rumps, giving them pear-shaped proportions.

On the other hand, most men and some women who become obese take on a rotundity—a tire of fat wraps itself around their middles, causing their figures to resemble apples on legs.

Dr. Ahmed Kissebeh, of the Medical College of Wisconsin at Milwaukee, says that 25 percent of obese men and women are apples, and 25 percent are pears. The remainder, he says, combine aspects of both.

However much the pears lament about their hips, they may have a good-health edge. Science is discovering that apples die at two to three times the rate of pears their own age. The apples fall prey more often to heart disease, high blood pressure, diabetes, gallbladder disease, gout, stroke, and—perhaps most frightening of all—cancer. Pears generally stay relatively healthy for years longer.

When women enter menopause and their hormone levels change, sometimes the fat shifts from below to above their waists, turning them from pears into apples with the same risks for the diseases that plague male apples. It's not only how much fat your body carries that affects your health—where it's draped counts, too.

"We are just learning how dangerous fat above the hipline can be," says Dr. Marvin Kirschner, who runs an obesity clinic at Beth Israel Hospital in Newark, New Jersey. "It's not as dangerous to be a pear." And the doctors are learning about visceral fat, which apples accumulate *inside* the abdomen. It clings to the intestines. If you have a lot of visceral fat, you're a major target for the diseases that strike apples. And because visceral fat lies deep in your body, you may not know it's there.

Besides its ill effects on the circulatory system, belly fat also may raise the risk of breast cancer in older women. Dr. Aaron R. Folsom and his colleagues at the University of Minnesota School of Public Health in Minneapolis studied 40,000 postmenopausal women. The obese apple-shaped women had twice the rate of breast cancer as women of average build. Dr. Folsom says that changes in female hormones caused by extra fat may set off the cancer. Studies suggest a similar tie-in with colon cancer in both men and women.

Seymour Abend, of Manhattan, knows just how unhealthy appleness can be. He had survived a heart attack.

At a height of 6 feet and a weight of 280 pounds, Mr. Abend then weighed 80 pounds more than the height/weight tables advised. Most of that extra poundage had settled in his trunk. He measured 53 inches around the waist. Unknown to him, pounds of visceral fat also clung to his intestines.

After his heart attack, Mr. Abend lost 13 pounds and lowered his cholesterol readings from 240 to 200. He takes medicine to control his high blood pressure and has reduced his risk of a second heart attack. He says he plans to join the Weight Watchers program.

Dr. George Blackburn directs the Center for the Study of Nutrition and Medicine at New England Deaconess Hospital in Boston. "We need to get to the apples more than the pears between the ages of 19 and 34," he says. "Fifty percent of all people who diet don't need to. Eighty percent of the people who need to diet—the apples—are not doing it."

All Obesity Is Risky

Even for pears, there comes a point when too much poundage takes it toll.

That fact comes from the Framingham Heart Study of 5,200 men and women living in Framingham, Massachusetts. It began in 1948 and is now researching two generations of subjects. Dr. William Castelli is the medical director of the project, which receives financial support from the federal government and support staff from Boston University. Says Dr. Castelli, "By becoming obese—even without developing the risk factors of raised levels of blood pressure, cholesterol, and uric acid—eventually you still pay a price. You still get more strokes and heart attacks. It just takes a bit longer for them to develop." In fact, he adds, in a study of men and women aged 30 to 40, it was found that such life-threatening conditions occur in about 8 years in obese men, about 14 years in obese women.

One study tracked women, aged 30 to 60, who weighed at least 30 percent more than recommended by the height/weight tables. After 26 years of study, data showed they suffered twice as many heart problems as did women of desirable weight. "Extra weight is one of the worst risk factors we have for disease," Dr. Castelli says. "We are one of the fattest countries on earth. We're committing national suicide."

A National Institutes of Health panel concluded that 15 percent of American adults carry enough flab to put them at risk for major health problems. Dr. Kirschner says that if you weigh 20 percent more than the height/weight tables recommend, you're at risk.

How Do You Know Whether You're an Apple or a Pear?

Dr. Kissebeh has an easy system. First, at the narrowest level of your waist and then at the widest point of your hips, use a tape measure to find how many inches wide you are. Write down the number of inches for each. Divide the waist number by the hip number. For women, anything below 0.75 is a pear, above 0.85 is an apple. For men, the cutoff points are less than 0.80 and more than 0.95.

A woman with a 25-inch waist and 36-inch hips scores a little under 0.70 (a pear), and a man with a 36-inch waist and 35-inch hips scores over 1.0 (an apple).

The Greater Peril of Appleness

The apple-pear theory emerged in the 1940s when a French physician, Dr. Jean Vague of the University of Marseille, noticed that, of his patients, the pears were far healthier than the apples, who suffered more often from diabetes and heart problems.

And, 30 years later, Dr. Kissebeh found the first chemical sign of the peril of appleness: Apples had more sugar in their blood than did pears after drinking the sugary potion of a glucose tolerance test. In addition, apples—even those who were otherwise healthy—had early signs of diabetes.

A study of 15,000 obese women revealed that the apples among them ran 10 times more risk of diabetes than the pears. Dr. Kissebeh also showed that the cells of the apple-shaped person seemed resistant to insulin.

Then scientists discovered that the apples had higher blood pressure than the pears. Next, studies revealed that belly fat disrupted the body's cholesterol balance. The more belly fat, the more artery-clogging low density lipoprotein (LDL) cholesterol in the blood.

It is unclear why belly fat—particularly *inside* the belly—does such damage. Marielle Rebuffe-Scrive, a French scientist who worked at Yale University, contends that it's easier for apples (especially men) to draw the energy from belly fat and the visceral fat inside the belly than it is for pears to draw energy from the fat on their hips or thighs. That's why, when apple men diet, their bellies flatten quickly—that fat melts away. But when pear women lose weight, their thighs and buttocks remain large.

Kimberly Cox, of Newark, New Jersey, measured 5 feet, 6 inches tall and tipped the scales at 230 pounds. By medical standards, she was close to morbid obesity, a level that is terrifyingly dangerous. It is life threatening, eventually leaving the patient with high blood pressure, arteriosclerosis, diabetes, some cancers, arthritis, obstetrical complications, and a high risk of stroke.

But Mrs. Cox says, "I'm basically healthy." Her doctor agrees. Her pear shape has protected her health. Before pregnancy, she measured 33 inches at the waist and 53 inches at the hips. Using Dr. Kissebeh's method of dividing her waist measurement by her hip measurement, Mrs. Cox comes out at 0.6—a definite pear—with all her excess weight on her hips and thighs.

Why the Difference?

There is growing documentation that your pear/apple condition depends on your genes and gender.

Dr. Rebuffe-Scrive says she has evidence that, along with other hormones in women, estrogen causes fat to deposit in the thighs and rump. Apple-shaped women, Dr. Kirschner has shown, produce higher male sex-hormone levels. A man is a true pear, he says, under certain medical conditions where there is a low level of male hormone.

Some researchers theorize that belly and visceral fats flow immediately into the liver. The consequent rush of fatty material prevents the liver from removing extra insulin from the blood. It also interferes with the cholesterol balance.

Thigh and rump fats do not burn up easily—*except* when the woman is either pregnant or breast-feeding. As a design for survival of the human species, this makes sense. Women store fat in the thighs and rear, preparing for the day when they have to bear and nurse their young but have too little food. Then they tap into their stored fat for fuel.

In most men and in the apple women, their male sex hormones direct extra fat to the trunk and innards. That makes sense, too. In prehistoric times, humans foraged for food and went for long periods with inadequate diets. It was essential to store energy for long, foodless treks. Using belly fat, which was quickly turned to energy, a hunter or gatherer could go for days with little food.

But few of us now go for days without food, and our tendency to store fat has become a liability.

Dr. Claude Bouchard, of Laval University in Quebec, Canada, has shown that the movement of body fat is partially controlled by inherited chemical systems. He performed a carefully executed experiment with 12 pairs of identical twin brothers whose average age was 21. Such twins, coming from one egg, have the same heredity.

Dr. Bouchard kept these men sedentary and overfed by 1,000 calories a day for 84 days. At the end, each of them had gained between 9½ and 23 pounds. They put on the fat in different places and different amounts. But when he compared each twin pair with the group as a whole, the brothers were more like each other than they were like the rest of the men. X rays revealed that, in the identical twins, body fat had been deposited in the same areas and amounts.

"There's good reason to believe that genes are involved," Dr. Bouchard says. Apples or pears generally reproduce in kind. However, he contends that obesity is only about 25 percent under genetic control. The eating environment in which you grow up accounts for 30 percent of total body fat. What determines the rest—45 percent—is unknown.

Dr. Albert Stunkard, of the Department of Psychiatry at the University of Pennsylvania in Philadelphia, worked with scientists in Sweden who have been accumulating data on twins reared together and twins reared apart. He also explored the genetic control of obesity in twins.

Dr. Stunkard examined the obesity patterns among 93 pairs of male and female identical twins reared apart and 154 pairs of identical twins reared together. Their ages ranged from 21 to 80. He found that, whether together or apart, the twins were more like each other than unlike. For men, the match was close 70 percent of the time; for women, 66 percent of the time.

Is there a gene for obesity? Dr. Bouchard and others are on the genetic trail.

Peeling the Pounds Away

Dr. Kirschner says only 10 percent of patients on calorie-controlled diets lost weight and *kept it off*. Very low-calorie diets—400 calories a day—do somewhat better under strict medical supervision. Dr. Kirschner's patients who followed a liquid diet regime that is available only through a doctor's prescription had 32 percent success in losing weight and keeping it off.

During the weight loss, blood pressure drops, the cholesterol system returns to a healthy state, arthritis is relieved (especially in the weight-bearing joints), and many diabetics no longer need injections of insulin.

Dr. Blackburn says that some patients who lost only 10 to 15 percent of their excess weight had, within 3 to 6 months, reversed the life-threatening symptoms of high levels of blood pressure, LDL cholesterol, uric acid, and high insulin.

Researchers, trying to find chemicals that will cancel the drive to eat excessively, have found some drugs that help. One being tested in Europe is dexfenfluramine. Scientists showed that, with the drug, patients lost an average of 10 percent of their body weight in 6 months and kept it off for a year. Without the drug, the patients lost 8 percent of their weight in the same period. Only 55 percent stayed on the diet without the drug, compared to 63 percent with it.

In this country, Hoffmann-LaRoche, the pharmaceutical company, is testing a drug that inhibits a key enzyme required for fat absorption, preventing some of the ingested fat from being absorbed.

In sum, discoveries about apples and pears, the genetic basis of obesity and the distribution of fat, as well as new drugs to cut the storage of fat, have opened a new route to the control of disease in obese men and women.

Start Exercising—and Stick with It

EXERCISING IS A LOT LIKE DIETING. YOU KNOW that losing weight and getting in shape is good for you. You've started a diet or an exercise program a dozen times. But, after a few weeks or months, you're sitting in front of the TV, munching corn chips and feeling guilty about not doing pushups or swimming or *something*.

Maybe one in three of us who starts exercising sticks with it for a year. The Centers for Disease Control in Atlanta report that only 10 percent of Americans exercise enough to reap important health benefits. Of those who need it most—the overweight, those with high blood pressure, and heart-attack convalescents—far too few will start, let alone stay with, an exercise program.

At last, scientists are uncovering the secrets of how to start working out and keep on doing it—for life. *Parade* can now offer you some of the best of the known techniques for making exercise into an enjoyable, lifesaving habit.

"If you want to live longer, exercise. It's that simple," says Dr. Ralph Paffenbarger, Jr., professor of epidemiology at the Stanford University School of Medicine in California. He studied 17,000 Harvard graduates and found that those who exercised more really did live longer. Perhaps best of all, if you follow a good exercise program, you'll look and feel 10 to 20 years younger.

However inactive they were in the past, almost everybody can exercise an hour or two a week and easily avoid injuries. Your own customized exercise program need not interfere with work or family life and might even enhance them.

Michael O'Shea, *Parade*'s fitness editor, has run successful training programs for years. "I've rarely seen anybody who couldn't do some sort of physical activity if he or she got the right exercise in the right way," he says.

So why do most people avoid exercise at all costs? Generally because the workout is uncomfortable. Many trainers will say, "No pain, no gain." In this case, the reverse is true: Pain is punishment. And psychologists have proved that habit formation relies on reward.

Try *Parade*'s Seven-Point Fitness Program, which prescribes enjoyment as the secret to perseverance. Here is its premise, simply put: To make it a habit for life, avoid pain and discomfort; exercise only for pleasure. Exercise at your convenience. Reward yourself in every way.

Follow *Parade*'s program, step-by-step, and you'll find yourself on the move—walking, jogging, swimming, biking, or lifting weights—and enjoying every active second of it.

The Seven Points

1. Make the Decision
Before you read further, follow these instructions from Dr. Rod K. Dishman, director of the Behavioral Fitness Laboratory at the University of Georgia in Athens. To allay fears that you'll look foolish while exercising and get only small returns for your time and effort, he suggests you fold a sheet of paper down the middle and write the pros for exercising on one side of the fold and the cons on the other. Try it.

Now look at your negatives. Did you put down "not enough time"? Are you so busy that you can't spare an hour or two a week? Often, in the morning, I met David Rockefeller, the financier and philanthropist, at my exercise club in New York. And I thought, "If he can find the time to work out, I surely can."

Examine each pro and con fully. At the end, write "I will exercise" or "I will not exercise." If you vote no, you can stop reading now.

2. Pick the Exercise
First, the workout has to be enjoyable and healthful, so choose exercises that are both effective and fun. They fall into three categories:

1. Aerobic: makes your heart go fast and your chest heave, benefits your heart and lungs, and fights fatigue and depression

2. Muscle-strengthening: helps in sports, facing emergencies, avoiding accidents

3. Flexibility: eases joint movement and muscle stretching, relieves the pains of arthritis, and helps avoid the cramps and cricks that come with the moving of weak muscles

There's a simple way—change your style. Instead of taking elevators, climb the stairs. Instead of driving, walk—at least the shorter distances. Or park your car halfway and walk the rest, but *stride* at a brisk pace. On weekends, get lively: Try roller-skating, swimming, cycling, or taking long, zippy walks.

Leonard Epstein, professor of psychiatry at the University of Pittsburgh School of Medicine, found that for children such changes work far better than formal programs. Both are equally effective in helping children lose weight, but the children who make activity part of their lives keep the weight off and keep on exercising. It could work for you.

3. Ask "How Much Exercise Should I Do?"

At first, do very little—not even enough to make you breathe hard. If you have been inactive all your life, a sudden burst of activity could prove dangerous. You might take a medically supervised stress test. Your doctor will put you on a treadmill or a stationary bicycle and monitor your heart, blood pressure, and breathing as you move faster. At the end of the test, an exercise prescription can be written just for you and your needs.

Usually, exercising healthfully requires you to keep your heart beating at a specific level during your workout. You can calculate the pulse rate that's right for you this way: Subtract your age from 225. Multiply the result by 0.6. If you are 45 years old, it works out like this:

$$225 - 45 = 180$$
$$0.6 \times 180 = 108 = \text{your training pulse}$$
$$\text{(heartbeats per minute)}$$

At this level of exercise, you should be able to talk without breathlessness and shouldn't feel that the exercise is too hard. As your body becomes conditioned to this level, you'll be able to increase the load so that your heart will beat faster without discomfort.

Eventually, your heart will beat slowly even under heavy loads. It will recover easily from exertion and go quickly to its resting rate. As a result, that resting rhythm itself will drop.

To get the full training effect, you have to exercise aerobically for at least 20 minutes three times a week. You will find that, by exercising more often and for longer periods, your heart's capacity to handle exertion will increase all the sooner. But to start, take care to stay within your comfort zone. When you begin weight training, for example, lift only as much weight for as many repetitions as you are perfectly comfortable. Don't worry; in time, you will be lifting much more—and more easily.

Michael Pollock, director of the Center for Exercise Science at the University of Florida's College of Medicine in Gainesville, has a 45- to 80-minute training program. It includes warm-up, stretching, moving, 10 minutes; muscular conditioning, 10 to 20 minutes; aerobics, 20 to 40 minutes; and cool-down (stretching, walking), 5 to 10 minutes.

4. Choose the Time and Place

Most experts favor mornings, before your workday begins. Once you're in the habit, you will enjoy it. Fresh from a night's sleep, you're ready for a workout.

Find an exercise place that you can get to easily. Working out at home with your own equipment is fine—once the exercise habit is in place. Millions have been spent on exercise equipment for the home, and much of it gathers dust.

5. Get a Coach or a Buddy

"A coach has the expertise to guide you mentally and physically," says Michael O'Shea. In fact, studies by John Martin, a psychologist at San Diego State University, revealed that a good trainer plus a few interest-enhancing techniques can double attendance in an exercise class.

If you can afford one, hire a private trainer. "If you exercise alone," Mr. O'Shea notes, "everything has to come from within. It is very easy to find ex-cuses not to go to the gym." The next best thing to a trainer is a buddy who works out with you.

6. Set Your Own Goals, Keep Your Own Records

John Martin says research shows you will be more likely to stick to your program if you set your own goals rather than accept goals established by another. He favors both short- and long-term goals but says the short-term goals work best. Some short-term targets: walking a half-mile, lifting 10 pounds five times. With cycling, running, or swimming, set goals for time rather than for distance.

Some typical long-term goals: swimming 30 laps, lifting 50 pounds, doing 12 push-ups, getting your resting heart rate down to 60 beats a minute.

Write down your goals, and design your own exercise program to achieve them. Learn to take your pulse, and record the result after each exercise. If, during aerobics, your rate is below the training level, increase the speed with which you exercise or the distance (or duration), or both. Once you are in the habit of keeping an exercise diary, it will become a powerful motivator for you to continue.

7. Reward Yourself

Make workouts enjoyable. Research shows that high-intensity workouts lead to dropping out and injury. Plan to reward yourself for hitting short-term targets. Think of something specific—go bowling, watch a favorite TV show. Then, when you meet that goal, give yourself that reward. Or arrange for someone special to do something nice for you.

You also can give yourself "thought" rewards and try to think of something pleasant as you exercise, rather than thinking about your effort. Dr. Martin calls this a "distraction" from your exercising discomforts. He also recommends listening to a radio or cassette while exercising, a pleasant distraction that cuts down the boredom. In his studies, those who learned to distract themselves pleasantly kept to the program much longer.

Caution: Get a medical exam before starting any exercise program, especially if you are overweight, smoke, have heart trouble or any chronic ills, have seldom exercised, or are over age 40.

It's time to get off your duff and start moving—for life!

Four Ways to Test Your Fitness

DOES A QUICK RUN UP A FLIGHT OF STEPS LEAVE you huffing and puffing? Can you touch your toes without suffering shooting pains in your lower back? Does an 8-hour workday leave you so exhausted that you cannot enjoy your after-hours?

If you answered yes to any of these questions, you may lack complete physical fitness. You may also be at extra risk for diseases.

Parade's Fitness Test can help you determine how fit you are and the areas where you may need improvement. The test was put together by Dr. Bernard Gutin, a professor of applied physiology at Columbia University's Teachers College in New York and the author of *The High Energy Factor*. Each part measures fitness in a particular area. You may be fit in one way but not in another. To improve your fitness, you will need an exercise or diet program, or both.

Do the tests in order. Do *not* take any part, however, without first consulting your doctor, particularly if you (1) have chest pain or feel dizzy or short of breath *before* you begin; (2) have heart disease, diabetes, emphysema, high blood pressure, epilepsy, panic attacks, osteoporosis, or any other chronic disease; or (3) suffer knee, ankle, neck, or lower-back problems or have other physical weak spots. Be sure to wear loose, comfortable clothing and sneakers. *Stop* at any point if you feel weak, have chest pains, feel dizzy, or have breathing difficulty.

Test 1: Are You the Right Weight?

If your excess weight is in fat rather than muscle, then, by definition, you are not fit. Being overfat puts you at risk for heart disease, high blood pressure, diabetes, and menstrual irregularities. Too much body fat also may predispose you to cancers of the colon and breast.

Height and Weight
Here are good, general height-and-weight guidelines from Dr. Gutin.

For Women   Your weight allowance is 105 pounds for the first 5 feet, plus an additional 4 pounds for each inch above 5 feet.

Suppose you are 5 feet 4 inches tall and weigh 135 pounds. Here is the calculation:

For the first 5 feet, start with 105 pounds.

For the next 4 inches, allow 4 × 4, or 16, pounds.

Your total weight allowance is thus 121 pounds.

This is the maximum allowed for you to be the right weight. In fact, you are 14 pounds overweight. (Your weight of 135 pounds minus allowable weight of 121 pounds.)

For Men   Your weight allowance is 123 pounds for the first 5 feet, 2 inches, then 4 pounds more for each additional inch.

Suppose you are 5 feet, 9 inches, and you weigh 170 pounds. The calculation:

123 pounds for the first 5 feet 2 inches.

Add 4 × 7, or 28, pounds for the next 7 inches.

Your total weight allowance is thus 151 pounds.

You weigh 170 and so are overweight by 19 pounds (170 [actual weight] − 151 [allowance]).

The hypothetical woman and man in these examples are "moderately" overweight. To be highly fit, lose those extra pounds.

Your own overweight calculation
A. ___ Height (inches)
B. ___ Weight (pounds)
C. 105 (women's allowance for first 60 inches) or
123 (men's allowance for first 62 inches)
D. ___ Weight allowance for next ___ inches (4 pounds × inches)
E. ___ Total weight allowance (C + D)
F. ___ Overweight (B − E)

Test 2: What Is Your Aerobic Fitness?

Aerobic fitness means that your heart, lungs, muscles, and circulation are working efficiently, releasing energy by using oxygen from the air. To maintain aerobic fitness, you must engage in high-energy activities like running, jogging, bicycling, and swimming for extended periods. People who are aerobically fit are less susceptible to fatigue at the end of a workday because their heart-lung system and muscles are used to sustained work. This test has two parts.

Step-Pulse Test

Find your pulse on your wrist or the side of your neck. Count the beats in 30 seconds: that's your pulse rate per half-minute.

Next, find a stairway. Bring your right foot up on the first step, then your left. Then, step down with your right foot: follow with your left. The rhythm is up right, up left, down right, down left. Time yourself with a sweep-second watch and complete two cycles every 5 seconds. Continue for 3 minutes. After you stop, sit down and find your pulse. Wait 30 seconds. Then count the number of pulse beats in the next 30 seconds. Compare with this chart:

	Women	Men
Good	45	41
Average	50	46
Poor	56	51

The 1¹/₂-Mile Walk/Run

Take this part only if you scored average or better on the Step-Pulse Test and only if you have engaged in vigorous activity (running, swimming, energetic walking) for the last few weeks. This test puts a strain on the unconditioned body.

Walk or run as quickly as you can for 1¹/₂ miles. Maintain a steady pace, unless you are in excellent condition. Be sure the terrain is flat and the weather cool, below 68°F. Your score is measured in minutes.

	Age 20–30 Women/Men	Age 31–50 Women/Men	Age 51–70 Women/Men
Good	13/10	14/11	15/12
Average	16/12	18/13	19/14
Poor	19/15	21/17	22/18

Test 3: How Flexible Are You?

Having a wide range of motion around your joints—that is, being flexible—is crucial for the health of your back, particularly for people who have arthritis.

Stretching

Sit on the floor with your knees straight. Bend forward slowly to loosen up your back and leg muscles and reach for your toes. Then reach out as far as you can and hold it for at least one full second. *Do not bounce.*

	Women	Men
Good	More than 3 inches beyond toes	More than 2 inches beyond toes
Average	Touching toes	1 inch from toes
Poor	More than 3 inches from toes	More than 4 inches from toes

Test 4: What Is Your Anaerobic Fitness?

Scientists call the ability to release energy from our muscles very quickly *an*aerobic fitness, because such energy does not require oxygen from our lungs. You need anaerobic fitness for relatively short periods of activity that require muscular strength and endurance, such as some racket sports, calisthenics, basketball, and softball.

This test measures how long your muscles can work at high intensity before they cramp. Cramping occurs when the muscles build up a waste product called lactic acid. The more efficient your muscles, the less buildup of lactic acid. And the more fit you are.

Sit-ups

Lie on your back on a mat or rug with your hands clasped behind your head, knees bent, the soles of your feet flat on the floor and ankles secured. Then do as many sit-ups as you can in 60 seconds. Adopt a steady pace. Rest in a lying position if you cannot continue, then start again until the whole minute is up.

	Age 20–30	Age 31–40	Age 41–50	Age 51–60
	W/M	W/M	W/M	W/M
Good	35/40	32/36	29/33	27/31
Average	24/30	22/27	20/25	18/23
Poor	18/20	16/18	15/17	14/15

Caution: If you can do only one, two, or three sit-ups, do not try doing a full sit-up for several weeks. As a preliminary exercise, try crunches. In a crunch, just try lifting your shoulders 1 inch from the floor. When you can do about 25 crunches, you may try sit-ups.

Once you reach your desired level of fitness in these exercises, you can maintain that level by exercising at least three times a week. If you want to raise your level of strength, flexibility, and endurance, find a local gym or workout organization. Consider using a trainer, at least at the beginning of your program.

You can substantially increase your fitness to an athletic level. Maintenance is the key.

High-Tech Medicine

WITHIN 3 YEARS, A TINY TV CAMERA HAS TURNED the world of surgery inside out, allowing doctors to see inside their patients' abdominal or chest cavities without having to cut them open. Surgery on the organs in either cavity now can be done without massively invading the patients' flesh, bones, nerves, and muscles.

With video surgery, there are only three or four small wounds, which generally heal without ugly scars and are small enough to be covered by a Band-Aid. Rather than having to spend an expensive week or more in the hospital and a painful month recovering, a patient often returns home the same day and is back to work in a week.

Because the doctor has not cut muscle or bone and has cut flesh so minimally, the convalescent suffers little of the postoperation pain that savages people who have undergone major abdominal or chest surgery performed in the traditional way. Consequently, no heavy doses of drugs for pain relief are needed.

Brian Mendelson, 53, of Reistertown, Maryland, owns an automobile repair shop in Baltimore. Here's how he benefited from the new video surgery in late 1990: "It was the day after Thanksgiving," he relates. "I had pains in the stomach—really bad pains. Two days later, I was almost dead. I could not walk, I had no strength. I was sweating. The pains were getting worse."

The cause of all this proved to be his gallbladder.

In search of help, Mr. Mendelson found his way to Dr. Robert Bailey, an assistant professor of surgery at the University of Maryland Medical Center in Baltimore. Dr. Bailey was one of the first physicians in the United States to try the new video surgery method. Through a small hole in Mr. Mendelson's midriff, Dr. Bailey removed the gallbladder.

Mr. Mendelson says he had little postoperative pain and adds, "I went back to work in 1 week. I had only four small incisions, but I've talked to other patients who had [conventional] gallbladder surgery that left them with 8-inch scars. They took at least 6 weeks to recover from their surgery."

After the French surgeon Dr. Phillipe Mouret published a report in 1989 stating how he had removed a gallbladder using video cameras, the rush was on.

Estimates are that 70 percent of all gallbladders now are removed by video surgery and that the total has now reached approximately 600,000 such operations each year in this country. Driven by patient demand, 25,000 American surgeons have learned the video technique in just 2 years. Rarely does the surgical community adopt a new technique so rapidly.

The operation seems simple, but it requires training and practiced skill. Several surgeons liken the hand-eye coordination demanded by video surgery to playing a medical version of a Nintendo video game. As the surgeon's hands manipulate the instruments inside the patient, the surgeon's eyes watch a TV screen displaying every move that's made for the operation.

Dr. Avram Cooperman, formerly the chief surgeon at St. Clare's Hospital in Manhattan and a video surgery pioneer, has removed a gallbladder in as little as 8 minutes. He says, half in jest, that the upcoming crop of surgeons, who grew up playing video games as kids, probably will cut the time in half.

Here's how the video docs perform gallbladder surgery.

With the patient anesthetized, four small holes are incised in the abdomen. Through the puncture nearest the navel, a plastic tube called a trocar is inserted. A pipe is then slipped through the trocar, and carbon dioxide is pumped into the abdomen, causing the skin and muscles there to rise, tentlike, over the internal organs. This makes room for the surgeon to operate.

Next comes the video camera, which in size and shape resembles a pocket-size cylindrical cigarette lighter. It sits at the outside end of a bundle of glass fibers that conduct light. To illuminate the dark interior of the tent, a high-intensity light beam travels down those glass fibers, as the images it makes visible travel up the fibers to the camera.

On the TV screen can be seen the organs of the abdominal cavity—the bowel, liver, and gallbladder. Everything on the screen is enlarged up to 18 times, making visible the nerves and small blood vessels that ordinarily can be seen only with difficulty.

Through the other openings made in the patient's abdomen, the surgeon inserts the tools for cutting, sewing, stapling, and the like. The surgeon can clamp the gallbladder, cut and seal the blood vessels attached to it, and then remove the gallbladder through the navel.

Today's video surgery method did not arise full-grown with Dr. Mouret's first gallbladder operation. As early as 1910, doctors were performing minor surgery through a tube inserted in the abdomen. But that method never caught on because, without the magnification provided by TV, it was like peeping through a keyhole. Gynecologists long have used the tube (called a laparoscope, because it crosses the soft part of the body between the ribs and the hips, termed *lapara* in Greek). With it, they can look at the ovaries or draw fluid from the fetal sac to test an unborn baby's cells for genetic data.

In 1976, Dr. Harry Reich, now of the Graduate Hospital in Philadelphia, removed a patient's ovaries using the laparoscope while he was on the staff at Nesbitt Hospital in Kingston, Pennsylvania.

"The big breakthrough then," Dr. Reich says of using the laparoscope, "was treating abscesses from pelvic inflammatory disease. It was preferable to using antibiotics, which often ended with blocked fallopian tubes."

Charlene Wahila-Kelley, a hair stylist from Endicott, New York, suffered from endometriosis. That is a condition in which endometrial tissue, which normally grows inside the uterus, also grows outside of it. It has been known to cover the ovaries, fallopian tubes, and intestines and to cause much suffering.

"In 1988, the pain began to be unbearable," Mrs. Wahila-Kelley recalls. She adds that it persisted until she had surgery this past summer. Now she is free of pain and says that both she and her husband agree it's "wonderful" to have her feeling like her old self again.

Dr. Reich performed a total hysterectomy, using the laparoscopy tube to detach her ovaries and uterus. He then removed them via the vagina. "I went into the hospital on a Tuesday and left on a Friday," says Mrs. Wahila-Kelley, "and

I probably could have gone home Thursday. I had no postoperative pain and no scar." She says her sister, Marlene Wahila, also of Endicott, had a traditional hysterectomy that ultimately required 200 stitches. Says Ms. Wahila, "I wish I'd been able to have the video surgery. It would have saved me—from missing 8 weeks of work and from a lot of pain."

Following the gynecologists, bone doctors have developed a procedure called arthroscopy (*arthro* for "joint," *scope* for "see"). Employing first an optical probe tube and then a TV camera mounted behind the tube, they are able to look into a damaged knee joint. To repair torn tissues, the surgeon makes two more holes in the knee, through which he inserts the cutting instruments. This has revolutionized knee surgery: instead of having to take the knee apart, the surgeon makes just three small holes, which heal quickly. Instead of 3 months of convalescence, patients are back on their feet in a week or so.

Abdominal surgeons quickly caught on to this new method as well, in Europe but not in the United States. In 1982, doctors in Germany and France began using video surgery to remove a patient's appendix. A German team from St. Josef Hospital in Linnich, near Cologne, has reported on 625 laparoscopic appendectomies.

The doctors declare this surgical method safe, leaving their patients with little or no pain, rapid recovery and minimal scarring. In the March 1991 issue of the journal *Surgical Laparoscopy & Endoscopy,* they reported that the barely visible scars "might be the decisive factor in [patients'] acceptance of the new method."

The list of surgeries that have switched over to the laparoscopic video method grows daily. It includes these:

• Lungs. Until now, the removal of a section of lung or the taking of a sample of tissue from the lung for microscopic examination meant a patient had to spend at least a week in the hospital plus a month or more recovering. The surgeon performed a thoracotomy, opening a window into the chest. To do that, the physician and his assistants cut a giant opening across the patient's back and chest. With special clamps, they spread apart the adjoining ribs and, if necessary, broke them. The resultant postoperative pain often swamped the patient.

Dr. Ralph Lewis heads the thoracic surgery department at the Robert Wood Johnson University Hospital and St. Peter's Medical Center in New Brunswick, New Jersey. Last September, Dr. Lewis performed video surgeries for a biopsy of a diseased lung and for the removal of a lobe of a cancerous lung.

"It's like looking for a penny under a subway grating," Dr. Lewis says of video surgery. "You stick your instruments and TV camera between the ribs, using the TV image to guide them. There is no need to break the ribs." He points out that, with this method, a surgeon can remove an accumulation of fluid from the chest or from around the heart of a patient. "I've had calls from heart surgeons who are interested in this procedure," Dr. Lewis adds.

• Prostate gland. The video laparoscope has been used in the removal of cancerous prostate glands. Again, this procedure saves the patient pain and recovery time, both while in the hospital and while convalescing at home.

Dr. R. Ernest Sosa, a urologist at New York Hospital in Manhattan, has used video surgery to battle prostate cancer. He removes the lymph nodes that drain the prostate gland. Those nodes move fluid around the body outside the bloodstream. If a cancer has spread, the lymph nodes are the first to get the deadly cells. With the nodes out, the microscope reveals whether they are cancerous.

"If the nodes are clean," Dr. Sosa says, "and the biopsy of the prostate shows cancer, we go in and cut out the organ or treat it with radiation, and the patient has an excellent future." He adds, however, "If the lymph nodes are cancerous, treating the prostate itself is insufficient." In that case, Dr. Sosa says, "We do not operate or radiate—we treat the patient with medication."

The medication stops the production of the hormone testosterone, on which four out of five prostate cancers depend for growth. Although this treatment slows the disease and improves the patient's quality of life, it unfortunately is not a cure.

- Colon, pancreas, liver. Dr. Cooperman and other surgeons already have used the video technique to remove sections of diseased large bowels from patients. There is one report of 20 total colon removals with no deaths. Patients are able to go home in 3 to 5 days, instead of the usual 10 days. Dr. Cooperman, well known for his skill in pancreatic surgery, also has taken liver samples using video surgery. And Dr. Reich of Philadelphia has used the video method to repair injured bowels and urinary bladders.

Dr. Karl Zucker, professor of surgery at the University of Maryland School of Medicine, also is a pioneer video surgeon and has developed a treatment for intractable stomach ulcers. With his video viewer, he finds and severs the vagus nerve, which normally triggers the release of acid in the stomach. The cut nerve cannot stimulate the release of excess acid. As a result, less acid flows out of the stomach, and the ulcers have a chance to heal. This can be done with a traditional operation, but Dr. Zucker says he prefers his comparatively painless procedure. He adds that it has worked in 19 of 20 cases.

Dr. Cooperman predicts that most surgeons will employ the video surgery method within 5 years. Until then, surgeons must master the new procedures it entails. Dr. Andrew Warshaw, associate chief of surgery at Massachusetts General Hospital in Boston, is both enthusiastic and cautious about video surgery, saying, "Patients are going to be at some risk for a while. There was a wave of injuries caused by laparoscopic gallbladder surgeries. This has gotten better, but each new technique will go through that."

Many surgeons have trouble, initially, comprehending in two dimensions what is going on in 3-D. For example, they may push their instruments too far or not far enough. Suturing is difficult—needle and thread may be 18 inches from the physician's fingers, after all, and visible only on a TV screen.

Some surgeons seem unable to adjust, and Dr. Warshaw says he fears that refusal by such doctors to put aside the new surgery and resume the conventional methods they have mastered could put their patients at risk.

"It is important," he says, "for surgeons to know when to quit and not consider it a defeat." Otherwise, he notes, the defeated ones are the patients.

How does a patient know whether a video surgeon is competent? Experts say that once a doctor does at least 25 such surgeries, you can feel sure of that physician's abilities. But, certainly, 100 surgeries are even more reassuring.

Surgeons often complain of a technology lag, saying too few instruments are designed especially for video surgery. Instrument companies are working to fill their quite specific needs. Under development is a direct-vision optical trocar that allows the surgeon to view the punctures at the very moment they are made.

Meanwhile, several estimates indicate that the savings from video surgery average about $1,000 per patient.

Multiply by $1,000 those 500,000 gallbladder operations being done every year, and you'll find the savings total $500 million. Even with inflation, that's not exactly peanuts.

A World without Disease

IMAGINE A NEW WORLD, A WORLD IN WHICH disease no longer kills or maims. Cancer is cured—even prevented before it invades and destroys body tissue. All bodily infections, from malaria to viral pneumonia, are eliminated or effectively treated. And every inherited disease, from Down syndrome to diabetes, is cured in the womb so that the individual is born healthy.

Imagine in that same world of the future that there is ample food to feed all people because crops also resist disease, grow under bad weather and soil conditions, and provide more nourishment than any of today's fruits, vegetables, and grains. And that hardier, disease-resistant cows, chickens, and other livestock turn feed into milk or meat more effectively.

A science fiction tale? Not at all. We may be well on the way to such a remarkable world because scientists have a new tool—the science of genetic engineering. It enables scientists to uncover, rearrange, and make clones, or copies, of genes—the stuff that makes all living things what they are.

What Are Genes?

Genes are the chemical blueprints of all living things. They determine whether an organism will grow into a plant, an animal, a bacterium, or a human being. They also determine sex, the color of your eyes and hair, and, in part, how intelligent you are.

Genes do their work inside the cells, the tiny building blocks of bodies are constructed. If you looked at a cell under a microscope, you would see a murky, colorless bag of chemicals.

Under higher magnification, you would see that the cell had an information center comprised of the nucleus, protein-manufacturing units, and energy production points. The genes are in the nucleus. They contain all the information the cell needs to carry on its protein and energy production.

Now let's go deeper and take a closer look at the genes. You would see long, spiraling double strands of atoms. (This is the DNA, or deoxyribonucleic acid, the master chemical of genes.) The sequence or layout of those atoms contains all the instructions the cell needs to function, just as the sequence of beads on an abacus determines numerical value.

Tracking Genetic Disease

Genes control the chemistry of every cell of all plants and animals. A gene that is missing, malformed, or out of place profoundly distorts the chemical activity of the cell, and often of the entire organism. In humans, such genetic defects can lead to disease or deformity, such as Down syndrome, sickle cell anemia, cystic fibrosis, diabetes, atherosclerosis, Tay-Sachs disease, and others.

Scientists now know that about 100,000 genes are inside each human cell. They have isolated 21,500 of these genes and identified the specific jobs they do. For example, scientists know the chemical structure of the genes that make insulin, a hormone whose lack causes diabetes.

Cancer Genes

Indeed, genetic engineers already have claimed one tremendous advance—the discovery of cancer-causing genes called oncogenes (*onkos* is Greek for "mass," as in the massing of malignant cells in a tumor). Each of us probably carries one or more of these genes in every cell in our body. Undisturbed, oncogenes are harmless. Then, one day, something comes along that triggers the oncogenes. They make a chemical that causes cells to divide and multiply uncontrollably, forming millions of new cells that invade and choke our organs. A cancer.

The first human oncogene, for bladder cancer, was discovered in 1981. A year later, Dr. Robert Ellsworth of the Ophthalmic Oncology Center at New York Hospital–Cornell Medical Center identified the gene that controls the growth of cancer cells in the retina, causing a disease called retinoblastoma. In total, scientists have discovered about 20 oncogenes; there may be 10 more. What does that mean? For 100 years, doctors believed that cancer was not one disease, but many different diseases. Now they know that most cancers are probably caused by one or more of the 20 oncogenes.

Researchers have yet to unravel exactly what turns on an oncogene, how to prevent it from turning cancerous, or, once it has turned cancerous, how to turn it off. Once they do, they can cure and prevent cancer.

Dr. Paul Marks heads the Memorial Sloan-Kettering Cancer Center in New York, the largest private cancer institution in the world. He was my classmate when we both went to high school in Brooklyn. Neither of us could then imagine the scientific wonders of today. Now, as we spoke about oncogenes, he could hardly contain his optimism.

"Gene manipulation will provide fundamentally new approaches to the prevention and cure of cancer," he said. "When? I am an optimist, but it will take a while. I can't say this year or the next 5 years. In your lifetime or mine? I expect so. I hope so."

Creating Natural Drugs

Genetic engineering is already bringing relief to some people and hope to others. Fred Kostaras, of Levittown, Pennsylvania, has diabetes. He injects himself every morning and evening with a genetically engineered form of insulin that is the exact molecular duplicate of human insulin. Tracy Moreno, 10, who was growing too slowly, gets regular injections of growth hormone, cloned in the laboratory from human genes. Now, says Dr. Selma Kaplan, of the Pediatric Endocrine Unit at the University of California, San Francisco School of Medicine, Tracy is not fated to go through life as a 4-foot, 10-inch adult.

And there is hope for Marion Bennett, of Cheraw, South Carolina, who was stricken with melanoma in 1973. Despite surgery, the deadly skin cancer spread throughout her body. She is counting on injections of genetically engineered interferon to pull her through. Interferon is part of the body's natural defense system in combating illness.

To create insulin, human growth hormone, and interferon, genetic engineers have taken a page from the beer brewer's manual. Brewers use yeast to make beer because the yeast cell has a gene that controls the manufacture of alcohol. In the same way, genetic engineers can use yeast or bacteria—two simple germs—to create "natural" drugs. To make insulin, for example, they first isolate the gene for insulin from human cells. They splice the insulin gene into the yeast or bacteria genes. Those fast-growing microbes then turn out the human chemical, in this case, insulin. And because bacteria and yeast are easy to grow and reproduce so quickly, they can turn out limitless supplies of once scarce human hormones or chemicals.

Genetic engineers most recently cloned antihemophilic factor, the substance that helps blood clot, which hemophiliacs lack. Other "natural" drugs that may soon be genetically engineered include the following:

- Endorphin—a natural morphine-like compound that controls pain and mood
- Interleukin—a protein that regulates the body's immune system

- Human serum albumin—another protein available from blood that is used by doctors to replace blood loss from surgery or injury
- Streptokinase and urokinase—two enzymes that work within the blood system, dissolving blood clots in the body, particularly the heart, brain, and lungs. Both are available now
- Tissue plasminogen activator—a protein that dissolves blood clots, working at the site of the clot without affecting the blood supply
- Erythropoetin—a natural human protein that stimulates the production of red blood cells

Genetic Counseling

Because they know the genetic formulas for several genes, scientists can hunt down and diagnose certain genetic abnormalities in the tissues of the human body.

Doctors already screen for genetic defects prenatally (i.e., before birth) thanks to amniocentesis. In the diagnostic procedure, the doctor removes a sample of amniotic fluid from the mother's womb, into which cells from the fetus have been shed. He then checks these cells for genetic defects.

One day, doctors will routinely screen adults to see whether they carry faulty genes. They also will be able to detect a person's susceptibility to certain diseases such as hardening of the arteries, gout, and diabetes, even though the illness may not develop until years later.

At the University of California, Irvine, Drs. G. Wesley Hatfield and Moyra Smith recently cloned three different genes that mutate in certain people, which prevent the proper metabolism of alcohol. If pregnant women have this problem, even small amounts of alcohol will cause severe developmental defects in the unborn child, a condition known as fetal alcohol syndrome.

Doctors also hope to replace missing genes. One way to insert a missing gene is to splice it into the genes of a virus. The virus infects all the body cells and drops the missing gene into them.

Splicing genes into viruses is also being used to make vaccines. Scientists at the New York State Department of Health used this technique, which is also known as gene transfer, to make experimental vaccines against herpes and hepatitis viruses.

To make a herpes vaccine, for example, they isolated a gene from a herpes virus. They transferred that gene into a harmless virus called *vaccinia*. The vaccinia then "looked" enough like the herpes virus to stimulate the production of antibodies against herpes. When the vaccinated person later was exposed to a real herpes virus, he was protected by those antibodies. The scientists used the same technique to create the hepatitis vaccine.

Wiping Out World Hunger

Scientists also see the possibility of changing the genetic endowment of animals and plants alike, making them more efficient and disease-resistant producers of meat, milk, and grains by transplanting in them the genetic properties of hardier life forms. Only recently has it become possible for genetic engineers to put foreign genes into living animals. For example, researchers at the University of Pennsylvania School of Veterinary Medicine successfully transferred a human growth hormone gene into a fertilized mouse egg. After the mouse was born, the human hormone helped it grow to twice the size of a normal mouse!

Agricultural scientists, meanwhile, are hoping to transfer the disease-resistant properties of one plant to another. At the University of California, Irvine, scientists already have developed bacteria that aid plants in resisting frost. Now they are introducing genes into other bacteria that will enable plants to take nitrogen out of the air and fix it in the soil, so that plants can grow without expensive fertilizers.

The Watchdogs

If scientists find the power to change the genetic makeup of plants and animals, the possibility exists of changing the heredity of human beings, of removing or putting genes into fertilized human eggs, and then allowing those eggs to mature into adults with new traits. Ideally, one could imagine changing humans so that they would be less susceptible to disease, more intelligent, stronger, and faster. We would have "humans by design."

In any case, the brave new world of genetic engineering has arrived. The first products are helping diabetics, slow growers, and cancer patients. The scientists are convinced that much more is to come. The genes are doing good deeds.

The Wonders of High-Tech Medicine: A Fantastic Journey

METAL AGAINST YOUR FLESH. CHEMICALS swimming in your blood. Plastic disks resting in and on your eyes. Radioactivity stirring in your heart. Laser sun guns zapping cancer.

As a health reporter, I have been a traveler with doctors and scientists on their voyage of discovery.

I have seen an infant's life saved because a laser burned away choking tumors. I watched a surgeon install a new plastic valve in a man's heart. I saw a physician put plastic pebbles in a man's brain to correct a tangled knot of blood vessels.

After five decades of high technology—chemistry, physics, engineering, and biology—and its revolutionary impact on medicine, still I marvel. High-tech medicine saves lives that once would have been hopelessly lost; it also offers better lives to those crippled by disease. We have hundreds of examples.

A diabetic woman I know pricks her finger with a needle and puts the resultant drop of blood on a sliver of paper, slips the paper into a machine the size of a pocket radio, and red numbers appear. They tell how much sugar is in her blood. For the first time, she can keep track of what her body is doing, control her diet exactly, and keep her blood sugar normal. That means, powerful studies indicate, that she won't suffer the complications of heart attack, kidney disease, or blindness. She can safely have a baby.

A girl—a prize-winning flutist—is pushed off a New York subway platform into the path of a train. She survives, but the steel wheels cut off her hand. A policeman gathers up her hand. At Bellevue Hospital, Dr. William Shaw and a team of doctors reattach her hand under microscopes with threads and needles finer than hairs; the surgeons repair blood vessels, tendons, muscles, nerves, and skin. The young girl gets her hand back, and it works.

Surgeons have put back severed arms, legs, fingers, feet, even a scalp.

There's more on this incredible journay: A vaccine that prevents hepatitis. Computers that help doctors make better diagnoses. New drugs that help the heart. An electrical stimulator that straightens spines. Hormones to strengthen immunities.

Fiber Optics

In the dark room, peering through a tube inserted near the navel of Linda Tejada's pregnant belly, Dr. Karen Filkins says, "I can see the mouth, and there's the jaw. And the eye. It's perfect."

Dr. Filkins has inserted a flexible rod into her patient's womb to look directly at the unborn fetus, checking for deformity.

Six years earlier, Mrs. Tejada had given birth to Rolli, a boy with defective jaw, head, and eye. Now, at University Hospital in Newark, New Jersey, she wanted to find out about her new baby. Five months later, she gave birth to Priscilla, unblemished in any way.

"I would not have become pregnant again if I had no way of finding out if my baby was going to have Rolli's problems," she told me. Her son has undergone several operations.

To examine Priscilla, Dr. Filkins relied on fiber optics: thousands of tiny glass fibers, each 0.0004-inch thick. Each fiber carries a narrow pencil of light. Even with the fiber bent 90 degrees, doctors can see around corners and illuminate the womb.

With fiber optics, doctors operate on unborn babies. At Yale Medical School, they have drained a blocked bladder that could destroy the kidneys. Others have transfused new blood to the fetus.

Fiber optics give doctors a direct view of an adult's stomach, lungs, large bowel, kidney, and gallbladder. Physicians have removed gall and kidney stones without surgery. And in the large bowel, they find early cancer and clip it—without operating.

In the future, scientists want to look directly into the beating heart to see the valves. They probably will.

New Organs, New Lives

Sixteen years ago, Robert Brown clung to the edge of life. At 40, because disease had destroyed his kidneys, poisons piled up in his body. A lumber salesman with four children and a wife, he was kept alive by having his blood washed.

"I had no life," he says. "I lived a day-to-day existence. But everything is beautiful now."

Drs. David Hume and John Merrill at Boston's Peter Bent Brigham Hospital transplanted a kidney from a dead person who was not related to Mr. Brown.

Mr. Brown knew the risk was high: he had one chance in six of dying on the table, and most kidneys were rejected. White blood cells would surround the alien flesh, attack it, kill it. Often the patient would die too.

Bob Brown became a member of the club: long-lived survivors of a kidney transplant from an unrelated person.

Thanks to new and better drugs, surgery, antibiotics, and new ways to fight rejection, more people today survive with new organs. The current 1-year survival score: 95 percent for kidneys, 80 percent for hearts, and perhaps 75 percent for livers.

"We've made tremendous advances in the past couple of years," says Dr. Merrill. "Kidney transplantation may be the greatest medical advance in the last 25 years."

Cyclosporin A, a chemical found in a soil fungus, has been the most effective and safest rejection fighter yet. As it holds down the number of white blood cells that kill foreign tissue, the body adjusts to its new organ.

Cyclosporin A has generated new enthusiasm for heart transplants. While thousands of kidneys have been transplanted, only about 300 hearts have made the transfer, most of them at Stanford University.

And for children born with damaged livers or adults with liver disease, new livers for the first time mean new life. Dr. Thomas Starzl, of the University of Pittsburgh, who pioneered in liver transplants, has saved several dozen children and adults.

Dr. Merrill says that the surgery is safer than ever, the death rate dropping by 75 percent. New treatment for rejection could make kidney transplants "take" 100 percent of the time. Many believe that high-tech medicine will make a transplant as safe as a tonsillectomy and will promise, in Bob Brown's words, a "beautiful" life for thousands.

The big drawback is a shortage of organs. Hearts and livers, which must come from healthy persons who die in accidents, are especially scarce. That's because most people killed in accidents die before they reach a hospital prepared to take a heart, kidney, or liver. Relatives often refuse to allow organs to be taken from a loved one. The number of hearts taken stood at 2,000 for years, while the need is at least 10,000.

Superman's Eyes

I was flat on my back in bed, my legs up in the air pedaling a bicycle suspended from the ceiling. A huge white object, like a quarter of a beer barrel, was pressed against my chest.

"Keep pedaling," the technician called. My breath came hard. I could feel my heart pounding.

"We have a good picture," announced Dr. Jeffrey Borer, of Manhattan's New York Hospital.

It was a black-and-white movie of the inside of my wildly beating heart, and it looked like a hunk of putty being squeezed by a fist.

But Dr. Borer pronounced my heart perfect. He helped develop the technique that uses a nuclear camera to detect heart diseases that escape other methods. (Fourteen years later, I did have a problem: narrowed coronary arteries left over from my days of eating huge amounts of animal fat.)

Dr. Borer's camera works by detecting radioactivity in the heart. Before I did my upside-down exercise, I got an injection of radioactive chemicals.

The nuclear camera is one of a dozen incredible machines that allow doctors to peek inside the human body without cutting it open. It is as if the eyes of Superman had come off the comic strip and into the laboratory.

Besides viewing the heart, they can see inside the brain, stomach, small intestine, liver, kidney, and a mother's womb to see the unborn infant.

• The sonogram: It sends inaudible, high-pitched sound waves into the body. A detector picks up the waves as they bounce off the internal organs.

On a television screen, you make out the fuzzy outlines of a fetus's head, arms, legs, and eyes.

• The CAT-scan: This is a super X-ray machine with a computer to interpret 100 X-ray beams as they bore through your body. On a TV, you see all the parts.

• The PET-scan: You swallow or are injected with special radioactive chemicals. The computer locates those chemicals in your body.

So far PET has detected the center of epilepsy, checked blood flow in the brain of a stroke victim, and tracked cancer growths.

• Neutron activation: The scientists shoot neutrons at you. The neutrons—subatomic particles—make some of your atoms radioactive. The scientists can tell whether your bones are growing.

• Nuclear magnetic resonance: Your head is placed between the poles of a giant magnet. The atoms in your head emit radio waves. From the waves, a computer then produces a picture of your brain.

A Laser Sun-Gun

Dr. Lawrence Yannuzzi peers into a horizontal microscope. At the other end, a clamp locks Tom Ward's head so that he cannot move it. His left eye is open.

A flash of red laser light cuts into Mr. Ward's left eye. In a trillionth of a second, it travels through the cornea, the window of the eye; through the lens; through the eye's central bowl of clear jelly; through the retina, the living "photo film."

The beam halts at the back inside wall of the eye. Dr. Yannuzzi sees a white dot appear on the wall. It is smaller than a pinhead. The light beam has burned the back wall.

Dr. Yannuzzi is treating macular degeneration, a disease that blinds more elderly people than any other. No one knows the cause. It had already wiped out the sight of Mr. Ward's right eye.

At 62, Mr. Ward is a retired banker who has become a painter and etcher. Without vision, his life would crash.

In his microscope, Dr. Yannuzzi detects a tangle of tiny blood vessels clinging to the eye's back wall. They cluster under the macula, a yellow spot on the retina. As if they were a balloon, the vessels lift the macula. If it's lifted too far, the living film will go blank.

The laser destroys those dangerous blood vessels by burning them. With pinpoint accuracy, Dr. Yannuzzi burns more and more of the back wall until only a flat scar remains under the macula. Even without anesthesia, Mr. Ward feels nothing.

"I can paint," Mr. Ward says now. "I can do the fine work of etching. I have a tiny blind spot where the laser hit. But I can drive and do almost anything."

He is lucky. The laser helps at most 13 percent of macular degeneration victims. Dr. Yannuzzi, director of retinal services at Manhattan Eye, Ear, and Throat Hospital, introduced the krypton laser, which helps even more by burning closer to the center of sight, the centralis. Eye doctors are testing other lasers and surgical techniques.

The National Institutes of Health has approved laser treatment of macular degeneration.

The Scalpel

For surgeons, the laser has become a scalpel, reaching with its hot light beam where steel cannot go. At the University of Utah, doctors have used lasers in the following ways:

- In the brains of children, to burn away growths—tumors and cancer—that are close to vital centers
- In the eye, to make tiny drainage channels that relieve the water pressure of glaucoma. Unrelieved, the pressure destroys the optic nerve.
- In the bladder, at the end of a bundle of glass fibers, to destroy cancers without bleeding
- In the stomach, to stop bleeding ulcers
- In the large bowel, to vaporize little sacs called polyps, which can turn into cancer
- In a woman's abdomen, to remove the invading purple tissue of a disease called endometriosis, which causes severe pain and infertility
- On the teeth, to seal them against cavities
- In a baby's throat, to open a closed channel so the infant can breathe
- In a woman's throat, to stop the bleeding of 400 tumors
- On the face, to remove big purple birthmarks called port wine stains

The laser works because the surgeon can pinpoint its hot beam to within a thousandth of an inch. And as it burns, the laser closes up blood vessels so there is no bleeding. Worldwide, doctors have adopted the laser as a scalpel to save lives and to remove deformities.

New Joints

Unlike plants, humans move. We walk, dance, run, throw, grasp. And when we cannot move, we feel less than human. We are prisoners in our own bodies.

Once these prisoners had no hope.

Now medicine, engineering, and chemistry have joined to give them the gift of motion. Locked fingers pick up pins. Hobbled knees stride confidently. And rigid hips lift up from wheelchairs to leap out into the world.

My father, now 84, was crippled by a shriveled arthritic joint. Seven years ago, surgeons constructed a new knee of steel and plastic in his left leg. Today, he strolls along the boardwalk. He even dances at weddings.

If arthritis attacks the lining of the joint, it cannot move. You get stiffness, swelling, and pain. By afflicting hips, knees, and fingers, arthritis has disabled 7.3 million Americans.

In 1962, a British surgeon created and inserted the first artificial hip of plastic and steel. There was then the danger of germs invading the hip, of doctors putting it in the wrong place, and of the device coming loose from its mountings. But an explosion in technology has changed all that.

Mrs. Ann Ridilla, of Wilkes-Barre Pennsylvania, was born with dislocated hips. "For 55 years, she walked like a crab, all hunched over," says Dr. William H. Harris, chief of hip and implant surgery at Massachusetts General Hospital in Boston. "Five years ago, we gave her new hips. She's walking straight as an arrow."

But problems remain. Germs still invade one new joint out of 100 within 3 years, even with massive doses of antibiotics, and occasionally the artificial hip comes loose. But meanwhile, engineers have created new joints that don't easily break, and they have improved the moorings of the parts. The loosening rate of knees, which take a stronger pounding than hips, has also been cut.

Physicians have also freed the frozen fingers of victims of rheumatoid arthritis. Dr. Alfred Swanson of Grand Rapids, Michigan, and Dr. John J. Niebaur of San Francisco have created finger joints out of plastic called silicone. The replants are easily replaced. Soon, doctors may be able to replace elbow joints too.

Thousands have been given the gift of motion, which, for some, is close to the gift of life.

Plastic Eyes

When contact lenses came out, millions of people threw away their glasses. In a few months, many were sorry. The contacts hurt. Every day, you had to take them out of your eyes. And, much too often, you were down on your knees like a grazing sheep looking for a lens that had dropped onto the floor.

Now, thanks to plastic engineering, contact lens wearers can leave their plastic disks in their eyes for up to 1 week, playing sports and sleeping with them in.

The new lenses are called extended-wear contact lenses, and more than a half-million Americans now wear them.

"You can't tell they're in your eyes," says Barry Maddox, a restaurant buyer in St. Louis. "It's almost as if I have no eye problem." Since he was 13 years old, Mr. Maddox had worn thick, unattractive eyeglasses.

The old contact lenses didn't let much oxygen through to the cornea, the outside window of the eye. Without oxygen, the cornea could swell up. So engineers created a plastic that soaked up water like a sponge. The water lets the oxygen through to the cornea.

"It's like wearing a teardrop with a lens," says Dr. Louis Wilson, director of the contact lens clinic at Emory University School of Medicine in Atlanta. Many eye doctors now prescribe daily disposable lenses.

Big drawback: they cost between $300 and $500 a pair.

Stretching the Body's Power to Grow

AT AGE 9, ANGELICA RODERICK STOOD, WHEN she could stand at all, at 3 feet, 7 inches. Most of the time she kept to her wheel-

chair because the bones of her lower legs did not sit properly in her knee sockets. Angelica, now 11, was born with a disease that curved and slowed the growth of her leg bones.

Ten thousand miles from Angelica's home in Queens, New York, was the Russian bone doctor who discovered a cure for her condition 29 years ago. They met briefly in the United States in 1987.

The doctor is Gavriil A. Ilizarov, who created a method that has straightened and lengthened bones for thousands. They include midgets, athletes with twisted limbs, persons with a short arm or leg, victims of accidents, and cancer patients with chunks of bone missing.

"It is the answer to some people's prayers," says Dr. Victor H. Frankel, president of New York's Hospital for Joint Diseases Orthopaedic Institute. In 1986, Dr. Frankel became the first surgeon in this country to use the Ilizarov method.

Dr. Ilizarov has gone beyond inventing a new technique by making a fundamental discovery. He has found a way to make old bone grow as if newborn. In the end, the new bone is as strong as the original bone.

"It is remarkable," says Dr. Frankel. "If you stretch the limb very slowly after dividing the bone, you get not only new bone but also longer muscles, tendons, and nerves. I've lengthened some kids' height by 7 inches. Ilizarov has gone 12 to 14 inches. We have filled in gaps of bone 4 to 5 inches in length."

Dr. Ilizarov's technique should not be confused with another remarkable achievement: Dr. Michael Lewis at Mount Sinai Medical Center in New York has invented a titanium alloy replacement for bone, which is extended as needed by the surgeon. If a child loses a leg bone to cancer, for example, Dr. Lewis can implant his device, maneuvering it to "grow" as the child grows.

In October 1987, Frankel's colleague, Dr. Wallace Lehman, who is head of pediatrics at the Orthopaedic Institute, began stretching Angelica's leg bones, using the Ilizarov technique. First, Dr. Lehman cut open each leg, exposing the bone. With a chisel, he carefully cracked a narrow ring in the outer shell of bone.

Dr. Ilizarov discovered that if, at this point, the broken bone is put under tension—if pulled—it will grow. New cells will be produced to fill the gap. And as long as you pull on it, the bone will grow. That's a revolutionary and breathtaking biological principle.

He invented a "fixator." Imagine two metal rings circling the leg, separated by about 6 inches, like the hoops at the top and bottom of a barrel. Three rigid rods—long screws—hold the hoops fixed. The rods can be lengthened and the rings pushed apart simply by turning the screws.

Lehman then attached wires to the rings and to Angelica's bones, above and below the broken area. By turning the screws, the bones are put under tension. The screws are advanced by 1 millimeter ($1/25$th of an inch) a day. In 25 days, the bones are extended 1 inch.

By June 1988, Lehman had stretched Angelica's legs by 5 inches and had straightened their terrible curves. She also grew 4 inches on her own. At age 11, she is now 4 feet, 5—an inch taller than her mother, Antoinette Roderick, who also stopped growing as a child.

"Children can be very cruel to other children with deformities," says Mrs. Roderick. "I hope Angelica won't suffer what I went through. Her legs are perfectly straight and gorgeous."

The bone stretching was painful for Angelica, although not everybody experiences pain to the same degree. "Now I'm walking great," she says. "My legs don't hurt very often anymore. I'm glad I did it."

Ten years ago, no Western doctor had heard of Ilizarov. Now 500 surgeons have studied his methods in the United States, even more worldwide. I met Dr. Ilizarov when he visited the States, but the interview was brief, and he was quiet and withdrawn.

Dr. Vladimir Golyakhovsky works with Frankel at the Orthopaedic Institute and knew Dr. Ilizarov in the Soviet Union. He told me of Dr. Ilizarov's early years.

In 1947, 4 years after his graduation from medical school, Dr. Ilizarov went to Kurgan, a little town in Siberia about 1,500 miles from Moscow, to work in a small, old hospital. There, he got his idea of using the fixator to set severely shattered bones. In 1951, he made his first one out of metal scraps.

Dr. Ilizarov discovered the stretching principle after a patient came to him in 1960 with a short stump of leg bone. To elongate the bone with a graft taken from the hip, the doctor broke the stump, put it in the fixator, and told the patient how to elongate the instrument himself. Then Dr. Ilizarov went on vacation.

On his return, Dr. Ilizarov took X rays, expecting to find a hole between the two ends of the bone. To his amazement, there was no gap: new bone had filled it in! He followed up with many experiments and proved the validity of the bone-stretching principle.

But the Soviet medical bureaucracy thought him a fake. His being Jewish did not help matters. In 1967, fate intervened when Valery Brumel, a 1964 Olympic champion (winner of the gold medal for his high jump of 7 feet, 1.75 inches) and a hero in the Soviet Union, broke his leg bones in a motorcycle accident. Infection spread.

Luckily, Mr. Brumel found Dr. Ilizarov, who stretched the affected bones and created a new ankle. A year later, Mr. Brumel high-jumped 6 feet, 11.75 inches. This news created a sensation in Russia. Gavriil A. Ilizarov soon became as famous as Valery Brumel.

Dr. Ilizarov headed a modern, 800-bed hospital in Kurgan, where doctors from all over the world have gone to learn his technique. Italian doctors brought it West in the early 1980s. Dr. Frankel learned it from the Italians in 1985.

When she was 19, Cheryl Tucker of Selden, New York, was in a motorcycle accident that crushed her right leg. Her infected injury would not heal; she was left with a 1-inch opening in the bone. After 4 years and 11 bone grafts, doctors wanted to amputate.

"I went nuts," Ms. Tucker says. She came to Dr. Frankel, who put her in the fixator. After 9 months, the ends of the bone touched and grew together.

"I bowled 180 last week," says Ms. Tucker. "Today, I'm free of wheelchairs, crutches, and canes. I want to return to school."

Anthony Tarabocchia Jr., 13, of Moonachie, New Jersey, went to Italy to have his leg bones extended in 1985. He was born a dwarf, destined to be no more than 4 feet tall. Desperate to help her son, Mary Tarabocchia learned of successful Dr. Ilizarov operations in Italy. When Anthony was nearly 9, he asked for the surgery.

"Everyone is taller than me," he told his mother. "I can't do things on own—I can't go to the bathroom or sit on a couch. I can't reach light switches." In 1985, Italian doctors began the procedure (completed in New York by Dr. Frankel in 1987) to extend his lower leg bones by 7 inches. In 1986, the physician also lengthened Anthony's arm bones by 6 inches. Three years later, Dr. Frankel has begun stretching the boy's thigh bones 5 inches to bring his body into proportion.

Eric Kershenblatt, 27, an attorney in Atlantic City, New Jersey, had a left arm that was 6 inches shorter than his right. When he was 9, surgeons had removed a bone cyst and unavoidably had cut away the growth plate of the bone.

Life was not easy with arms of unequal length. Mr. Kershenblatt says, "Tying my shoelaces was harder. There were a lot of little things that add up to disability. I love baseball, and I could not field balls to my right side."

Dr. Frankel began using an Ilizarov fixator on Mr. Kershenblatt. Since then, his bone has grown 6 inches. Now both arms are of equal length, and the fixator soon will be removed. Mr. Kershenblatt works with the apparatus and turns the screws himself daily. He cleans the wires with peroxide to avoid infection.

The application of the Ilizarov system grows each day. Dr. Ilizarov has shown that other tissues will grow under tension. He has created large skin flaps to cover holes created by burns or injury.

For Dr. Gavriil Ilizarov, the success and recognition are made all the sweeter by his patients' triumphs over what once were considered hopeless conditions.

When Poison Cures

A BOTULISM OUTBREAK CAN TERRIFY A CITY. Botulism is caused when food becomes contaminated by the bacteria that pro-duce botulinum, a deadly toxin. It kills most of its victims. The symptoms—arriving in a rush—include muscular weakness, paralysis, and the impairment of vision, swallowing, and speech. Survivors often suffer from brain damage. Fortunately, botulism outbreaks are rare.

Now science is turning evil to good, using the botulinum toxin to relieve the muscle spasms triggered by conditions as severe as stroke or as simple as a furrowed forehead. Most of us have had brief spasms, maybe a painful "charley horse." But for some, the agony is chronic. And it was untreatable—until now.

Muscles come in pairs. If equal in strength, they balance each other's force. If one is stronger, it contracts and stays in spasm. Injection of a minute amount of the toxin equalizes the muscles. Botulinum toxin is being used for many conditions caused by muscle spasms, including several that affect vision.

Injection of the toxin brought back precious sight to Marjorie Daley of Yonkers, New York. She had been unable to function since 1982, when her eyelids began to squeeze shut intermittently. This condition is called blepharospasm (*blepharo* is Greek for eyelid).

"I couldn't drive or read," says Mrs. Daley. She found help in 1986 at Columbia-Presbyterian Medical Center in New York City, where a tiny amount of the poison was injected into the convulsed muscles that control eyelid movement. "Within 24 hours," she recalls, "I could keep my eyes open and sleep at night. My eye wasn't jumping all the time."

"Botulinum toxin relieves the effects of muscle spasm, regardless of the under-lying disease," says Dr. Mitchell Brin, a neurologist at Columbia-Presbyterian. "Before, we had no way of relieving such horrible deformity, which could occur in any part of the body."

The treatment was conceived by Dr. Alan Scott, a San Francisco ophthalmologist. He was seeking a nonsurgical treatment of strabismus (*strabos* is Greek for squint-eyed), or weak eye, which can cause eyes to cross or a weak eye to look to the side; the stronger eye focuses as desired. Dr. Scott knew the weak eye wanders when its stronger muscle pulls it over too far, preventing it from working in tandem with its normal partner. His brainstorm: poison the weak eye's strong muscle and make it equal in strength to its weak muscle.

After first working with animals, he tried the toxin on a human; the strabismus disappeared. Since then, the Food and Drug Administration has approved botulinum toxin for blepharospasm, strabismus, and related facial muscle spasms. It is sold as BOTOX by Allergan, a company in Irvine, California.

In 1981, soon after Dr. Scott published his findings, Dr. Howard Eggers of Columbia-Presbyterian injected the toxin into the right eye muscles of a patient suffering with strabismus for 22 years. Over 5 months of injections, the eye retained correct positioning.

Dr. Stanley Fahn, chief of the Movement Disorders Clinic at Columbia-Presbyterian, heard of the toxin's effectiveness and had Dr. Brin work on other spasms. Dr. Brin and Dr. Andrzej Freidman, visiting from Poland, first treated torticollis, or "wry neck."

Jack Newhall, 61, of Bethlehem, Pennsylvania, recalls the onset of wry neck in 1978. "My head started turning to the left. A pain began. My head started to pull down, nearly to my left shoulder. The pain was so bad! It never went away." After 10 years of torture, he found Dr. Brin. "I got the shots," he says. "In 9 days, the pain was gone. My head was up straight. It was a miracle."

BOTOX is being tested widely for numerous disorders, including these:

• Large-muscle spasms. Usually these are side effects of a disease—stroke, head trauma, multiple sclerosis, spinal-cord injury, or cerebral palsy. They mostly affect the arms, legs, and neck. Dr. Brin has treated 16 patients for large-muscle spasms. Each improved, including Alyce Pollack of Fort Lee, New Jersey, who walked with crutches until November 1989, when her legs "just locked together." In February 1990, Dr. Brin injected her thigh with BOTOX. "I had immediate relief," she says. "I walked with my crutches again." Dr. Brin says BOTOX could help other conditions that lead to cramps of large muscles. "Say, in the first few days of a stroke, one gets a spastic arm. If treated early, the arm could be saved immediately, with no therapy required later."

• Dysphonia. This condition, in which a muscle cramp in the voice box keeps vocal cords open or shut tight, prevents speech. It struck Bill McNarney, 53, of Des Moines, Iowa, in 1986. By the end of the year, he says, "I sounded strangulated. I could not talk on the phone." In 1988, he got help through Dr. Christy Ludlow, a speech pathologist at the National Institutes of Health (NIH) in Bethesda, Maryland. Doctors at NIH injected the toxin into Mr. McNarney's cramped vocal-cord muscle. "By the summer and fall of 1990," he says, "I could make phone calls." Says Dr. Ludlow, "We've seen functional recovery in 14 percent of our patients—no full cures yet."

• Stuttering and oral spasms. Dr. Ludlow and Dr. Brin have treated stuttering originating deep in the throat. They've also reduced oral spasms—involuntary moving of lips, tongue, jaw, and mouth that impedes chewing and swallowing.

• Tremors. Such shaking of hands, head, limbs, or body may result from Parkinson's disease, caused by a brain malfunction, or from essential tremor, of unknown cause, which may run in families and affects about 5 million Americans. Dr. William Koller, chief neurologist at the University of Kansas Medical Center in Kansas City, Kansas, and Dr. Joseph Jankovic at Baylor Medical School in Houston are testing BOTOX against tremor along with Dr. Brin. "If it works," Dr. Koller says, "it will help a lot of people."

• Cerebral palsy. Dr. L. Andrew Koman, professor of orthopedic surgery at the Bowman Gray School of Medicine of Wake Forest University, Winston-Salem, North Carolina, tried BOTOX on 12 children with cerebral palsy. They had resorted to walking on their toes because their calf muscles were cramped. All but four benefited significantly, but, says Dr. Koman, "We need more study."

• Writer's cramp. This condition occurs when you use your hands too much and can be very painful. Dr. Mark Hallett, of the National Institutes of Health, has used BOTOX on more than 50 patients (writers, musicians, and others who steadily use their hands), and, he says, 80 percent have improved. "Writer's cramp," he says, "is a lot more common than realized. The disorder does not go away. But four of five patients show improvement."

• Furrowed brow. Some of us frown so hard and so long that a furrow develops on the forehead between the eyes. It can be filled in with collagen, but, warns Dr. Jean Carruthers, an ophthalmologist at the University of British Columbia, blindness is a risk. With "major surgery," she says, some physicians cut out the spastic or cramped muscles that support the furrow. She has eliminated the furrow instead by injecting the cramped muscles with BOTOX.

For data on more than 25 centers doing botulinum toxin research, write to the Movement Disorders Resource Center, The Neurological Institute, Unit 33, 710 W. 168th St., New York, NY 10032.

What a Laser Can (and Cannot) Do

THE AMERICAN MEDICAL ASSOCIATION REVISED its ethical guidelines in 1975 to permit advertising by doctors. Taking advantage of this opening, some physicians have lifted the laser to the status of cure-all and come-on.

Ads in newspapers and on billboards, radio, and TV—as well as doctors appearing as guests on TV and radio talk shows—often make outrageous claims for use of the laser's intense, oscillating beam of light. These toutings harken to the days of snake-oil salesmen and horse-drawn medicine shows.

In skilled hands, the laser has touched and helped heal many areas of the human body. Although, lately, it too often is promoted as a treatment for everything from cancer to ingrown toenails, the laser actually has real curing power and true pain-relieving potential. But much of the advertising reeks of hype to get you in the doctor's door, so check the physician's experience with lasers. In the hands of an untrained doctor, the laser can be deadly. In the hands of an unscrupulous one, the only thing patients will be relieved of is their cash.

Dr. Barry Levine, an expert in laser surgery and chief surgeon at Montefiore Medical Center in the Bronx, New York, does not see lasers as limitless. "Lasers for hemorrhoids are a gimmick," he says, adding that he also doubts the efficacy of lasers for aiding migraines and knee and foot problems. Still, lasers are seen as treasures for many conditions, including glaucoma; torn retinas (surgery is being done to restore sight when a retina, the photographic plate at the back of the eye, has torn loose); nearsightedness (a new, highly regarded surgery is being tested); prostate surgery; and the removal of tumors, gallstones, and urinary bladder stones. These and other laser applications are described later in this chapter.

Basically, a laser is a high-powered light beam. It can deliver intense heat—hotter than the sun—to a spot the size of a pinpoint. It can weld cut arteries. Since lasers cut and weld at the same time, laser surgery is noninvasive and almost bloodless. Devised in 1960, the laser creates a focused, intense, one-color beam of light. Light from an incandescent bulb is widespread and a mix of many colors; in the heated filament of a light bulb, billions of atoms dance to

different temperatures and span the colors of the spectrum. In a laser, the electrons that circle each atom vibrate together to the same energy level. Released together, they emit light at the same energy and color, and the energy they release creates a temperature so high that it can vaporize skin, bone, or muscle. There are lasers of various energies, including the excimer laser, which can remove molecules from tissue without damaging the cells surrounding it.

Eye Surgery

Lasers have revolutionized this field and saved the sight of thousands.

• Torn retinas. Using a laser, a surgeon can spot-weld or seal a torn retina, the biological photographic plate, to prevent detachment and restore vision. Dr. Lawrence Yannuzzi has treated this condition at the Manhattan Eye and Ear Hospital in New York City, where he is director of retinal services.

• Abnormal growth of blood vessels of the eye. In cases of macular degeneration and some diabetes patients, blood vessels proliferate abnormally. If left untreated, they will leak, bleed, and scar, damaging vision. The laser cuts them back and seals them off. "Regrettably," Dr. Yannuzzi says, "we can't cure these diseases yet, but we can significantly reduce vision loss."

• Nearsightedness. Just 5 years ago, for the first time, the excimer laser successfully reshaped the cornea, the window of the eye. Within 1 minute, the laser sculpts the surface to eliminate, perhaps forever, the need for glasses in nearsighted patients. The FDA approved this procedure in 1995.

• Glaucoma. Ophthalmologists are using a laser technique to relieve glaucoma—pressure in the eyeball. The pressure is the result of fluid building up in the eye and developing enough tension to kill the optic nerve and cause blindness. To prevent this, the surgeon creates a drainage system by using the laser to drill small holes in the iris, the colored part of the eye.

Tumors

Using lasers, surgeons have, with great precision, cut through tumors blocking a vital organ—not curing the patient but greatly relieving pain. Some cures actually have resulted from the removal of large benign growths. In patients too weak to endure major surgery, the laser can provide relief by burning away tumors that block the channels that take in air and liquids.

Dr. Mark Shikowitz works in the Otolaryngology (ear, nose, and throat) Department at Long Island Jewish Medical Center in New Hyde Park, New York. One of his many research projects includes testing a new therapy for treating laryngeal papillomas—benign tumors of the larynx, which cause choking. They are generated by the human papilloma virus. Repeated treatments often are needed; the polyps tend to recur, Dr. Shikowitz says. First, he explains, he gives the patient an intravenous dose of a special photosensitive dye. Within 48 to 72 hours, the normal cells release the dye. But the *tumor* cells retain it and die when a laser is shined on them. The normal cells live.

Ear Surgery

Dr. Shikowitz and others in this specialty are using lasers for treating hearing loss that results when otosclerosis paralyzes a small bone in the ear called the stapes. A laser can drill a hole to permit the implantation of an artificial stapes.

Throat Surgery

Lasers do well in removing tonsils and soft tissues in the throat that cause snoring.

Prostate Surgery

Yearly, 300,000 to 600,000 patients undergo surgery on the prostate gland. This gland often enlarges after a man reaches age 50, creating a need for frequent urination but allowing passage only of a weakened stream. Traditional surgery removes the blockage with a small cutting instrument introduced through the penis. With lasers, the obstruction is burned away.

Urinary Tract Stones

Many urologists use lasers to break up urinary bladder stones. Says Dr. Bryan Shumaker, director of Laser Science and Research for St. John Hospital and Medical Center in Detroit, "The laser produces a flash at a temperature of 100,000 degrees Celsius. Like a nuclear bomb, it creates a shock wave which slams into the stone, smashing it. But the tissue around the stone is unharmed."

Heart Treatments

Almost 400,000 patients undergo surgery in the United States every year to reduce the cholesterol plaque that has piled up to clog their coronary arteries—blood vessels that serve the heart muscle itself. An additional 400,000 patients have surgery to bypass such blockages. Scientists are searching for ways to keep the blood vessels from reclogging.

• Balloon angioplasty. A balloon is inserted into an artery, then inflated, in an effort to compress the plaque and push it back against the arterial walls. The goal is to widen the arterial channel and let the blood flow more freely. The result is circulatory relief, but 30 percent of the arteries clog up again within 6 months.

Migraine Headaches

Dentist Mark Friedman of Mount Vernon, New York, is conducting migraine relief research with a noncutting "cold" (low-power) laser. Dr. Friedman says pain relief results when he shines a laser on a region of the inner jaw that is tender to the touch for migraine sufferers. This method is experimental and is being assessed by the FDA.

Pigment Stains

Lasers also remove color blotches (port wine stains, cafe au lait stains) from the skin. Says Dr. Robin Ashinoff, head of laser service at New York University Medical Center in New York City, "We can remove the stains as early as birth. That's best—the surface is much smaller."

Tattoo Removal

High-energy lasers can, in time, burn away the colors that have been tattooed under the skin. A grayish blotch is sometimes left in its place. The method is controversial, and some skin specialists prefer surgical removal.

Hair Implants

To cover a bald region on the scalp, dermatologists take hairs from the patient's hirsute body regions and transplant them, rooting them into the pate. Praising the method is Dr. Walter Unger, an associate professor of medicine at the University of Toronto in Canada. He says that using a laser for this procedure produces a better, more natural-looking result than traditional surgery provides. The method is still experimental and under study.

To Beam or Not to Beam?

Decidedly, lasers can do great things, but remember also that there is much they cannot do. If a doctor proposes a laser treatment for you, insist that the doctor shows you (1) why it is preferable to traditional treatment and (2) that he or she is skilled with lasers and has patients who are satisfied with the results.

Then get a second opinion.

How Computers Are Helping

DOCTOR JONES EXAMINED HIS PATIENT AT THE hospital. Hastily, he scribbled a message on her medical record ordering the attending nurse to increase the patient's heart medicine. Then he left.

Fifteen minutes later, the nurse was complaining bitterly. She could not read the doctor's crabbed handwriting; neither could anyone else. And the doctor was somewhere between the hospital and his home. For all the nurse knew, the patient's life hung in the balance.

Similar incidents happen nearly every day in every hospital across this country, probably costing untold suffering and possibly hundreds of lives.

But at L.D.S. Hospital in Salt Lake City, Utah, a bedside computer system called HELP has all but eliminated such mixups. Now doctors and nurses can type their notes into a computer terminal. The computer's electronic record for each patient contains results of examinations, laboratory tests, and treatments—from drugs to surgery. The computer stores the patient's data for the doctor.

Responding to questions by a doctor or nurse, the computer displays on a TV screen the numbers that describe the patient's condition, including temperature, blood pressure, fluid loss or gain, lab results, diet, and diagnosis. At the push of a button, the doctor also can see these numbers charted on a graph. Printouts can be made immediately.

Sure, doctors and nurses still make some mistakes, but since computerization, their error rate has dropped dramatically. Says Dr. Doug Ridges, an L.D.S. cardiologist, "There's no question HELP improves the patient's care and the physician's efficiency. I can even use my computer in my office or in my home to check on a patient. I don't have to take a nurse away from my patient to hunt down a medical record."

Computers have started to enter medicine in a big way.

Says Dr. James Todd, a senior deputy executive vice president of the American Medical Association (AMA), "We here at the AMA are convinced the future of medicine and its advances will involve computers. Medical knowledge is doubling every 8 years. It will be impossible to keep up with that if we can't computerize the information. We think more and more doctors will use the machines."

It's estimated that almost half of all physicians now use computers, mostly for keeping track of finances. But other uses are moving up fast. Here are some ways in which computers will affect your health, directly and soon.

Diagnosis

Today's doctor faces a formidable task. There are thousands of diseases. Each may have a cluster of symptoms. Some show up as patient complaints—abdominal pain in an ulcer case. Others are noted during the doctor's examination—swelling of the ankles, perhaps, in a patient with congestive heart failure. Laboratory tests of blood or tissues reveal other signs—high blood-sugar levels in diabetes. In addition, there are X rays, stress tests, sonograms, and a dozen other diagnostic techniques. That adds up to thousands of facts that the doctor must filter through to diagnose the illness correctly. To complicate matters, diseases may have similar symptoms. Consider, for example, indigestion and heart attack.

A new computer program called DXplain can, in just a few seconds, propose a list of diagnoses based on the doctor's input into the system. The physician takes his or her pick. The doctor might use any of 4,700 medical terms: fever, arthritis, abdominal pain, anemia, and so on. DXplain helps narrow the possibilities and suggests to the doctor how he might focus on one diagnosis. The program also explains to the doctor how the diagnosis fits the patient.

Dr. Phillip Klein, a general practitioner in Parrish, Alabama, has been consulting DXplain via telephone and his personal computer since the American Medical Association put the program on its AMA/NET computer network.

"I can practice the same kind of medicine they practice in New York City, and I'm just a rural doctor," says Dr. Klein. "I had this 30-year-old patient with a racing heart and fearing a heart attack. I put all the data into DXplain. It came up with 10 or 12 diagnoses, most of which I rejected as way out west."

One of the computer's suggestions was mitral valve prolapse (MVP), a floppy heart valve. It makes your heart jiggle and scares you, but it won't kill you.

"I sent the patient to Birmingham for tests I couldn't do, and out popped MVP," Dr. Klein recalls. "She's well today. She knows she's not going to die."

Essentially, the computer puts an extensive medical library at the doctor's fingertips 24 hours a day. Although other computer-diagnostic programs are available, DXplain probably is the one most accessible to doctors.

The National Library of Medicine also is developing a program to diagnose rheumatism. It's called AI/Rheum (*AI* stands for artificial intelligence). Scientists have programmed the computer to think like an expert in arthritis.

In the end, the doctor is still responsible for the final diagnosis and treatment; the diagnostic programs are no more than fancy textbooks designed to help the doctor to think and to manage information.

Treatment

Like HELP, which is used by L.D.S. Hospital in Utah, CARE is used by Wishard Memorial Hospital in Indianapolis to check a patient's electronic medical record. As data from examinations, tests, and drug treatment pile up, the program may advise what treatment to try next, or it may warn against using the wrong treatment.

Another system now being tested, called ATTENDING, helps anesthesiologists find the optimal combination of drugs to use on a patient. The doctor enters the plan and the patient's characteristics into the computer. The program then weighs the characteristics and critiques the doctor's plan.

A program called ONCOCIN suggests possible cancer treatment plans. A cancer patient might be given as many as eight drugs, X rays, surgery, or all of these. At Mount Sinai Medical Center in New York City, Dr. Larry Norton developed the Norton-Simon Model computer program to find the best way to give drug therapy to breast cancer patients. Since then, such patients' survival rates have increased significantly.

The National Cancer Institute developed a program called Physician Data Query (PDQ) to put doctors everywhere in touch with the latest cancer treatments. With a computer, a physician can find the right therapy for a patient with any type of cancer. The computer also can list the names and addresses of cancer specialists and identify those who are doing the most advanced research on cancer treatment.

At L.D.S. Hospital, a HELP computer checked on the use of antibiotics before and after surgery had begun. These chemicals kill bacteria so they do not spread to other organs during surgery. The computer system revealed that patients who were given antibiotics *before* surgery developed infections only half as often as those given antibiotics *after* the start of surgery. As a result, the system now sends automatic "alerts" to doctors, reminding them to give antibiotics at least 2 hours before the patient gets to the operating room. Since the alerts, infections have decreased measurably.

At Canada's Misericordia General Hospital in Winnipeg, Manitoba, doctors tested a desktop computer in the Drug Interactions Advisor system, which alerts doctors to drug conflicts. For example, if doctors simultaneously prescribe tetracycline, an antibiotic, and Coumadin, a blood thinner, the blood may get too thin and hemorrhaging could occur. Dozens of such possibilities exist.

In a test of 100 patients, the Canadian physicians found that 51 had potential drug conflicts, and the computer advised changing treatment in 26 cases.

Doctor's Training

Physicians now can play computer games to keep themselves intellectually sharp.

A program called CYBERLOG, for instance, deals with one topic at a time—high blood pressure, fluid balance, diabetes. The doctor gets a printed manual plus a floppy disc for a personal computer. The program challenges the physician to solve simulated case problems. The program also gives the doctor the tools to solve real-life medical puzzles—helping determine the correct dose of insulin for a diabetic, for example, or which drug to use for a hypertension patient.

At Massachusetts General Hospital in Boston, doctors can study simulated medical conditions via telephone on AMA/NET. Medical students at Harvard practice on simulated "computer patients." Similarly, a program for a personal computer called MacDope—developed cooperatively by St. Bartholomew's Hospital in London, England, and McMaster University in Hamilton, Ontario, Canada—allows medical students to administer drugs to computer patients and study the results. DxTER, a privately developed program, provides simulations for medical professionals.

Dr. G. Octo Barnett, a professor of medicine at Harvard Medical School, is enthusiastic about computer teaching. But, he warns, "There is a lot you cannot learn on a computer: being compassionate, picking up the nuances of a conversation, reading the patient's face. Computers will never replace enlightened, humane instructors who provide role models and inspiration."

Information Searches

Doctors and medical researchers can use their personal computers to delve by telephone into the vast literature that exists in the National Library of Medicine, which holds 10 million items on diseases, body parts, and treatments.

Patient Education

Like doctors, patients now can play computer games to learn more about their illnesses and how to cope with them. The University of Minnesota in Minneapolis has developed a desktop system for helping patients with cystic fibrosis, a severe, often fatal lung disease. The patients' parents also can use the computer to learn how to deal with this illness. Similar programs exist for diabetes, heart attack, sexually transmitted disease, and drug abuse. One program at the University of Minnesota will evaluate your health risks based on your lifestyle, parents' diseases, and such factors as cholesterol levels.

In Louisville, distraught parents soon will be able to sit down at their own personal computers to get medical information instantly if their child is sick, thanks to Dr. Matthew Witten, who developed the pediatrics program there. Connected by telephone to the University of Louisville, a parent at home will type the child's symptoms onto the computer screen. Back will come information on what to do immediately, when to see a doctor, and when, simply, to wait.

In Tucson, people can dial a phone number at the University of Arizona for a health assessment quiz to determine their risks for a particular condition. Callers can choose a quiz on one of 10 subjects, from stress to cancer. A computerized voice on the Tele-Health System asks the questions, and callers answer by tapping their touch-tone telephones. The voice then gives each caller's risk score, based on the answers given.

Beyond these major trends, computer science is spreading widely and deeply into the medical community with new systems, either recently established or in the testing stages. For example, computers have made possible analyses of X-ray negatives so clear that pictures emerge of whole organs. Similar advances have been made with magnetic and sound-wave probes. A doctor now can "see" a cancer that only a few years ago was not visible.

The United Network for Organ Sharing, a nationwide computer system, now directs donated organs—kidneys, hearts, livers—to the right patients with the proper match of blood and tissue.

Many drugstores and hospital pharmacies are computerized to reduce errors in prescriptions. A computerized pharmacy can spot drug conflicts, check to see whether you are overdosed, and find your prescription if you have lost it.

Why More Children Survive

WHEN YOU ENTER THE BRIGHTLY LIT, SCRUBBED, white room, you think you're in a Star Trek space station. Blinking lights, computers, plastic tubing, attendants in white. You're in the infant intensive care unit at Philadelphia's Children's Hospital. Then you look closely. You see a pinkish-yellow little creature, hardly bigger than a kitten, lying on a tiny bed. The tubes, the lights, the attendants surround it; its scrawny chest heaves with effort.

Such a creature was Matthew Luccarella of Pennsville, New Jersey. His mother, Darlene, gave birth to him 2 months too soon, and he weighed only 3 pounds, 6 ounces. Matthew was a "preemie," a premature infant. By age 7, Matthew was growing normally and earning good marks in the second grade. "At his birthday, there are still tears," says his mother. "I get very emotional when he blows out the candles. Matthew means 'gift of God'—that's how he got his name."

Matthew typifies the incredible progress of the last 40 years in keeping all children alive and healthy. Since 1950, the death rate for children between the ages of 1 and 14 has dropped by half, and it's still going down. For infants younger than 1 year, the mortality rate has fallen even faster.

Much credit belongs to the vaccines and antibiotics that have conquered infectious diseases such as polio, diphtheria, tuberculosis, measles, whooping cough, chicken pox, and mumps—diseases that once swept through communities in epidemic proportions. High technology and brilliant medical skills have mitigated the deadly powers of birth defects and children's cancer. New techniques and discoveries are piling up faster and faster, saving more children, keeping them healthier, and warding off the killers of the past and present.

Saving the Preemies

As they did in Matthew Luccarella's case, doctors are saving tens of thousands of infants who are born too soon or too small. Dr. William Fox, director of the infant intensive care unit at Children's Hospital, says, "We're getting 60 percent survival in babies who weigh less than 2 pounds. Ten years ago, only 1 percent of these infants lived."

More preemies now survive because of ingenious advances in three crucial areas: diagnosis, feeding, and, perhaps most important, mechanical breathing. Such newborns often suffocated to death because their lungs, the last organs to develop, did not work well enough to absorb oxygen.

Diagnosis

Instruments can now detect changes in the preemie's heart rate, breathing, oxygen supply, and temperature. Sound-wave pictures of the inside of the body, known as ultrasound or sonograms, allow doctors to examine the baby's brain. Sonograms have revealed that the blood vessels of up to 40 percent of preemies burst and hemorrhage into the brain because of the too high pressure of the ventilators. Because the sonogram detects that bleeding, the physician—who sometimes walks a thin line between keeping the baby alive and causing brain damage—can take countermeasures.

Feeding

Preemies used to starve to death because their digestive system also had not reached maturity. They would throw up any food given to them. Now nurses feed preemies by vein with a special liquid mixture of protein, sugars, fats, and vitamins. This gives the intestines and stomach time to "grow up" before the baby is given ordinary food.

Scientists designed food pumps and feeding tubes (called catheters) so that the liquid food pours day and night into a large vein that feeds directly into the heart. The method is called hyperalimentation, meaning "superfeeding."

Mechanical Breathing

Doctors can now save most infants born with underdeveloped lungs. They place a tube into the baby's airway and connect it to a machine called a ventilator that pushes oxygen into the lungs. In addition, new devices measure how much oxygen seeps into the blood. So the doctors can adjust the ventilator to deliver the most oxygen at the least pressure. Matthew Luccarella—like President Kennedy's son Patrick, who weighed 4 pounds at birth in 1963—was born with a film of fluid covering his lungs. It's called hyaline membrane disease. Normally, an infant's body makes a chemical that removes the film. The two boys lacked the chemical.

In a week or so, with the help of the ventilator, Matthew's body made the chemical to clear his lungs, and he began to breathe on his own. Patrick Kennedy, without the ventilator, died 2 days after birth.

Feeding Sick Children

Hyperalimentation by itself has revolutionized the care of all critically ill children, not just preemies. Some babies are born with their stomachs and intestines outside their bodies. It takes three or more operations to repair this defect. Many babies starved between surgeries.

Now surgeons save four of five such infants because hyperalimentation keeps them alive between operations. Similarly, chronic diarrhea formerly killed more than three of four of the infants whom it attacked. Hyperalimentation now rescues nine of 10.

It helped 3-year-old Taina Gomez of New York City, who was born prematurely and could not absorb food taken by mouth after much of her small intestine unaccountably died. Now, a food pump pushes liquid nutrition into the big vein of her heart. But it costs $15,000 a month to keep Taina alive at home.

Dr. William Heird, of Columbia University's College of Physicians and Surgeons in New York City, who started Taina on hyperalimentation, says, "Some of these children may have to be fed this way for life. It's not clear that they can live this way but, for now, they are living."

Mending the Heart

New technology is helping surgeons repair what used to be deadly defects of the newborn's heart, such as holes in the interior chamber walls, big blood vessels that are connected to the wrong chamber, and bad valves. All carried high death rates; babies who survived were sickly.

Today, surgeons aim for complete correction of coronary defects rather than temporary relief. They operate on smaller and younger infants, cutting and stitching hearts the size of limes. The salvage rate: 75 percent.

Straightening Crooked Bodies

Orthopedic surgeons now aggressively attack crooked spines, or scoliosis, which may afflict between 5 and 10 percent of all teenagers. They have better surgical methods and braces and new ways to diagnose curved backbones early, before the spines twist into humps forever.

From the time she was 8, Nicole Kuper of Cleveland fought to straighten her spine, first with braces that she wore for 23 hours a day and later with surgery that put rods in her back. At 13, Nicole was still in a cast, but her curvature has straightened almost to normal. "I can't wait to go swimming and get on the track team," she says.

Conquering Children's Cancer

When I started reporting on cancer 30 years ago, children with acute lymphatic leukemia died within 18 months. Today, several drugs taken in combination have boosted the 5-year survival rate to 70 percent. Some cancer-stricken children are living long enough to bear children.

At Children's Hospital and the Dana-Farber Cancer Institute in Boston, a special group of baby leukemia patients has not had a relapse in years. That's a cancer cure, and for me it's absolutely breathtaking.

Even for the relapsed patient, there's hope. In a third of these cases, bone marrow transplants provide new, cancer-free blood. First, doctors treat the child with heavy doses of cancer-killing drugs. That treatment not only kills the cancer cells but also the patient's blood-forming system. To provide a source of blood cells, doctors transplant healthy marrow from the bones of a donor, usually a relative. If the marrow "takes," the leukemia is vanquished.

With cancer-killing drugs, the doctors have also achieved great successes in other types of leukemia, cancers of the lymph glands, and various types of rare tumors, all of which used to be incurable. Physicians now save up to 85 percent of these critically ill children.

Dr. David Nathan, who heads the cancer division at Children's Hospital in Boston, remembers when, not too long ago, "all of my patients died.

"Can you imagine," he says, "what this new success means? If we lose a patient now, there is enormous roaring and rage."

Saving Bubble Babies

In Houston, a 12-year-old boy named David has lived in a germ-free room since birth. When he goes out, he wears an astronaut's suit to keep the bacteria and viruses away. He lives in a bubble.

David suffers from one of the most mysterious and deadly of children's diseases—immune deficiency. He was born without the ability to fight off even the most common germs. If any microbe gets to him, it could kill him.

Bone marrow transplants, so promising for young leukemia patients, also are making headway against immune deficiency disease. Three-year-old Phillip Ryan Wissar of Miami was born with this disease. He got bone marrow from his brother Randy, 6. Doctors at Memorial Sloan-Kettering Cancer Center in New York City first removed certain white blood cells from the marrow that could attack Phillip. Randy's marrow grew in Phillip's body. Now, when Phillip gets colds and other infections, he defeats them. Dr. Richard O'Reilly, of Memorial Sloan-Kettering, says almost two thirds of immune deficient children now survive such bone marrow transplants.

Operating in the Womb

The great progress in treating children after birth has encouraged physicians to experiment with therapy *before* birth. "The fetus has become a patient," says Dr. Michael Harrison, codirector of the fetal treatment program at the University of California, San Francisco. "We used to be frustrated when we would get newborns who were too sick and too far advanced at birth to help," he says.

Thanks to ultrasound technology, doctors actually see and diagnose fetal defects in the womb such as enlarged bladders (caused by urinary tract blockages) and enlarged heads (caused by hydrocephalus, or water on the brain) and correct them before the mother delivers a sick baby.

Dr. Harrison performed the first intrauterine (within the uterus) bladder operation on an unborn child. To prevent urine from backing up and damaging the baby's kidneys, he opened up a hole in the mother's abdomen and uterus and inserted a small tube into the fetus's bladder to bypass the blocked urethra. Water on the brain is treated with similar fetal surgery.

The Ethical Dilemma

Physicians and parents now face excruciating ethical decisions. For example, very small preemies are more likely to suffer brain damage. Should doctors save an infant who will be a severely disabled adult?

"It's a very difficult issue," says Dr. Avroy Fanaroff, director of nurseries at University Hospital in Cleveland. "Fortunately, we don't run into the problem but once or twice a year."

Dr. C. Everett Koop, former U.S. Surgeon General, ruled in the early 1980s that any hospital that permits such infants to die would lose all government support. A federal court rescinded the rule, but the doctors still had a problem.

"We consult all the doctors and nurses and parents," says Dr. Fox of Children's Hospital in Philadelphia, "and if everyone agrees that the baby is too badly injured, we do not increase our treatment. We do not take anything away."

Dr. Fanaroff says, "We consult everyone, and if we get agreement, then we do not resuscitate such babies if their hearts stop. And we stop the ventilators. But it's rare."

Whodunit? Quick, Check the Genes!

GIVE A SCIENTIST TWO DROPS OF BLOOD, ONE from a man and one from a boy, and the scientist soon can tell you, with 99.999 percent certainty, if the man is the true father of the boy.

With the same precision, scientists can take a spot of blood or semen or a hair root from the scene of a crime and tell you whether those samples match others taken from an accused person. Even a few skin cells from under the fingernails of a murder victim can lead police to the killer.

All this is possible because, in 1985, the British biologist Alec Jeffreys invented DNA fingerprinting, a revolutionary system for identifying humans and animals. This method is fast being viewed as the major addition to the field of criminal and civil justice in a full generation of forensic science.

(Anybody who watched the O. J. Simpson trial for even a half day realizes that DNA fingerprinting has come of age.)

DNA is a complex chemical that carries all the information that your body needs to build a complete organism from the moment of conception when sperm and egg meet. Each of us inherited DNA from our parents, and they from their parents. No two people, not even identical twins, have identical DNA. Science has shown how to compare DNA taken from one person with the DNA of another. Like fingerprints, an individual's DNA has no identical counterpart.

Ever since it was first used for crime detection by the British police in 1987, law enforcement officials worldwide have been pushing to implement the technique in their own operations. Says Paul Ferrara, director of the Division of Forensic Science for the State of Virginia, "Hundreds, if not thousands, of cases have been solved with this technology."

Despite its name, the method has nothing to do with fingerprints. Both DNA samples and actual fingerprints can identify a particular person with few vestiges of doubt. With DNA fingerprinting—by using samples of your hair, blood, or other cells—scientists can pick you out of a crowd with such accuracy that the odds are a million to one in their favor. Similarly, they can single out a criminal who leaves the tiniest personal trace at the scene of a crime.

Just 2 years after Dr. Jeffreys made his discovery at the University of Leicester in England, he applied his DNA fingerprinting method and proved that a man suspected of murder and rape was innocent: DNA from the suspect's blood did not match the DNA from semen stains found on the victims, two 15-year-old girls.

Police tracked down the true criminal by asking for blood samples from 5,512 men in the neighborhood in which the crimes had been committed. One of the men, Colin Pitchfork, drew police attention by asking a friend to give blood in his stead. After he was arrested, Mr. Pitchfork's blood sample was taken. His DNA matched that of the semen stains.

"I was enormously surprised by the Pitchfork case," Dr. Jeffreys recalls. "When the police approached me, I told them I doubted whether it would work. I was wrong. Had the man not been caught, he would have killed again."

The technique is intricate and requires several chemical steps. In the final step, a "print" is represented as a series of horizontal bars resembling the bar codes imprinted on packaged goods sold in supermarkets.

DNA (deoxyribonucleic acid) is found in every cell of the human body. It contains the chemical instructions for all of life's processes. Each of us has DNA formations that are different from any-one else's. Scientists can pin down the distinctions in each DNA sample. And, finally, they can discern the parentage of a child of contested origin. The odds in favor of being right in such cases are said to be excellent—at least 100,000 to one. The process can take several days.

Says Dr. Richard Roberts, a scientist who discovered some of the chemical tools used in the process, "This is truly exciting. It carries us a quantum leap forward in criminal identification. There is a degree of precision not possible before." Dr. Roberts is assistant director of research at the Cold Spring Harbor Laboratory on Long Island, New York.

Dr. Jeffreys developed the technique and coined its name. His wife, Sue, is accorded accolades for suggesting it could be used to establish true parentage.

It was first used for this purpose in 1985, shortly after Dr. Jeffreys's new invention had been written up in a professional journal. The case involved a family from Ghana with British citizenship. One son went back to Ghana for a visit. On his return to England, authorities found fault with his passport and held him in custody. His lawyer, having read about Dr. Jeffreys's work, asked to have mother and son tested. When DNA fingerprinting proved their relationship beyond doubt, the boy was released.

"It has astonished me how rapidly the scientific community has used the technology, how rapidly it has been viewed positively by many young lawyers," Dr. Jeffreys says. "I thought the practical uses were years in the future."

Raoul Felder, a leading matrimonial attorney in New York City, says, "We still will have paternity suits, because some people will insist on going to trial—even if I have genetic evidence that is 99.99 percent certain."

We inherit our DNA from our parents—half from our fathers, half from our mothers. In the British immigration case, Dr. Jeffreys placed the bar charts of mother and son parallel to one another. This showed that the two shared DNA fragments. The other bars on the boy's chart represented his father's DNA.

Since then, DNA tests have vastly reduced paternity suits. Confronted with the DNA bar charts, either the biological father yields, or, if the charts show him not to be the father, the mother yields. In such a case in 1989, Coleman Young, the mayor of Detroit, conceded that he was the father of a child after he saw the genetic evidence.

In 1988, DNA testing uncovered a baby switch. Records show that Arlena Twigg was born in 1978 to Ernest and Regina Twigg at Hardee Memorial Hospital in Wauchula, Florida, and died of a heart defect 10 years later. But genetic tests taken before her death proved that the Twiggs were not the child's biological parents.

Records also show that Kimberly Michelle Mays was born to Robert and

Barbara Mays in the same hospital at about the same time as Arlena. The Twiggs tracked down Robert Mays. He agreed to take the DNA parentage tests only if, whatever the results, the Twiggs promised they would not seek custody of Kimberly, barring unusual circumstances (such as proven abuse or neglect of the youngster). The DNA tests revealed that the Twiggs actually were Kimberly Mays's biological parents.

"This technology has solved a mystery for the Twiggs, creating a lot of heartache and a lot of joy," says John Blakely, the family's attorney. "It has enabled them to find their daughter." He adds that his clients are trying to gain the right to see Kimberly more often.

Eric Lander, associate professor of biology at MIT's Whitehead Institute in Cambridge, Massachusetts, is among those urging caution to law enforcement agencies now rushing to incorporate DNA fingerprinting into their police procedures. He says the method Dr. Jeffreys has devised may be flawless in theory but is not always so in practice, due to mix-ups that might occur in the laboratory.

The Federal Bureau of Investigation now has its own DNA lab. "Over the past 30 years, we have been doing a lot of research on biological evidence," says John Hicks of the FBI's laboratory division. "We know that somewhere in that stuff is the key to helping solve crimes. DNA profiling is the breakthrough we've been looking for."

The FBI is training technicians from police labs throughout the country in DNA fingerprinting. It also encourages the use of universal standards, something Mr. Lander says he favors.

Several states now are taking blood samples from convicted rapists and other violent criminals. Their DNA profiles will be stored in a data bank for use by police across the United States. Using DNA fingerprinting, for example, detectives could trace a rapist convicted in Utah who later rapes in Ohio by matching the DNA "prints" on file with those in traces found on the victims. Statistics show that two of three criminals are arrested within a 3-year period for repeating their offenses.

Civil liberties groups warn that innocents might be convicted in the rush to apply the new technology. "DNA evidence is based on probabilities, not on exact matches," says Janlori Goldman, who leads the Privacy and Technology Project for the American Civil Liberties Union. "Juries tend to be overwhelmed by the technology. It is a complex science, not easy to reduce to simple terms."

But criminology is not DNA's only arena. Dr. Svante Paabo, a researcher in Munich, Germany, formerly at the University of California at Berkeley, has DNA-fingerprinted a 7,000-year-old human brain found in a Florida swamp. He discovered that its DNA is a type unique to American Indians and Asians. "This might be a link to the ancient origins of native Americans," Dr. Paabo says.

An even greater endeavor is the Human Genome Project. An international cooperative effort of scientists, it will try to map human DNA and the location of every gene it contains. That could lead to the improved detection, prevention, and treatment of all genetic diseases. It also will help with criminal identification: if scientists can pinpoint the gene for eye color, for example, a DNA analysis will tell the criminal's eye color. Further clues might tell a suspect's age and other characteristics. Although pessimists believed that the entire genome solution would go well into the next century, it looks as though new techniques have speeded the process. The complete genome could be known by the year 2000.

For DNA fingerprinting, the future has just begun.

Miracle Medicines Coming Our Way

IN 1953, IN ONE OF THE GREAT MARBLED meeting halls of the National Academy of Sciences in Washington, D.C., a young, thin, nervous man in his 20s told the most learned American men and women of science his astounding story of research into the hidden chemistry of life. An older scientist, who had undertaken to be my mentor, whispered to me, then a young reporter, "This is the greatest biological discovery of the 20th century." And he was right.

That young man was James "Double Helix" Watson, an American who, with Francis Crick, an Englishman, gave the first correct description of DNA, the basic chemical of heredity. They said DNA consisted of two long chains of clusters of atoms spiraling like the strands of a twisted rope. The spiral, or double helix, taken from a human being contains the chemical blueprint to build a human being. Rat DNA has the manufacturing data to make a rat, and so on for all the animal and plant species we know. Their discovery triggered one of the greatest bursts of creative research in history. After nearly 40 years of diligent labor by thousands of researchers, we are now enjoying the payoffs, including these:

- We're uncovering the chemical basis of mystery afflictions like muscular dystrophy and cystic fibrosis.
- We're getting new and miraculous treatments for cancer, heart attacks, strokes, diabetes, hemophilia, AIDS, and dwarfism, to name a few.

- We're creating biotechnology, a new multibillion-dollar industry to fashion those treatments.
- We will see medicines for mental disease; rare, deadly, inherited ailments like Huntington's chorea, which killed folk singer Woody Guthrie; multiple sclerosis; arthritis; and even the common cold.

David Baltimore, Nobel Prize winner, says, "We've seen these blockbuster products come out amid tremendous scientific activity. It is extremely exciting. By the year 2000, we'll have a whole new set of medicines. The situation is self-renewing."

Carolyn Schmidt, an interior decorator from Darien, Connecticut, contracted an infection that destroyed her kidneys' ability to clean toxic waste from her blood. Three times a week at home, Mrs. Schmidt hooks herself up to a machine that pumps her blood through a filter to remove the offending chemicals—and save her life. Finally, an artificial form of the hormone/protein erythropoietin (EPO) is injected into the venous line returning the blood to her body.

Healthy, working kidneys produce EPO, which prompts the body to make red blood cells. Her kidneys can't do this, so Mrs. Schmidt's blood becomes anemic—lacking in red blood cells. Before using this artificial EPO, she had blood transfusions, which are dangerous and expensive.

"I used to get tired and cold very easily," Mrs. Schmidt says. "I forced myself to keep going. When I used EPO, I didn't get short breath. I had red lips again. I bloomed. EPO makes the difference between sick and healthy. It really is a miracle drug."

EPO is connected directly to Watson and Crick's discovery in 1953. Scientists figured out that sections of the big DNA molecule correspond to genes—chemicals in the hearts of cells that control cell functions. We are made up of billions of cells, and our genes determine our size, shape, coloration, and much of how we think and feel. Genes also underlie many human diseases.

When Watson and Crick unlocked the chemical door to the secret of genes, scientists rushed in to unravel the secret code of DNA: the genetic code. Different stripes of DNA—which makes up the genes—tell the cell's chemical factory to put together different proteins.

The basic technique: Isolate the DNA fragment of the special gene; make copies; inject the copies into certain bacteria, yeast, or mammalian cells; collect and purify this soup, which contains the needed protein. It's called biotechnology. Such manipulations have revealed the genes—the chemical formula of the actual fragment of DNA—for muscular dystrophy, cystic fibrosis, Elephant Man's disease, and Tay-Sachs disease, a hereditary affliction that destroys children's brains.

The technology has also created Humilin—human insulin for diabetics, whose pancreas can't make the hormone.

Without insulin, the body's cells cannot burn sugar. Without insulin, a diabetic sinks into a coma and dies.

Until Eli Lilly and Co. marketed Humilin in 1982, diabetics relied on insulin from cows and pigs. Often their immune system rejected the foreign insulin, but not the human insulin.

Lilly also makes human growth hormones, now injected into thousands of American children whose pituitary glands can't make the growth-stimulating chemical. Without the hormone, they stay small. (Our genes determine our height. If a child has a normal pituitary gland, injections of artificial growth hormone won't increase height. So don't plan to produce a clan of basketball stars.)

Doctors at the North Shore University Hospital in Manhasset, New York, had remarkable but short-lived results with the hormone. Drs. W. Ted Brown and Fima Lifshitz injected the chemical into two children with progeria, a genetic disease that rapidly ages children's bodies. At the chronological age of 15, they are 90 years old biologically. They suffer heart attacks and strokes. They remain under 4.5 feet tall. Their pinched faces look like masks. No hair grows on their heads. About 20 of these children are known worldwide.

Kevin Brown was 5 when his parents brought him from Cleveland to Dr. Brown. His biological age was somewhere around 40. Later he suffered a mild stroke. A few months later, Jessica Davis, 6, came to Dr. Brown from a sub-urb of Pittsburgh. Given daily injections of growth hormone at home, both children grew 1.5 inches in 3 months.

"We don't know if we have lengthened their lives in any way yet," Dr. Brown says. "But we're excited, because this is the first positive result we have had." Because this research is very demanding, progress moves slowly.

Doctors also have had great success using growth-stimulating hormone in otherwise healthy children who lack the natural hormone. A trip to Disney World proved a bitter disappointment for Ryan Fleckner of Huntington, New York, because he was not tall enough to go on the rides. Soon after, Dr. Lifshitz prescribed injections of growth hormone three times a week, and Ryan grew about 7 inches in a few short months. Again the complexity of the work has held back faster progress.

Dr. Daniel Rudman and his colleagues at the Medical College of Wisconsin at Milwaukee injected growth hormone into 12 men, ages 61 to 81, for 6 months. The artificial chemical increased their muscle mass, decreased the fat content of their bodies, and thickened their skin. The hormone appears to reverse these aspects of what was thought to be the inevitable process of aging. Again, it is too early to tell.

Physicians already have genetically engineered the hormone/protein interferon A. They can give big enough doses to treat effectively the unusual blood cancer called hairy-cell leukemia. Interferon also cleans up genital warts, believed to be a forerunner of cervical cancer. And it fights back—but does not cure—Kaposi's sarcoma, a cancer found in many AIDS patients.

Then there's TPA, an artificial enzyme that cause clots in blood vessels to dissolve. It activates tissue plasminogen, a naturally occurring enzyme that exists only in inactive form. The genetically engineered version of TPA stops heart attacks by melting clots in the blood vessels feeding the heart.

There are now two genetically engineered vaccines. One is for hepatitis B, which can cause cancer of the liver. The other prevents hemophilus influenzae B, the bacterial infection that causes meningitis in children. (Do not confuse this with common influenza, which is caused by a virus.)

Scientists are working overtime to develop a vaccine against AIDS, a biological nightmare. Once the AIDS virus, called HIV, enters your body, it attacks the very white blood cells (called T cells) that are meant to protect you against infection. During the infection's various phases, the virus changes its protein overcoat several times. This means that if white cells make a chemical to fight one type of AIDS virus, it won't fight all AIDS viruses. Scientists hope that some day one protein will be able to fight all the AIDS viruses.

The biological industry has at least 100 more products in the pipeline undergoing feverish testing. One of the major artificial products, colony stimulating factor (CSF), may hold the secret of new and powerful cancer treatments. CSF is found naturally in the blood, but only in tiny amounts. Bioengineering has created several varieties of CSF, in unlimited amounts.

Because high doses of anticancer drugs destroy the bone marrow, doctors can use only small doses that are less toxic. But CSF saves the bone marrow, which lets the physician give the biggest jolt of anticancer drug possible. Doctors hope this will result in millions of cancer cures. It is still being tested against breast cancer; researchers expect results some time in 1998.

Various universities, institutes, and pharmaceutical companies have been working on these proteins:

• A new Factor VIII helps stop the bleeding of hemophilia. The old Factor VIII, derived from pooled human blood, was contaminated by the AIDS virus, and a quarter of the nation's 20,000 hemophiliacs now carry the deadly virus. The new Factor VIII does not carry the AIDS virus.

• Interleukin, a hormone similar to interferon, treats advanced cancer. Interleukin, a blood hormone similar to interferon, treats advanced cancer and AIDS. Interleukin can turn certain white blood cells into killer cells that seek out and destroy cancers. As of this writing, the killer cells act sporadically, curing some patients but leaving others to die.

Other proteins are undergoing initial testing for these purposes:

- To speed the healing of wounds and eliminate chronic leg or body ulcers
- To protect corneal transplants taken from recently deceased individuals and transplanted to a person who has damaged the window of the eye
- To prevent organ poisoning in infants, who are receiving transplanted kidneys
- To suppress the rejection of transplanted organs by the body's immune system (one such protein, OKT-3, is now widely used)

Scientists are also moving into gene therapy for diseases caused by bad or missing genes. Missing genes are now said to account for several cancers, including colon cancer.

Researchers at the National Institutes of Health took white blood cells from a young girl born with severe combined immune deficiency syndrome (SCIDS, also known as "boy in a bubble disease"). She was a sitting duck for any virus or bacterium that came along. She lacked the gene that makes an enzyme needed to keep white cells alive. The scientist took the normal gene she lacked from another human's DNA and implanted it into the white cells they took from the girl. They then reinjected the white cells into the patient. At this writing, the youngster has produced a normal number of white blood cells for the first time in her life. But more time must pass before the experiment can be evaluated. Some scientists have criticized the experiment, saying that not enough is known about gene transfers in humans or their long-range effects.

Jeremy Rifkin, president of the Foundation on Economic Trends, has urged more caution in the whole genetic engineering enterprise. "In their mad dash for profit," he says, "companies and scientists have given short shrift to problems that could have profound impact on human health. The more powerful technology that allows us to intervene in living creatures, the more powerful the long-term disruption. We are changing the genetic blueprint."

Scientists are busy making the total human DNA molecule. They want to find the structure and location of every gene in that strand. The map of genes is called the genome.

Some scientists estimate that it will take 15 years and $3 billion to pinpoint each of the 100,000 DNA genes. They fear the genome project will take money from smaller but critical basic research projects—the kind that Watson did as a young man.

Scientists favoring this project argue that having a complete map of genes will reveal the genetic component of every disease. They could then ferret out the genes for intelligence, mental diseases, susceptibility to infection, even emotional reactions and behaviors.

In 1996, new techniques were developed for identifying genes and their structure. A growing number of biologists think that the time will be cut short in approaching the full structure of DNA from human beings.

Even without the genome project, science was well on its way to many exciting developments. We can be sure of one thing: we cannot foresee all of the biological marvels yet to come.

Mental Health

Closing In on Mental Illness

HEREDITY OR ENVIRONMENT: WHICH PLAYS THE major role in the development or disordering of a personality? The question is an old one, leading to a heated argument that rages still. In recent times, we have heard a lot of blame being heaped on the environment—especially on the family. In other words, most of us have learned that *psychological* forces cause mental illness. Now science is actually finding ways to pinpoint our potentially trouble-making *biological* forces.

David Wieder had nearly everything going for him when he was a youngster. He was nice-looking and came from a well-to-do family in University Heights, Ohio, a suburb of Cleveland. But, by the age of 12, he had begun having trouble with his schoolwork. By the age of 16, he had begun to hear the wind talking to him. "The wind would echo my thoughts," he says. If he thought, "Gee, it's a nice day," the wind would repeat the thought. He became fearful, afraid to go outside. He didn't know the time of day or the place he was in. Of course, the wind wasn't talking to him. It was all in his head.

Finally, at 17, David was hospitalized, and his long bout with schizophre-nia began. His parents took him from doctor to doctor. "Guilt overwhelmed us," says his mother, Anne. "We asked ourselves, 'What did we do wrong?'" In fact, his parents' behavior was blameless and had not caused their son's illness. It lasted 14 years. David, presently stabilized, works and lives on his own.

Scientists are exploring evidence indicating that some of the 2 million persons who suffer from schizophrenia in this country do so because their parents' genes combined in an unfortunate sequence to produce it.

Dr. Herbert Pardes, president of the American Psychiatric Association, says that the last decade has been an extraordinary time of discovery for psychiatry. "We have been learning that the genetic factor plays a far greater role in some cases of schizophrenia than we'd ever thought before." He adds, "There also is evidence of physical or chemical disturbances in the brain. Size of the temporal lobe, for example, has been found to be smaller than normal. Schizophrenia often attacks adolescents while their brains and bodies are undergoing great change. Or chemical systems—the dopamine system, for example—are out of balance."

Practically speaking, the new findings about the brain mean that more and more doctors will treat mental illness with medicine—with chemicals. Happily, new drugs have appeared in the last few years to quiet the torments of patients suffering from severe mental illness.

In addition to schizophrenia, scientists have identified specific brain-and-biology problems in obsessive-compulsive disorder (OCD), manic depression, panic attacks, and Alzheimer's disease.

In OCD, the patient has obsessions that he cannot stop: fears of dirt, for example, or fears of his own violent impulses. The patient also feels compelled to repeat endlessly the same rituals. Hand washing is a common one. Scientists now contend that a chemical disturbance in the brain creates the OCD symptoms.

Martin D'Amico, 33, president of a real estate management corporation in Waterbury, Connecticut, found himself checking and rechecking simple things.

"I locked the door so many times, I broke the handle," Mr. D'Amico recalls. "I pushed on the emergency brake of the car so hard, I had to pull with both hands to release it. I broke light switches, checking them so often."

Mr. D'Amico ultimately found his way to Dr. Wayne Goodman, who runs the OCD Clinic at Yale University in New Haven. Dr. Goodman prescribed fluvoxamine, a drug that affects chemicals in the brain.

"I took the drug for 3 or 4 weeks before I noticed anything," Mr. D'Amico

says. "It creeps up on you like a shadow. The edge was taken off. I didn't have to do the rituals so urgently."

Despite the growing emphasis on biology and bodily chemistry as a cause of mental illness and the increasing use of drugs to equalize that chemistry, psychological techniques still relieve many patients. They include helping the patient in the following ways:

- Teaching methods for mastering emotional control (e.g., learning to control anger)
- Teaching how to get along with others
- Teaching how to look at yourself and others realistically
- Teaching how to form good new habits and get rid of bad old ones

While Martin D'Amico took his prescribed medication and benefited from it, a psychologist also helped him to explore and practice ways to avoid his compulsions, his rituals.

"She told me to just try to turn off the light switch one time and walk away from it," Mr. D'Amico says. "I would have to say to myself, 'I know I turned off the light.' By practicing, I was starting to get control. I felt like I had been given eyeglasses for the first time."

Psychologists also can teach parents of schizophrenics how to handle their children in ways that could help lower the number of breakdowns they might have. A $10 million study by the National Institute of Mental Health showed that, for less severe forms of depression, psychological treatment has cleared the symptoms just as effectively as drugs have.

Dr. T. Byram Karasu, professor of psychiatry at Albert Einstein College of Medicine in the Bronx, New York, puts it this way: "We cannot treat a mental illness only biologically. We need to address the person, his ability to work, live, love. No drug can generate motivation, desire, ability to love and be loved."

The most exciting possibility for breakthroughs in biological understanding and scientific progress comes from the study of chromosomes and genes. Chromosomes are bundles of chemicals found in your cells. Each chromosome has a thin thread of DNA—deoxyribonucleic acid—running along its entire length. Also running along the chromosomes are the body's approximately 100,000 genes. Genes are the carriers of genetic information, passed on from generation to generation. They are composed of DNA. DNA is made up of four basic molecules. For simplicity, let's just call them A, B, C, and D. Too small to see under a microscope are many millions of molecules—AACD-BACC—running helter-skelter along the chromosomes in continuous strings. The genes are long segments of the four molecules' "letters." The sequence of the letters acts as "words" that "spell out" the chemical formula or structure of, say, a particular protein, a larger molecule that controls the chemistry of a cell.

Under a microscope, you can see the cells of muscles, the brain, skin, and other organs. All are distinctive. Skin cells look like tiny boxes, nerve cells look like long thin pipes stemming from a central body, and muscle cells resemble sausages. If a gene is damaged or missing, a cell ends up with damaged or missing protein. The sad and unlucky result very well could be a damaged organ—even, quite possibly, the brain.

The discovery that the *sequence* of those molecules sets up the chemistry of your cells—and therefore of your body and your brain—is the greatest biological discovery of the 20th century.

Susan Dime-Meenan, 34, probably has a disrupted chemistry of the brain. Since age 13, Ms. Dime-Meenan, now a court reporter in Evanston, Illinois, has suffered from manic depression. In 1982, at 4 feet, 9 inches tall, she weighed only 68 pounds. "I stopped eating and sleeping," she recalls. "I spent $27,000 on clothes in 1 week. You feel nothing can stop you. You feel extremely good about yourself—lots of confidence."

That's the manic phase of the illness. Then there's the crash. Ms. Dime-Meenan would become apathetic, listless. Others become depressed and joyless, with overwhelming feelings of doom. Some commit suicide. Perhaps 5 million Americans now suffer from various forms of depression.

In 1987, scientists reported that they had isolated a spot on one chromosome (we each have 23 pairs of chromosomes) that contained a gene for manic depression. Since then, scientists have tried to confirm the finding. A second spot has also been identified. But not known yet are the gene—the sequence of ABCD—and the protein the gene makes.

"It's like saying we know the gene is in one of the 50 states," Dr. Pardes says. "We know which state, but we don't know the street address."

If scientists could find the precise spot of the gene and learn its ABCD makeup and which protein it makes, they would be able to do far more for manic-depressive patients. Right now, doctors have many drugs, including lithium salts, to calm the mania and/or relieve the depression. Scientists developed the treatments by hit-and-miss methods.

Susan Dime-Meenan takes such drugs. She also lives a satisfying life. "Now I feel balanced," she says. "This is how people are supposed to feel. I don't get peaks and valleys anymore."

But the drugs neither work for everybody nor work all the time; patients may have setbacks. The gene revolution could herald the creation of medicines that target and correct the exact chemical defect in the brain. In other words, a cure seems possible.

"We are virtually certain there are several different genes and nongenetic causes for manic depression," says Dr. Kenneth K. Kidd, professor of human genetics, psychiatry, and biology at Yale University School of Medicine. So scientists have their work cut out for them: finding not just one gene, but many, and then counteracting the effects of each gene.

Much the same can be said about research on schizophrenia. Two years ago, scientists said they had found the gene for the disease. But the research on this is still in its infancy.

The new biology is giving weight to findings made two generations ago. The late Dr. Franz Kallmann, of the New York State Psychiatric Institute, followed up on cases of identical and fraternal twins, one of whom had suffered from either schizophrenia or manic depression. His studies pointed strongly to a damaged or missing gene as the cause of both diseases.

Identical twins, born of one egg, have identical genes inherited from the sperm and egg of their parents. Fraternal twins, born of separate eggs, share some, but not all, of their genes. Dr. Kallmann found that if one of a pair of identical twins had either disease, there was a 68 percent certainty that the other also would inherit that mental problem. If one of a fraternal pair was affected, the other twin ran only a 15 percent risk of the disease.

More recent studies of adopted children show the same family inheritance. If one of an adopted child's biological parents had schizophrenia, there would be a high probability of the child having it too, despite being raised by a family without mental problems. The healthy psychological environment would not cancel out the genetic disease.

In addition to the study of genes, scientists have explored the brain and found that, basically, the system is chemical. Picture this: The ending of one nerve (A) in the brain lies close to the ending of another (B). There is a gap between them. When nerve A fires electrically, its ending releases chemicals into the gap. They travel to nerve B, where the chemicals then trigger another electrical discharge. Billions of nerves "talk" to each other in this way. Thoughts, then, are both chemical and electrical.

Scientists know that in the case of some mental problems, the chemical transfer between nerves has gone awry. There may be too much of one chemical or not enough of another. Or the receiving nerve cannot absorb the right chemicals. Scientists cannot pinpoint the specific defects in schizophrenia or manic depression—yet. They have only tantalizing clues.

But progress has been so great that many scientists predict tremendous advances, including drugs that restore chemical balances in the brain.

Another development, computer-assisted tomography, or the CAT scan, "sees" the brain with a special three-dimensional X-ray picture. Such pictures have shown distortions of the brain in schizophrenia.

Even more detailed images now come from magnetic cameras, called magnetic resonance imaging, or MRI.

Positron-emission tomography, or the PET scan, does much the same. The patient is given a mildly radioactive chemical tracer, which travels to the brain. Outside, a camera detects and photographs the radioactivity. The scientist can then look at the photo and trace the chemical's movements, noting where it went and what it did.

Dr. Lewis L. Judd, a former director of the National Institute of Mental Health, exults over the new imaging methods. "We can see the brain as it is functioning," he says. "We can see how medication works. We can show specific abnormalities of schizophrenia, manic depression, and panic attack."

Dr. Judd points out that there is much to celebrate and estimates that the discovery that lithium salts control manic depression has saved the nation $39 billion. The new biological psychiatry promises even more—not only in dollars but also in healthy lives.

You Can Find Help for Depression

EVERY OCTOBER SINCE 1992, THOUSANDS OF Americans have made a move to improve their lives by going to a free screening for depression, one of the most common and deadly diseases in America. Left untreated, depression ends in suicide for one in seven with the illness, says Dr. Douglas G. Jacobs, the Harvard psychiatrist who created the screening project.

Sponsors of the National Depression Screening Day each year invite 100,000 people to show up at more than 1,800 sites nationwide. Sites include hospitals, clinics, schools, churches, military stations, and even shopping malls.

Of those who attend the screening each year, nearly half have taken the short depression test printed in *Parade*'s annual article on depression. Use the new test printed here to help decide if you should be screened.

As of 1996, Dr. Jacobs calculates that 8,000 depressed Americans probably would have died by their own hands had they not attended a screening. "Their symptoms were so severe," he says, "that the attending physicians recommended immediate treatment or hospitalization." The screenings also save many others from the terrible day-to-day effects of milder forms of depression.

The National Institute of Mental Health found that 80 percent of those screened each year are "clinically depressed," Dr. Jacobs says. Data also show the most prevalent symptoms were psychological—such as a sense of hopelessness or joylessness—rather than physical.

"We had always expected depressed people to report mostly body symptoms like fatigue, weight loss, sleep troubles, and restlessness," Dr. Jacobs explains. "I hope that doctors will now be paying more attention to the patient's mental state. The most important and deadliest

---

A Simple Test for Depression

1. I find it easy to do the things I used to do.   Yes___ No___
2. I feel hopeful about the future. Yes___ No___
3. I enjoy the things I used to enjoy. Yes___ No___
4. I find it easy to make decisions. Yes___ No___
5. I feel useful and needed. Yes___ No___

If you answered no to most of these questions, there is a high probability that you are depressed and need help. The more NO answers, the higher your probability of being ill.

If you agree with the statement "I have felt so low that I've thought of suicide," you must seek professional help immediately—don't wait for the screening day.

sign is a patient's statement that he or she wants to commit suicide."

Depression is not hopeless. New and old treatments work better for depression than treatments for most other mental diseases. Powerful antidepressants may be used to keep the illness at bay. Psychotherapy, the "talking cure," is effective for many. Even if the patient is on the threshold of suicide, medication and psychotherapy are effective. For those patients who do not respond, there are alternative treatments, including the modern form of electroconvulsive therapy—a safe treatment for the most serious forms of depression.

You may want to pass along the depression test to friends or relatives. If you need help approaching them, Dr. Jacobs suggests that you write a note something like this:

Dear _____:

I care about you, and I am concerned that you are not yourself lately. I don't like to see you unhappy. I read in *Parade* that in each October there is a National Depression Screening Day. I'll be happy to go with you. Professionals will be there to help you. You don't have to stay sad. I hear depression is an illness with very effective treatment. This is my way of saying I care.

If you feel that it's too long to wait until October, you can alter the note to say "I would be glad to go with you to see a health professional." Leave the rest of the note as it is, leaving out the screening program.

For a copy of the free booklet "Let's Talk Facts about Depression," write to the American Psychiatric Association, DPA/PM96-1400 K St., NW, Washington, D.C. 20005.

Help for Your Mind

RIGHT NOW, HOW DO YOU FEEL? I DON'T MEAN physically. I mean your feelings, your mood, your thoughts. Happy or unhappy? Calm or angry? And how about the people around you, your family and friends—are they feeling good or feeling bad?

You may use other names for feeling bad, such as blue, depressed, anxious, or nervous. They're all different names for emotional distress.

Whatever you call it, you are not alone. Scientists at Johns Hopkins University in Baltimore conducted a study to find out how many people were mentally ill. They discovered that about one third of the 3,481 persons surveyed said they had at some time sought help for a mental or emotional problem (or a drug or alcohol problem). They found help by talking to a friend, a relative, a mutual help group, or professional.

The data also indicate, says Dr. Ernest Gruenberg of the Baltimore study, that one person in nine said he or she feels the need for professional help now.

Many problems come from an overload of stress. You lose your job, for example, or your spouse to death or divorce, or someone you love becomes seriously ill. A new baby is born, or a new job means moving and starting over in another town. You feel troubled, inadequate, unable to cope.

Not everyone who feels bad has overwhelming problems. Some people suffer from irrational fears, or phobias. They can't enter an elevator or a tunnel, for example, without panicking. When the reaction to stress or anxiety is severe, it can lead to nervous collapse or to alcohol and drug abuse.

Chemical imbalances in the body also contribute to serious conditions such as manic-depressive syndrome, psychosis, or schizophrenia.

We've included a short "stress" quiz to help you determine the state of your mental health. If you feel down in the dumps for days, you can be helped by safe, effective treatments used by mental health professionals today. They can relieve the anguish caused by mental problems. We include therapies based on the time-honored cure of "talking," different forms of behavior therapy, and mood-altering drugs. If you're suffering, the treatments are there for you.

Who's Who

Many different kinds of mental health professionals are trained to help you.

Psychologists receive at least a 4-year college degree. Many states license psychologists and require a Ph.D. (hence, the title "Dr.") or a master's degree. Psychologists may specialize in emotional and learning problems, guidance, or testing IQs. About 80,000 psychologists practice in the United States today.

Psychiatrists are medical doctors who specialize in mental illness. They are the only mental health professionals who can prescribe drugs, including tranquilizers, or other medical procedures. The American Medical Association says that there are 30,000 licensed psychiatrists in the United States.

A *therapist* can be either a psychologist or a psychiatrist, or neither. "Therapist" is a general term that can include social workers; marriage, family, or guidance counselors; or anyone trained to do counseling, such as clergy. Beware of therapists who have no formal training.

Should You Seek Help?

You can't sleep, perhaps, or you're unable to eat. You depend heavily on tranquilizers or barbiturates. These are a few signs of mental distress.

Here is a short version of a National Institute of Mental Health test prepared by Dr. Baqar Husaini of Tennessee State University. For each question, ask yourself, "How many days this past week have I . . . "

1. Thought my life is a failure?
2. Not been able to shake off the blues even with the help of my family or friends?
3. Felt fearful?
4. Felt lonely?
5. Felt people were unfriendly?
6. Had crying spells?
7. Felt sad?
8. Felt people disliked me?

Every time you answered 0 to 1 day, score 0; 1 to 2 days, score 1; 3 to 4 days, score 2; 5 to 7 days, score 3. If your total score is 7 or higher, you might want to seek some professional help.

Talking Can Cure

"I'm no good," a young mother sobs. "My home life is too much for me."

By getting this woman to talk about her feelings, her psychologist relieves her distress. He uses psychotherapy, sometimes called the "talking cure." Clergy use a form of psychotherapy to counsel. So do social workers, doctors, teachers. Psychotherapy helps three of four persons.

Psychotherapy has many forms, all stemming from psychoanalysis, invented by Sigmund Freud in the 1890s. Dr. Freud found that hidden thoughts—the unconscious—shape behavior. And childhood experiences with our parents create unconscious thoughts. By exposing your unconscious to you, Freudians say they help you gain control over your behavior. They delve into your past to reveal the injuring events in your life. Such events include physical and sexual abuse by your parents, siblings, and other relatives. Usually, they say, by working through these events (i.e., remembering them and dealing with them now), you can feel better about yourself. Keep in mind that early childhood memories may be deeply distorted.

Dr. Carl Rogers invented a form of psychotherapy called *reflection*. The therapist "reflects" back to you your thoughts and feelings. You say, "I feel depressed because I have nobody to talk to." The therapist replies, or reflects, "You feel that if you had someone to talk to you would feel better." By examining that feeling as it is reflected back to you, you can change your thoughts and behavior.

Dr. Rogers was one of the first psychologists to subject his theory to scientific analysis. He proved that his clients were able to make personality and behavioral changes that help reduce anxiety and depression

What Do They Mean?

You often hear, "Oh, he's neurotic," when what the observer probably means is that the person is high-strung. Or someone says, "She's just paranoid" to explain his friend's fears about losing her job. But neurosis and paranoia are real mental disorders with identifiable symptoms. Here are some mental health terms that are commonly misused.

• Anxiety/fear. Anxiety occurs when you are paralyzed with fright but don't know what you are afraid of. Many emotional disturbances begin with anxiety. Your fear may be specific, like a fear of snakes or mice. I know one young woman who is so terrified of mice that she cannot stand even seeing the word in print.

• Psychosis. This disorder is characterized by defective or lost contact with reality. Psychotics often "see things" and "hear voices." Their behavior is often bizarre; they may, for example, believe that God is telling them to murder someone.

• Neurosis. This emotional disorder is caused by a conflict of which the person is unaware. For example, you want sex but also want to please your mother, who said sex was bad. This unconscious conflict produces a neurosis that could affect your sex life. You may go out of your way to avoid any sexual contact.

• Paranoia. This is a severe personality disorder in which a patient feels persecuted or has ambitions of grandeur. A paranoid person may believe that spies are out to get him or that God has picked him to lead the world. Paranoia is often a feature of schizophrenia.

• Manic-depressive syndrome. This condition is marked by mood swings between uncontrollable elation and activity,

on the one hand, and withdrawal and depression, on the other.

• Schizophrenia. This group of disorders can cause delusions, hallucinations, or aggressive and antisocial behavior.

Behavior Therapy

Several years ago, I put a pigeon named Harold into a cage equipped with an electrically controlled feeding trap. By tapping a button, I could open the trap door and let the bird take a corn kernel.

Whenever Harold moved to the right, I'd open the trap door. He would snap up the released corn kernel. Then I'd wait until he turned more to his right. Another bit of corn. Again and again, I fed Harold until he turned completely in a circle.

Without a word, I had changed Harold's behavior using a technique developed in the 1940s by Dr. B. F. Skinner at Harvard University.

Psychologists have since modified Dr. Skinner's behavior modification method for use in the counseling room, where they call it behavior therapy.

Today's behavior therapists "positively reinforce," or reward, the behavior they want to encourage. With my own grandson, Ethan, I came closest to treating a human being with the technique used on Harold, the pigeon. I toilet-trained Ethan in 1 day with a method invented by Dr. Nathan Azrin of Nova University in Fort Lauderdale, Florida. I fed Ethan little salted crackers and fruit juice every time he came close to using the toilet. I added lots of love. In a few hours he was toilet trained. (My experience taught me that it is easy to change the mood of 2-year-old children simply by toilet-training them at 18 months, thereby avoiding the conflict between parent and child. The behavior of children in the "terrible twos" can drive parents to distraction.) Many parents scold or spank their children to train them. Such punishment, or negative reinforcement, also brings about the desired behavior. But negative reinforcement breeds hostility; therefore, professional behavior therapists don't use it.

A troubled family can transform itself with a kind of behavior therapy called *family contracting*. Each person promises to stop disruptive behavior or to help the others do so. Each parent and child selects a reward, approved by the others. Everyone keeps score. Those who change their behavior get the rewards.

Unlike a psychotherapist, a behavior therapist who treats phobias does not care what originally scared you. Instead, the therapist relaxes you, then has you *imagine* the feared situation (e.g., riding in an elevator, holding a cat, or swimming).

Dr. Aaron T. Beck, of the University of Pennsylvania, builds up the confidence of depressed patients with a form of behavior therapy called *cognitive therapy*. It deals with what people *think* they know.

For example, suppose you think, "I am worthless and no use to anybody.

Who will ever want to marry me?" That's what you *think* you know. When you are depressed, everything looks bad.

The cognitive therapist would have you write down all of your qualities, good and bad. ("I am not beautiful. I am not tall. But I *am* friendly. I *am* smart.") This therapy confronts you with a balanced, more realistic look at yourself. After several sessions of such exercises, moderate depression lifts. Dr. Albert Ellis, a New York psychologist, discovered this method in parallel to Dr. Beck.

A Revolution in Psychiatry

In the 1950s, 600,000 Americans languished in state mental hospitals. Today, many seriously afflicted mental patients live outside institutions. State hospitals hold only 130,000 patients.

The revolution in treatment of the mentally ill began in 1954 with a drug called Thorazine, which relieved the psychosis associated with schizophrenia and manic-depressive syndrome. Other drugs followed. Lithium and Elavil modify the extreme mood swings of manic-depressives; tranquilizers such as Librium and Valium relieve anxiety.

Psychiatrists today prescribe any number of mood-altering drugs. And thanks to sophisticated new blood tests that measure how much of the drug has entered the patient's body, doctors can administer safe doses.

In addition, psychiatrists are treating psychotic, depressed patients prone to suicide. When suicide seems imminent, the physician may recommend electroshock—or, the term they prefer, electroconvulsive—therapy (ECT). Doctors have modified "shock treatments." They send electricity into a patient's brain. Unprotected, the person's body arched in epileptic-like tremors. In some cases, ECT ended with a broken spine. Physicians now have markedly reduced the amount of electricity. They also use general anesthesia plus a muscle relaxant to prevent muscle spasms. The body, asleep, remains still.

Scientists believe that the electricity alters the brain's chemistry, clearing depression. Proponents say ECT has cutthe suicide rate dramatically, with few side effects except a temporary loss of memory. Surprisingly, ECT is safer than drugs.

Consider Your Options

Sometimes a close friend or relative has to tell you that "you're not quite yourself" and need help. More often, only you are aware that something is wrong, but you don't do anything about it because you believe it is shameful to have an emotional problem, or you think that you should be able to heal yourself. If you are a man, you're even more likely than a woman to shy away from professional treatment.

Besides making an emotional commitment, getting professional help for mental distress requires a financial commitment as well. Psychotherapy is expensive. Depending on where you live and what kind of therapist you pick, you'll spend between $20 and $100 an hour, one to five times a week, for a year or more. (In an emergency, some psychotherapists can get results in 6 weeks.) If you want to cut the cost, try group therapy. For some people, it is even more effective than private one-on-one therapy because they learn from the others in the group. Behavior therapy, which is a short-term treatment, will probably not cost as much as psychotherapy, though the hourly rates may be the same.

You can find less costly help in community mental health centers and social service agencies. A local hospital or university may have a clinic. Or contact your church or synagogue.

And, of course, there are countless self-help groups. Alcoholics Anonymous is the most famous. But other groups help gamblers, overeaters, drug abusers, bereaved parents, and people with all sorts of personality and emotional problems.

Many counties have mental health agencies that can put you in touch with local self-help groups. Or they will give you the number of a hotline you can phone if a crisis arises.

People in emotional turmoil often find it difficult to make the phone call that will get them the help they need. That's why having a friend you trust is so important. A friend can do for you what you cannot do for yourself.

The National Self-Help Clearinghouse, 33 W. 42nd St., New York, NY 10036, can send you a list of clearinghouses across the nation.

You *Can* Fight Depression

YOU FEEL SAD, ALMOST LIKE CRYING. SOMEtimes you do cry. Mostly, you feel hopeless, overwhelmed, unable to move or work. Your problems weigh on you like so many stones on your chest. And you see no way of lifting those weights. Those feelings may persist without letting up for weeks or even years. A psychiatrist would say that you are depressed.

Up until a few years ago, doctors could do little to lighten the burden of depression. But now they have a variety of treatments to raise even the most depressed from the pits of despair. And that's good news for the 10 million Americans who each year slide into the blackness of depression. Unfortunately, most remain untreated and continue to suffer. Many die by their own hand.

A new federally sponsored program helps the millions of untreated depressives among us. To help you understand this disorder better, Dr. Lewis L. Judd, formerly of the National Institute of Mental Health, has answered the following questions for readers.

Many people believe a depressed person puts on an act. With just a little willpower, they say, he or she could be cheerful again. Is this true?

Depression is neither an act nor a failure of willpower. It's a real disease, just as a heart attack is real. Depression produces physical, emotional, and cognitive symptoms. Without treatment, depression can last for years and even end in suicide. With treatment, as many as nine of 10 people recover.

How can you tell whether a person is really generally depressed or saddened by some specific event, like a death in the family?

Everyone gets the blues or feels sad from time to time. If the symptoms grow too strong and last too long, the line is crossed from sadness to depression. The dividing line may seem fuzzy, but if four or more symptoms persist for more than 2 weeks, you should seek professional help.

We know that depression takes several disguises or forms. How can you tell which is which?

Some people suffer only one episode of depression in a lifetime; others may fall victim to depression many times. In still others, depression weighs so heavily that they can't function at all. In many, the symptoms appear constantly and for a long time, but in milder form. Many patients go through cycles of deep, depressive "lows" and soaring manic "highs." Their moods sweep from one pole to the other, so doctors call it "bipolar disorder" or "manic-depressive" illness.

Are more people depressed these days than they were in the past?

We do not know for sure, but it is not likely. With increased awareness and much better diagnostic methods, we are more accurately identifying and treating more depressed people. As a result, it may seem as if there are more depressed people, when actually we are much more alert to the disease now.

Depression often leads to suicide. How common is suicide among the depressed?

If not properly treated, one of seven severe depressives eventually will commit suicide. That's a higher death rate than from most other serious diseases. More men—particularly older white men—than women commit suicide. We don't understand the gender differences. We can, the statistics indicate, prevent suicide with quick diagnosis and treatment.

Are men or women more susceptible to depression? And what about different ages?

Although more men who suffer from depression commit suicide, twice as many women suffer from major depression but do not resort to suicide. Again, we don't know why. Bipolar disorder affects equal numbers of men and women. As for age, depression afflicts far more people under the age of 45 and fewer of those over the age of 65. However, depression in the elderly is serious and needs careful treatment. Depression can emerge in adolescence, but it usually first appears in patients in their early 20s.

Does depression run in families?

In the past 10 years, research has proved that depressive disorders appear in families, especially the manic-depressive/bipolar disorder. Some scientists have identified genes that they say are common to patients with depression.

Does something go wrong with the brain chemistry to cause depression?

Yes. Abnormalities have been found in the chemical signals between nerves in the brain. Those chemicals are called *neurotransmitters*. Depression-relieving drugs seem to correct neurotransmitter faults.

Is brain chemistry the only cause of depression?

No. Physical illness, abnormal hormone systems, and certain medicines can bring on depression. Distressing life events—the loss of a loved one or a job—could trigger the symptoms. You may be at risk if you depend too much on others for help in your life or if you don't think much of yourself.

Are women more susceptible to depression during menopause? Does menstruation affect depression?

Depression actually *decreases* among women between the ages of 45 and 60. As for menstruation and depression, we still are researching this.

Do men suffer depression more in their 40s, when they realize they may not have reached the youthful goals they had set for themselves?

Depression does peak among men between the ages of 25 and 45, but we have no evidence that it arises from failed youthful expectations. However, the 40s are the years in which negative life events occur frequently. Such negative events can initiate depression.

Many people seem to become more depressed in the winter or around the holidays. Why?

Recently, scientists discovered that some people actually do become depressed during the winter months, a condition they call seasonal affective disorder (SAD). The absence of bright daylight causes chemical changes in the brain. We have been able to treat such patients successfully with artificial bright light that has all the colors of sunlight.

As for holidays, many people get nostalgic and think about old times around Christmas, Easter, and other special holidays and anniversaries. However, the memories may be distorted or totally fake. Especially for people who live alone or who are having problems, such thoughts can contribute to feeling blue. No data exist that tell us with certainty that people become clinically depressed more around holidays than at other times. However, a person who is already sick with depression no doubt will have a hard time during holiday seasons.

Many medicines now bring people out of depression. Could you sort them out for us?

This is the most exciting and hope-filled part of the depression story. Among the new drugs now available, we can find at least one or two that bring a depressed patient back to normal. We could not do that a few years ago.

Three groups of medicines are available: tricyclic antidepressants, monoamine oxidase inhibitors, and lithium. All three alter the brain's chemicals. They restore to normal the depressed patient's mood, appetite, energy level, outlook, sleep patterns, and concentration. The tricyclics are the basic weapons against major depression, with the monoamine oxidase inhibitors as backups. Lithium works most effectively against bipolar disease.

What are the side effects of antidepressive drugs? Can they be avoided?

The most common side effects include dry mouth, constipation, dizziness, and drowsiness—usually all mild. While taking monoamine oxidase inhibitors, patients should avoid certain foods (cheese, among others) to avert serious side effects.

Can psychotherapy, often called "the talking treatment," help depressed people as much as medication can?

In patients who are not too severely depressed, psychotherapy seems to work as well as medication. But in major depression, symptoms generally are relieved more rapidly by drugs than by psychotherapy. Most people do best when doctors treat them by combining drugs with psychotherapy.

Does shock therapy really work? Many people claim it destroys brain cells and memory.

If a severely depressed patient threatens suicide or doesn't respond to drugs, we rely on electroconvulsive therapy (ECT), commonly called shock therapy. It is effective and quick acting. Because better medicines are available now, ECT is used less and less. But new techniques also make ECT safer than it used to be. It now produces less of the temporary confusion and less memory loss than it once did.

How can a depressed person's family help?

The very nature of depression keeps the victim from seeking help. Family and friends can help most by encouraging patients to get the right treatment or even by taking them to the doctor. Overall, support, love, patience, and encouragement help far more than do blame, lecturing, and argument.

Where can a family get help?

The first line of defense is the family doctor, clinic, or health maintenance organization. Next, psychiatrists, psy- chologists, family therapists, and social workers can work with the patient to give the "talking treatment." But of these, only psychiatrists, who are medical doctors as well, can prescribe drugs. Many mental health centers, hospitals, and universities have depression programs.

The National Institute for Mental Health has begun a new program on depression. What's involved?

Everyone should know the symptoms of depression and the effective treatments for it. The goal of the project (called Depression/Awareness, Recognition and Treatment) is to help depressed persons get treatment and return more rapidly to normal activities, and perhaps even to save their lives. We are using every means of communication to put the message across.

Where can readers write for more information?

Write to D/ART Public Inquiries, 5600 Fishers Lane, Room 10-85, Rockville, MD 20857.

The Symptoms of Depression

If you suffer four or more of the following symptoms for more than 2 weeks, you may be depressed and in need of professional help:

Persistent, sad, anxious, or "empty" mood

Loss of life satisfaction

Hopelessness or pessimism

Guilt, worthlessness or helplessness

Can't give or accept affection

No interest or pleasure in daily activities, including sex

Insomnia, early wakening, or late sleeping

Weight gain or appetite change

Physical aches and pains

Excessive crying

Restlessness, irritability, or overactivity

Low energy, fatigue, or slowed thinking

Can't concentrate, remember, or make decisions

Thoughts of death or suicide, suicide attempts

Are You a Prisoner of Your Fears?

SUDDENLY, FOR NO REASON, YOUR HEART RACES, you cannot breathe, and you feel you are about to die.

The diagnosis: panic attack. Fear of unknown origin. You feel trapped, with no exit. Several different types of anxiety produce different symptoms. Some forms of anxiety incapacitate the victims. They cannot work, sleep, or have a social life. Some psychiatrists say a little anxiety keeps us better tuned to the world around us. With a tingling sense of fear, we are ready to meet that world. Excess fear paralyzes the victims.

But the National Institute of Mental Health estimates that, sometime in their lives, 24 million Americans suffer from some form of anxiety so intense that it interferes with work or family life, making it one of the most common mental illnesses in the country. The severe form of anxiety is a panic attack. Dr. Robert Hirschfeld, chief of anxiety disorders at the institute, has good news. "This is the age of anxiety," he says, "but we now have excellent drug and mental treatments."

Psychologists often solve panic attack problems by teaching patients how to breathe and relax. But a drug proved effective for a 38-year-old New Jersey mother of two who wants her name withheld. Doctors prescribed Xanax. It worked. "I can lead a normal, productive life," she says now. "The anxiety is still there, but the medication keeps it in check."

Yet many Americans suffer in silence because they do not realize that help exists. And panic attack is just one type of anxiety. Scientists have learned that anxiety comes in many forms:

• Agoraphobia—a fear of open spaces. With this illness, patients often refuse to leave home. Many doctors believe that in panic attacks and agoraphobia, something has gone wrong chemically with the brain. The drugs Xanax and Tofranil reduce the anxiety of agoraphobia.

• Specific phobia—a fear of something in particular, such as elevators, furry animals, the number 13, heights, flying, train travel, or small rooms. A friend of mine, who was in every other way normal, feared snakes. No amount of reasoning could shake that fear. Dr. Aaron T. Beck, professor of psychiatry at the University of Pennsylvania in Philadelphia, guides phobics to apply reason and logic to the situation so they can see that they are overreacting.

Once Dr. Becker nails home the idea of overresponding, he teaches them how to relax while he exposes them to the scary object with drug-free therapy. It works.

• Social phobia—a phobia in which victims avoid what they perceive as embarrassing situations, such as public speaking, social dancing, and dining in restaurants. The drug Nardil helps 70 percent of patients. Dr. Beck says his drug-free therapy helps nearly 100 percent of his anxiety patients, about 80 percent of panic attack patients. His claim is controversial.

• Obsessive-compulsive disorder—a behavioral combination of an obsession and a compulsion. An *obsession* is a thought you can't get out of your mind. A *compulsion* is a behavior you know is strange but can't stop. Obsession can lead to compulsive behavior. For example, if you are fearful of germs and you constantly think about avoiding bacteria, you may go through elaborate self-cleansing behavior. In experiments in the United States, obsessive-compulsive anxiety was removed in half the patients taking clomipramine or fluvoxamine.

• Posttraumatic stress disorder—once called "battle fatigue." This disorder is seen in people traumatized by awful accidents, abuse, or violence. Both psychotherapy and drug treatment help. Some patients cannot rid themselves of playing the horrific scene over and over again. Such behavior interferes with work and other social relations.

• Generalized or free-floating anxiety—a condition in which victims feel symptoms of anxiety most of the time with no known cause. Valium and other drugs with benzodiazepine (including Librium) mute the symptoms. BuSpar, a new medicine, seems to work as well as Valium minus its side effect of drowsiness and its potential for addiction. Tranxene also appears to relieve anxiety.

For more information on phobias and other forms of anxiety, write to the Anxiety Disorders Association of America, 6000 Executive Boulevard, Suite 513, Rockville, MD 20852. For a list of professionals in your area, please send a check for $3.

Hope for Ulcers

Is there an ulcer personality? Some specialists swear that anxiety produces stomach acid that leads directly to ulcers, or lesions, in the stomach or duodenum—the tube leading to the small intestines. But proof is hard to find.

These days, 85 percent of ulcer patients find relief in drugs that control the amount of acid in the stomach. Stomach acid, which increases when you're anxious, adds to the risk of sores rising on the surface of the stomach or duodenum. Although 7,000 Americans die each year from such ulcers, physicians often prescribe tranquilizers such as Valium. Doctors also urge patients not to smoke (cigarette smoking slows the healing of ulcers and hastens their recurrence) or drink (drinking alcohol may increase the risk of healed ulcers opening up again). In 1990, scientists discovered that a bacterium causes stomach and duadenal ulcers. The treatment now is antibiotics to kill the germs plus antiacids.

Test Yourself

1. Do you have these symptoms: a sudden racing of the heart, difficulty catching your breath, sweating, dizziness, lightheadedness?
Yes___ No___
2. Have you visited an emergency room or doctor more than twice in the last 6 months, fearing a heart attack, but, after a medical examination, no problem was found? Yes___ No___
3. Do you suddenly fear something terrible will happen? Yes___ No___
4. Do you avoid long car rides or travel on buses, subways, airplanes?
Yes___ No___

5. Are you afraid to leave your home without being accompanied by someone you know very well?
Yes___ No___
6. Do you avoid crowds or open spaces, such as shopping malls, parks, airports, train stations? Yes___ No___
7. Do you feel tense and anxious and unable to relax most of the time?
Yes___ No___
8. Do you spend most of your time worrying that bad things will happen?
Yes___ No___
9. Do you get extremely anxious when you are the center of attention?
Yes___ No___
10. Do you often feel you must get drunk or take tranquilizers before social occasions or performances?
Yes___ No___
11. Are there things that you feel you must do repeatedly—such as wash your hands, check the alarm clock or the front door—despite your best effort to resist? Yes___ No___
12. Do thoughts that you can't stop but that make no sense to you keep running through your mind?
Yes___ No___

If you answered yes to any of these questions (particularly to question 1), you may be suffering from some form of anxiety. Perhaps a visit to a physician, psychiatrist, or psychologist can help you identify your problem and gain relief.

We Can Cope with Schizophrenia

AT FIRST YOU DON'T PAY ATTENTION. YOU MAY hear it as a voice through a closed door of another room, and it sounds real. A single word: "Run!" or "Speak!" or "Quiet!" But soon you hear many words—commands: "Jump in front of the car." You *think* you are hearing real voices, but they're only in your mind.

If these are your symptoms, you have schizophrenia—a disease of the mind. A disease that confuses you. You cannot distinguish real voices—perhaps that of your mother calling you—from the imagined voices of your mind. You cannot plan or decide; you cannot change your thoughts. Your thoughts have captured you.

Schizophrenia is not a split personality—a mistake many make—but a disease, probably due to a biological dysfunction affecting the development of the brain or, as some theorize, a chemical reaction in the brain that destroys rational thought.

One percent of the population, or approximately 3 million Americans, will develop the disease in their lifetimes, estimates the National Institute of Mental Health; each year brings 300,000 new cases. It disables more people for a longer time than cancer. On any day, schizophrenia confines 100,000 Americans to hospitals. The illness hits young people, usually from the ages of 15 to 25,

lasting 30 to 40 years. And it costs taxpayers about $30 billion a year in medical treatment, disability payments, police and welfare work, and lost productivity. As the population increases, especially among the young, schizophrenia cases also increase.

At last, researchers are making progress in understanding its causes, treatment, and prevention. Dr. Samuel J. Keith, chief of the Schizophrenia Research Branch at the National Institute of Mental Health in Rockville, Maryland, takes a cautious view. "I would predict that the future will be a slow chipping away at this disease," he says.

Some of the researchers' discoveries may help schizophrenics like United States Air Force veteran Jim Dollard, of Albany, New York. The eldest of six children, Mr. Dollard has been hospitalized 17 times. Since its onset 17 years ago, the disease has twisted Mr. Dollard's brain and tortured his parents.

In many ways, his symptoms are typical: he hears voices, has hallucinations. The voices might tell him to do strange things. One order commanded him to rush out into automobile traffic. He sees imaginary spirits—black and white, angels and devils.

Mr. Dollard also has delusions. He believes that people are watching him, that psychiatry has taken over his mind. Other schizophrenics believe that their thoughts are broadcast for all to hear or that computers or radios are inserting ideas into their minds.

Mr. Dollard's thoughts won't let him work. They barely allow him to exist in his own room. He shows other symptoms. For example, he cannot easily solve the problems of ordinary living. Many schizophrenics can't even shop for groceries. Sometimes, when a schizophrenic is in a period of recovery and life deals a bad turn—say, the loss of a job—the stress may lead to all the symptoms returning in full force. The person then suffers a schizophrenic episode. He or she may not stay clean and wander the streets, shouting at others. Researchers estimate that schizophrenia afflicts half of all the homeless living in the streets.

Clues to a Cause

For 100 years, scientists have searched vainly for schizophrenia's cause. Today, some contend that it results from a chemical imbalance in the brain. But they have yet to identify a specific chemical mistake.

Scientists have, however, pinpointed one chemical defect in the brain that does not cause schizophrenia but might cause some of its symptoms. The problem lies in a faulty dopamine system. Dopamine is one of numerous chemicals in the brain that pass between the ends of nerves, allowing them to signal one another.

Dr. Arnold J. Friedhoff, director of the Millhauser Laboratories at New York University Medical School in Manhattan, has concluded that a healthy dopamine system allows us to manage mental stress. If we face severe stress, such as entering a new job or school, the brain *lowers* the dopamine signals to help us cope. But, when stressed, most schizophrenics' nerves are not quieted by their dopamine systems. Their brains go into overdrive; thoughts rush in and out from all directions; they hear sick voices.

Sarah and Harold Edwards of Syracuse, New York, have a son, Ben, who has been sick for 11 years. Ben, now 29, believes there is something like a computer in his head that tells him what to do. "All his past thoughts and present experience merge in a mental logjam," says Mrs. Edwards. "He's bored, scared, and angry. And he can't work or think."

Treating Schizophrenia

Around the mid-1950s, doctors discovered drugs that control the dopamine system and lower its activity. The best known of these is chlorpromazine (trade name: Thorazine). It doesn't cure schizophrenia, but it lessens the hallucinations and delusions. However, chlorpromazine slows the patient down, sometimes creating a slow-moving, slow-talking zombie effect. In a few patients the drug produces involuntary movements of the lip, tongue, and limbs. Usually, the movements stop if medication is reduced or stopped, but in a few patients this doesn't help. (Some studies show that in some types of schizophrenia, lithium salts can quiet the manic or excited phases. The studies are just now defining exactly who is helped by this drug.)

These drugs are the only real treatments doctors have. In the 1920s, they tried tooth removal to treat schizophrenia; in the 1930s, injections of horse serum; in the 1940s, enemas. All failed. In the 1950s, big doses of vitamins were tried, and the megavitamin trend persists, even though the American Psychiatric Association declared in 1971 that there was no evidence from studies that vitamin therapy did any good. Dr. Morris Lipton of the University of North Carolina Medical School at Chapel Hill headed the original studies and says nothing since has changed this.

For about 40 percent of schizophrenics, the brain drugs don't work. Dr. Friedhoff says that, although the drugs lower the dopamine levels as far as possible, the brain can't function properly.

The Two Faces of Illness

All this has led psychiatrists to identify two kinds of schizophrenia patients: those who respond to the drugs, with control of the dopamine system, and those who don't. Responsive patients show the outward signs of the disease—hallucinations, delusions, and strange behavior; the non-

responders are withdrawn, unemotional, seemingly devoid of feelings of pleasure.

For decades psychiatrists have held that many types of schizophrenia exist and that it may be the result of many different, separate diseases.

Dr. Richard J. Wyatt, chief of the Neuropsychiatry Branch of the National Institute of Mental Health, at St. Elizabeth's Hospital in Washington, D.C., draws this parallel with mental retardation: "A hundred years ago, we said that low IQ meant mental retardation. Since then, we've found a whole series of diseases that cause brain damage leading to a low IQ and retardation. Identifying the symptoms of schizophrenia is like having the results of an IQ test. I suspect that we'll find a number of diseases that make up the schizophrenia syndrome."

Scientists have discovered certain kinds of brain damage in some schizophrenics but not others and have found a low blood flow in the thinking part of the brain in some schizophrenics. A doctor in England found evidence of a viruslike particle. A U.S. physician found strange antibodies in the spinal fluid.

During the 1940s and 1950s, many psychiatrists believed angry relations between members of families caused schizophrenia in their children. As a result, many parents were tortured by guilty feelings of taking the blame for their child's illness. Most experts now reject that theory as unproved. Once again, however, evidence reveals that, even though families' behavior does not cause schizophrenia, the way families act toward their sick family members can prevent or trigger a relapse. In London, Dr. Julian Leff and his colleagues have identified family characteristics that affect schizophrenic patients. If a family's responses are warm and loving, for example, a relapse is prevented; but if they are hostile, critical, or overinvolved, the patient suffers more frequent episodes.

These findings set off a series of studies to learn whether doctors and social workers can train families to change behavior and ease sick family members. Nina Schooler, assistant chief of the Schizophrenia Research Branch at the National Institute of Mental Health, heads its multicity project. "People with schizophrenia are sensitive to stress, particularly interpersonal stress," she says. "We are working to educate the family to protect the patient against it."

Researchers also are trying to learn whether a patient can manage on less medication. The daily dose is reduced, or drugs are given to a patient only when the family detects the signs of odd behavior that warn of an oncoming episode.

Sarah Edwards estimates that, for the first 6 years of Ben's illness, the family spent $250,000 on his medical treatment. Ben now lives alone; his disease is stabilized. At his sister's wedding, says his mother, "It was hard to believe he was not OK. He is not so frightened as he once was and can control his own life."

Out of the need for family support has grown the National Alliance for the Mentally Ill, a group of parents and other relatives who teach themselves the facts of schizophrenia and where to find help. They learn that:

- schizophrenia is probably a brain disorder,
- drugs don't always quiet symptoms,
- most victims have their first episode in their late teens or early 20s,
- it attacks boys more than girls, and
- there is no cure—yet.

The family sessions help. "I get understanding from people who know what I am talking about," Mrs. Edwards says. "I ache so. I share my problems with people who are worse off."

Community Outreach

For schizophrenics who have no families or whose families have abandoned them, a few community programs offer help. One of the best, in Madison, Wisconsin, is the Program of Assertive Community Treatment (PACT), for young schizophrenics.

Dr. William H. Knoedler, who heads the program, says, "We don't wait for people to come to us; we go to them." The PACT doctors, nurses, and social workers reach out to teach the sick young people, on the streets or in their homes, how to cope with life. They also prescribe drugs to control symptoms.

"We don't discharge people for not coming to their treatment," says Dr. Knoedler. "We're available for them every day, 24 hours a day, and we're prepared to do this for life."

Dr. Knoedler tells of John R., who first experienced the disease at the age of 21. John believed that people on the street were causing him to be homosexual. He lived in the streets. By 1980, PACT got him to take medicine; he formed friendship ties with the group staff and began working as a computer keypuncher.

Studies of PACT show that, in its first 2 years, the treatment program actually costs a little less than the usual method of hospitalizing schizophrenic patients every time they get sick. It is also more humane.

Very few such community treatment programs exist. In most states, the money saved doesn't go back to the local government that set up the project but to the state. With so little incentive, local governments do little.

Until science understands schizophrenia's cause and then finds a cure or a means to prevent it, more and more troubled souls will be roaming our streets in need of help.

For more information about schizophrenia, write to the National Alliance for the Mentally Ill, 1901 N. Fort Myer Dr., Suite 500, Arlington, VA 22209.

It Quiets the Torment

IMAGINE: EVERY DAY, EVERY HOUR, YOU HEAR a voice in your head, saying, "You're stupid and ignorant. People can't stand the sight of you. Everybody hates you."

If you hear such a voice, the chances are that your brain is sick with schizophrenia. If so, the following probably happens to you as well:

• Your thinking skips from one topic to another without reason.
• Bizarre scenes (e.g., a dead person controlling your life) play themselves out in your head.

• You can't concentrate on simple tasks.
• You can't make friends or keep them.
• Your emotions stay flat and joyless.
• Untreated, you wander aimlessly along, talking and reacting to persons and situations visible only to you. Your strange actions frighten people off.

All these symptoms would indicate that schizophrenia has you in its grip. But a remarkable new drug called clozapine promises to help treat this terrible disease afflicting as many as 2 million Americans. It is not a cure, but many doctors and researchers consider it the best treatment to come along in 20 years.

Dr. John Kane heads the department of psychiatry at Hillside Hospital, the psychiatric division of Long Island Jewish Medical Center, in Glen Oaks, New York. He tested clozapine in schizophrenic patients unresponsive to other drugs. Of those drug-resistant patients taking clozapine, 30 percent showed improvement in functioning independently and had a reduced need for hospitalization.

The findings have made Dr. Kane and other brain specialists hopeful about the future of hard-to-treat patients. Until now, he explains, "Treating patients for schizophrenia has always been difficult. They are always ill or in the hospital. They can't function in the community."

Back in 1984, a form of schizophrenia struck Shannon Flynn, then a high school senior and honor student. "I had strong urges to cut myself, to punish myself," she recalls. "I was suicidal, paranoid. I thought people were reading my mind. I was afraid to look people in the eye. I was depressed, agitated. I paced the floor."

Ms. Flynn was treated with several medications. They enabled her to finish high school and graduate from Georgetown University in Washington, D.C. In July 1991, however, the symptoms returned. Her medicines were no longer effective. Ms. Flynn was so sick, her family had to hospitalize her. And treatment with clozapine began.

"Clozapine stopped the agitation, the paranoid feelings, and stopped making me want to hurt myself," Ms. Flynn reports. "My mind is a lot clearer."

She went back to her family. Ms. Flynn got a job as a research assistant at the National Institute of Mental Health in Bethesda, Maryland. "I will try to live independently," she says with determination.

But there is bad news buried in the good. Clozapine sometimes causes a potentially lethal toxic effect on the body's white blood cells. It happens to one patient in every 100, says Dr. Kane. If caught in time, stopping the drug usually can reverse the condition in 2 weeks. But when the disturbing mental symptoms return, the patient does not dare take clozapine again.

In 1973, Gilbert Honigfeld, director of scientific affairs at Sandoz Pharmaceuticals of East Hanover, New Jersey, started researching clozapine. Two years later, reports from Europe told of the drug's blood problem: it was killing patients. This discovery nearly stymied Sandoz's introduction of clozapine in the United States. Because a small number of patients had done well with the drug, however, they continued to receive it under a compassionate-need program. Their success eventually led to the resumption in 1987 of full-scale research in the United States.

At that time, with the knowledge of the Food and Drug Administration (FDA), says Mr. Honigfeld, Sandoz developed a weekly blood test to "ensure patient safety." It also probably afforded protection from lawsuits. Each week, a medical technician visited the patient, took a blood sample, and, if test results were satisfactory, handed out the next week's pills. Sandoz kept the drug on hold while the FDA studied results of the blood-monitoring program. In 1989, the FDA approved the use of clozapine by schizophrenia patients for whom all other treatments have failed. Cost to the patient: $8,900 a year—probably for a lifetime.

Protests rained down on Sandoz, which markets the drug under the trade name Clozaril. The National Alliance for the Mentally Ill (NAMI), an organization of patients and their families, said the expensive weekly blood-testing program would shut out the poor. State Medicaid officials refused to cover the costs.

In 1991, Sandoz announced that doctors, clinics, and hospitals could arrange for their own blood tests. Patients would be required simply to show their doctor or pharmacist proof of the satisfactory results of the weekly blood test before getting the next supply. The Health Care Financing Administration then ordered all state Medicaid programs to cover the expenses for their patients and said it would pay some of the states' medical costs.

Roch Thibodeau Jr., of Burlington, Vermont, got his clozapine under Medicaid. Schizophrenia had destroyed his ability to earn a living. When his illness began, Mr. Thibodeau first took older drugs, including Stelazine (trifluoperazine). Stelazine was a major breakthrough in treatment in the 1950s, along with Thorazine (chlorpromazine).

While the medicines kept him going and controlled the symptoms of the disease, young Mr. Thibodeau experienced severe side effects. "He suffered terrible dry mouth, blistering reactions to the sun, slurred speech," says his father. "He could not sit still. He could not focus." These side effects led Mr. Thibodeau to stop taking his medications. As a result, his schizophrenia again took hold.

When he started taking Clozaril in 1989, the symptoms all but disappeared. Side effects were not a problem. He began working 20 hours a week at a bus station kiosk, selling newspapers and light snacks. Now he works for a hospital, delivering supplies to various departments.

"Before Clozaril, I could not have done that," says Mr. Thibodeau. "I had a real struggle. I could not handle stress or function. I have a lot more motivation now."

Now, more than 60,000 patients have taken clozapine. Laurie Flynn, Shannon's mother, says, "Clozapine is the closest thing to a miracle that you will ever see. You see an amazing return of a patient's sense of humor, interest in life, and ability to relate to others." She adds that the drug probably would help many of the nation's schizophrenics, "but, for most of the people for whom this medicine would make a remarkable difference, it is unavailable."

Mrs. Flynn, who is the executive director of the National Alliance for the Mentally Ill, charges that the number of Americans taking clozapine is only a fraction of the 250,000 who have not responded to other drugs for schizophrenia and who thus qualify for a prescription. "The drug still costs $7,000 to $9,000 a year, including the blood tests," she explains. Although Medicaid can help the very poor, it is not available to those who earn just enough to stay afloat.

"Schizophrenia rapidly impoverishes families," adds Mrs. Flynn. "You run right out of insurance. It is a tragedy."

While critics say clozapine's cost generally puts it out of reach, Gilbert Honigfeld of Sandoz declares, "Compared to the cost of hospitalizing patients, $10 to $15 a day is a small investment. The cost is a fraction of the funds spent on diseases other than mental illness." And it is far less than the social and moral cost of leaving patients untreated.

Part of the price problem stems from the long research delay. If Sandoz is to recoup its research expenses on Clozaril, it must act quickly. After the company's patent runs out, anyone will be free to make and sell the drug and reap the profits.

Scientists see clozapine as a clue to even better drugs. In particular, they are looking for a chemical cousin to clozapine without the blood problem. Two candidates are being pursued.

Robert Kniffin, a spokesman for Janssen Pharmaceutical of Titusville, New Jersey, reports that the company is test-ing a new compound called risperidone (brand name: Risperdal). He says it already has been given to 2,000 patients.

In its 1991 annual report, Merck & Co. of Whitehouse Station, New Jersey, announced that remoxipride (brand name: Roxiam) is in the final stages of testing. "Roxiam," states the report, "may have fewer side effects than other available treatments."

Scientists still are puzzling over how clozapine and its cousins work. They contend that clozapine regulates the flow in the brain of molecules called neurotransmitters. They appear at the junctions of nerves. One nerve ending releases a neurotransmitter. It flows across the junction and causes an electrical discharge in the next nerve. Scientists have found a dozen neurotransmitters. Among those affected by clozapine are dopamine, serotonin, and norepinephrine.

Dr. Herbert Y. Meltzer, professor of psychiatry at Case Western Reserve University School of Medicine in Cleveland, explains how clozapine affects the flow of dopamine: It maintains a normal level of the neurotransmitter in areas of the brain that control emotion and motivation. With too little dopamine comes the disease's flat emotional response; with too much dopamine come excitability and delusions.

Patients taking older drugs complain of feeling medicated, sleepy, and zombielike. Those taking clozapine report feeling more like their healthy selves. This reaction indicates that, with clozapine, they will have less need for institutionalization, avoiding the hospital "revolving door" situation.

Dr. Meltzer is investigating the possibility of using clozapine to treat schizophrenia from its onset.

Since 1989, clozapine has caused blood problems in several hundred patients, and a few have died. In addition, about 1 percent of patients suffer seizures if the dose is too strong for them. But most of the other side effects, including weight gain and excessive salivation, are infrequent and mild. And, unlike other schizophrenia drugs, clozapine does not trigger involuntary movements of the face and mouth—a condition that persists in some patients even after they stop taking those drugs.

Scientists say clozapine will lead to a better understanding of schizophrenia. They now theorize that the tendency to schizophrenia is inherited or caused by a prenatal viral infection.

Clozapine has raised the hopes of both doctors and patients. It may one day do for schizophrenia what penicillin did for infections.

For more information, write to the National Alliance for the Mentally Ill, 200 North Glebe Road, Arlington, VA 22203, or call (800) 950-NAMI

Lighten Up Winter Sadness

MILLIONS DREAD THE COMING OF WINTER, NOT because it's cold but because the darkness of the night lasts too long. Daytime also carries a somber cloak. Many respond with moodiness, and some with frank mental depression that needs treatment. The treatment: sitting in front of bright, artificial light radiating from a box.

It may sound like quackery, like something out of science fiction or ancient myths, but, in fact, it does work. By shining intense light on the eyes of people suffering from deep depression in the winter season, psychiatrists have lifted the spirits of uncounted patients.

This light treatment, called phototherapy, has real effects on the minds of human beings. It has opened up a new way to treat the depression that affects millions of Americans from September, when days begin to shorten, through the winter and into March, when they begin to lengthen again.

A team of scientists at the National Institute of Mental Health in Bethesda, Maryland, began to focus on the link between mood and illumination. Dr. Norman E. Rosenthal, a chief psychiatric researcher at the institute, was one of them.

"There is not only winter depression—people get depressed in summer, too," says Dr. Rosenthal. "We think for summer it's the intolerance to heat. But we're not sure."

In the United States, Dr. Rosenthal estimates, 10 million people get clinically or dangerously depressed with the coming of winter. A smaller number become depressed with the advent of summer. All are suffering from what doctors now call seasonal affective disorder, or SAD.

Helen Smith, a housewife from New York City, says she finally realized she was starved for light. "Since puberty," she recalls, "depression was constant. I had no focus or goals. It took me 7 years to finish college. You can't just pick yourself up and make it better. Depression robs you of everything."

The families of people like Helen Smith often believe that the patient can simply overcome the depression by an act of will. But the person no more can eject the depression from the mind than you can cure cancer by thinking about it. Mrs. Smith's doctor sent her to Dr. Michael Terman, director of the Winter Depression Program at the New York State Psychiatric Institute in Manhattan.

"I've kept journals since the age of 9 or 10," says Mrs. Smith. "September 15 was always the day in my journals when I would crash. But I did not see the pattern until I met Dr. Terman." He took her off depression drugs and had her sit in front of a light box with six fluorescent tubes for 3 to 4 hours each morning and for 2 hours before bedtime. As she sat, she read, did needlepoint, or wrote in her journal. Within 3 weeks, she was feeling really good, she reports.

"I've had three winters depression-free," Mrs. Smith exults. "I have a future. I have a family now. I belong to the human race." Since being treated by Dr. Terman, she has married and has a baby girl. As do most SAD patients, she says she still hungers for light. "But now," she adds, "half an hour in the morning is all I need."

In less than 10 years, scientists have recognized that SAD is a mental disorder and that light plays a big part in its origin and treatment. The progress began when Dr. Rosenthal, then a young physician from South Africa, went to work in 1979 with Dr. Thomas A. Wehr, who was studying biological clocks in animals at the National Institute in Bethesda. The biological clock triggers many daily activities, each at about the same time every day—hunger, going to sleep and getting up, among others. Generally, your biological clock lags behind real time. With no cues from daylight, traffic noises, or temperature changes, you would feel sleepy later and later each day. Eventually, you could end up 12 hours out of step with real time.

In 1979, Dr. Al Lewy, now professor of psychiatry at Oregon Health Sciences University in Portland, and Dr. Wehr began work on a hormone called melatonin, released by the pineal gland in the brain. Their studies revealed that light plays an important role in triggering and setting the biological clocks in animals. Other studies showed that exposure to light stops nighttime production of melatonin in the pineal gland. Dr. Lewy, Dr. Wehr, and their colleagues have found that nighttime melatonin production in humans can be stopped with 2,500 lux-intensity light. (*Lux,* Latin for light, is the unit of measure for brightness.) This suggests that such brightness could be used to reset human biological rhythms.

It was their melatonin work that brought Herb Kern to the National Institute in 1980. He asked Dr. Lewy to measure his melatonin levels. Mr. Kern, an engineer, had an undiagnosed case of SAD. He had kept records on his mood changes for 15 years and had told his doctors that, as the days got shorter, he "just wanted to crawl into a hole and hibernate." Mr. Kern recalls, "I finally latched on to the thought that sunlight was the key. When the days got longer in summer, the wheels of my brain would spin again." But, he says, his doctors didn't listen to him.

Dr. Lewy suggested lengthening Mr. Kern's winter days by sitting him in a room under bright fluorescent lights for 6 hours—three before dawn and three after sundown. Within days, Kern reported feeling as if springtime were around the corner. He still takes 2 hours of light treatment at 6 A.M. from fall to spring. "Since using the lights, I have been able to manage my depressions very nicely," he says.

The doctors spent the next few years focusing on the effects of light on mood and wanted to extend the study with more patients. Dr. Rosenthal told a reporter from the *Washington Post* about Mr. Kern and another patient. When the article was printed, thousands inquired about treatment. That was the first hint that SAD was a common disorder. With a selected group of patients, the doctors showed that light relieves wintertime depression. They also found that the brighter the light, the shorter the SAD treatment. Since then, studies worldwide have demonstrated the same, and the American Psychiatric Association now lists seasonal mood swings as a form of mental disease.

In New York, Dr. Terman has a new computerized approach: creating an artificial dawn. In phototherapy, "we were turning on very bright light suddenly after the patient wakes up," he says. "But when the eye is adapted to the dark while sleeping, it is 'looking' for a gradual transition to dawn. We put computer systems in a patient's bedroom to gradually turn on a light from very dim to bright, like a sunrise. Within a few days, we got results equal to any effect of bright-light therapy. The patients wake up spontaneously, refreshed."

Dr. Terman says he tried it, because he detects seasonal changes in energy level and sleep in himself: "I maintained a summer sunrise throughout winter and was not groggy. It is a natural alarm clock."

Scientists already have shown that exposure to light can reset the biological clock if work shifts change or jet lag strikes. Some people have delayed sleep—biological clocks that won't let them go to sleep before 2 A.M. Others have advanced sleep and can't keep their eyes open after sundown. Light treatment can reset both.

To get an idea of the intensities of the light sources used for treatment, think of a bright, sunny day. The light falling on your eyes is equal to 100,000 lux. A standard light box puts out between 2,500 and 10,000 lux. Dr. Terman's dawn light: 250 lux.

There also are experiments with a visor, as on a baseball cap. This special visor has small battery-powered lights, and the illumination falls directly on the eyes. You cannot look away. Early results suggest that this device works at least as well as the panels of light, whether the light output is 600 lux or 32,000 lux.

Although these light sources are commercially available, all the experts warn against buying them without first consulting a psychiatrist trained to recognize SAD. (Take the test at the end of this article.) Diagnosing SAD can be tricky. The same symptoms may arise from other types of depression. Also, prescribed durations and intensities of light may vary. For some patients, light therapy doesn't work at all. Dr. Rosenthal says they may need other treatments: drugs, psychological therapy, relocation to a warmer winterless climate. He adds that studies show fewer cases are found the closer you go to the equator (perhaps 10 percent of New Hampshire's population may have SAD, but only 1.5 percent of Florida's) and that women with SAD outnumber men by 7 to 2—possibly, scientists say, because of hormonal differences.

Dr. Wehr says that children suffer from SAD and respond to the light as adults do. "It has a tremendous impact on their ability to function in school," he observes. "They start out the school year fairly strong, thinking they will enjoy it. In November, it starts to fall apart. They sleep 12 hours a day. They're not creative; they've lost the spark. Those with winter depression are slowed down. Their behaviors include overeating, oversleeping, and sluggishness." Other SAD symptoms include anxiety, irritability, an inability to tolerate stress, and withdrawing from others.

And then there's the summer SAD, a condition less studied than its winter form. Dr. Wehr says summer SAD patients have decreased sleep and loss of appetite and weight. "They are more agitated," he adds.

One of Dr. Wehr's patients, Helen O'Lone, a homemaker from Rockville, Maryland, suffered from depression all year. "But July was one of the worst months for me," she says. "The whole world seemed black. I had no appetite.

My sleep was restless, agitated." Dr. Wehr prescribed Prozac, an antidepressive drug. "Now I feel the best I've ever felt in my life," Mrs. O'Lone says. "I love to do water exercises and swim."

Do You Need to See a Doctor for the Treatment of SAD?

When winter comes, do you experience any of the following?

1. Needing more sleep
2. Eating more
3. Gaining weight
4. Losing energy
5. Socializing less
6. Feeling less cheerful
7. Having difficulties in coping with life as a result of these changes

Dr. Norman E. Rosenthal says if you answered yes to number 7, you would do well to check with a qualified psychiatrist.

For more information, write to the National Institute of Mental Health, Room 7C-02, 5600 Fishers Lane, Rockville, MD 20857.

The Deadly Emotions: They Can Shorten Your Life—If You Let Them

WE ALL KNOW THE TYPE—THE PERSON WHO stands at the elevator door and jabs at the button three, four, even five times when the car fails to arrive quickly enough. In conversation, this individual finishes your sentences for you or glances constantly at the time. People like this feel that they've got the world to conquer. And you're very cautious about what you do or say with them, because they can ignite like firecrackers into anger.

Thirty years ago, scientists first identified such individuals as exhibiting "Type A" behavior: in a hurry, impatient, often angry. They also found persons with "Type B" behavior: laid-back, calm, slow to anger, good listeners.

The researchers found that Type A's more often fell victim to heart attacks; Type B's less so. But the researchers could not figure out how the personality connected with biology. What was there about Type A behavior that killed you? They had no answer, then.

"We have strong evidence now that hostility alone damages the heart," says Dr. Redford Williams. One of the researchers who helped pinpoint the destructive effects of hatred, Dr. Williams is a professor of psychiatry at Duke University Medical Center in Durham, North Carolina.

"It isn't the impatience, the ambition, or the work drive," Dr. Williams says. "It's the anger. It sends your blood pressure skyrocketing. It provokes your body to create unhealthy chemicals. For hostile people, anger is a poison."

Psychologists and psychiatrists have always told their patients to "let anger out" because, they said, if you hold it in, you can become depressed or develop ulcers. Dr. Williams gives quite another prescription: Avoid *feeling* angry in the first place, and you won't need to suppress your anger.

Bruce T. Bowling, publisher of *Firehouse* magazine in New York City, clearly exhibited Type A behavior.

"I couldn't catch up," Mr. Bowling says. "I'd walk into my house, the Chinese food in one hand, mail in the other, scanning it as I went to the bathroom. I felt if I could do four things at the same time, I'd save time."

Mr. Bowling meted out large doses of hostility to those around him. "Waitresses were never fast enough," he says. "Taxi drivers drove me crazy. I would purposely undertip them. New York City, I used to think, will do me in."

In 1988, all his hostility took its toll. Just back from a firefighters' convention, Mr. Bowling felt the classic pains in his shoulders, arms, and neck. At the hospital emergency room at 3 A.M., they told

him: heart attack. He was lucky. He survived. Each year, half a million Americans don't.

Dr. Meyer Friedman is a cardiologist at Mount Zion Hospital in San Francisco and one of the codiscoverers of Type A behavior. He contends that hostility, impatience, and anger powerfully affect your body. Dr. Williams, on the other hand, says you can be impatient with impunity, so long as it doesn't lead to anger. It's the anger that gets you. The issue is not settled, but more and more experts agree that both anger and hostility can be hazardous to your health.

Originally, Dr. Friedman and his collaborator, Dr. Ray Rosenman, identified three parts of the Type A behavior:

1. Intense striving toward many poorly defined goals
2. Preoccupation with time and an obsession with getting things done faster
3. Free-floating hostility

To be hostile means that you want to hurt or punish somebody. Anger, Dr. Friedman says, can be the same thing or less—a feeling of displeasure toward yourself. Both hostility and anger rile your heart and body. To have "free-floating hostility" means that you are angry, or on the point of anger, much of the time, with or without major cause.

Dr. Williams says hostility has three stages, and he gives this example: You are in an express line at the supermarket checkout with a sign saying, "No more than 10 items."

Stage 1: You distrust others. You count the items in the baskets of the people in front of you. You *expect* somebody to cheat and thereby take advantage of you.

Stage 2: You *feel* angry when you find somebody cheating. The guy in front of you has 12 items.

Stage 3: You *show* the anger by saying something nasty to the "cheater."

According to Dr. Williams, all three stages can damage you. In one study, high levels of hostility found in healthy men at age 25 were seen as predictors that they were up to seven times more likely to get heart disease or die by age 50.

In another test, young men with and without high hostility levels worked on a complex mental task. Blood pressure in both groups rose at about the same rate. At one point, a psychologist began to harass the test takers. In the nonhostile men, blood pressure remained steady. In the hostile men, however, the pressure went through the roof.

Other studies show that hostility can spur the release of a hormone called epinephrine, which makes your heart beat fast and your blood pressure rise. High blood pressure leads to damaged arteries and heart attack.

Dr. Williams says those who cynically mistrust other people are most at risk. Dr. Friedman says hostility comes from unbridled greed, low self-esteem, or insecurity—feelings that you will be hurt, might fail, or won't be loved. Whatever

its source, doctors agree that hostility is a factor in heart attack.

There is some controversy, however. Two large studies failed to demonstrate the heart risk of Type A behavior altogether. Dr. Friedman says the scientists did not use methods that evaluate and measure Type A. In another study, heart attack victims with Type A behavior survived longer than those with Type B. But these studies were inconclusive. They did not include those people who died quickly. Many of whom could have been Type A reaped the tragedy of their emotions.

It could be, says Dr. Richard Brand, professor of biostatistics at the University of California at Berkeley, that Type A men follow doctor's orders more closely than Type B's do, by watching their diet, exercising, and stopping smoking, all of which would protect them against a second attack. Other doctors say that Type A's follow orders for only a week or so, then resume their old habits.

Along with Dr. Carl Thoresen, professor of psychology at Stanford University in Palo Alto, California, and Dr. James Gill of the Institute for Living in Hartford, Connecticut, Dr. Friedman worked out a method for reducing the Type A traits. When they succeeded with men who'd had a heart attack, Dr. Friedman says, the risk of a second heart attack was nearly halved. The researchers were able to modify the Type A behavior of almost 50 percent of the men and women in the group.

"We try to change their belief systems," Dr. Friedman says. "These are successful people, and we have to show them that no one does a creative job if in a hurry or angry. We teach them to do nice things for people, that charm is not a weakness."

It's much harder than it sounds. Adults have formed habits of a lifetime. Driving a car, Type A's scream at other drivers—even with the windows closed! They argue bitterly about small points. They constantly correct others in their work or speech or both. They drive themselves and others to perfection. But they themselves cave in to criticism.

With a specially trained team, Dr. Friedman treats Type A's in the Milton Friedman Institute at Mount Zion Hospital. He first concentrates on getting patients to realize what they are doing and saying through self-observation. Though it sounds easy, few people can do it.

The Scottish poet Robert Burns said it best (in translation):

> *Would that some power the gift*
> *give us*
> *To see ourselves as others see us!*

The Type A's also learn to practice physical and mental relaxation. They examine their thought processes to get rid of illogical thoughts that lead to hostility. They practice avoiding confrontations with coworkers and family members.

Myles Share, ran Lou G. Siegel's Restaurant, one of the biggest eateries in the garment center in New York City. The garment center is flooded with Type

A's. A year before, had you stepped into the kitchen, you likely would have found Mr. Share yelling at the cooks, the waiters, the dishwashers—anybody at all.

"I was a madman, a raving lunatic," Mr. Share recalls. "I would scream at them. I would make people feel useless, and I looked like an ass. If people didn't live up to my standards, I would publicly humiliate them."

Mr. Share knew he was rapidly spiraling downhill. Still a young man, he had moderately high blood pressure. He realized that his personality was killing him, making him hate the business that his father had built. He couldn't control himself.

Then Mr. Share consulted Dr. Reed Moskowitz, director of Stress Disorder Medical Services at New York University Medical Center in Manhattan. Dr. Moskowitz agrees that hostility can poison the body. He taught Mr. Share how to relax, breathe properly, and think logically.

"We taught him that people will do the best they can, but they also will make mistakes," Dr. Moskowitz says. "Look at your thoughts. Are you expecting people to be perfect?"

When I met Mr. Share several months ago, at both Dr. Moskowitz's office and the restaurant, I found a charming and relaxed young man. Waiters and busboys smiled at him.

"I enjoy coming to work," Mr. Share now says. "I am more patient. I take the time to teach, show, support."

Dr. Meyer Friedman and his team taught tough-minded lieutenant colonels how to reduce their Type A behavior at the United States Army War College. Some officers feared that the course would diminish their toughness.

Colonel Fred R. Drews, former director of the Army Physical Fitness Research Institute, says the reduction of Type A behavior benefited not only the officers but also the Army. Drews's successor, Lieutenant Colonel Paul T. Harig, shared his view of the course.

Bruce Bowling, the magazine publisher, enrolled in a Type A reduction program at New York Hospital. He says he is less prone to anger now, although he admits that he slips once in a while.

Despite all the positive evidence that reducing Type A behavior can save lives, most doctors pooh-pooh the treatment. They demand stronger data than Dr. Friedman's study offers. Scientists at Harvard and Yale applied for a $1 million grant to do a hard-nosed evaluation, but the National Heart, Lung, and Blood Institute turned them down.

The director of the institute, Dr. Claude Lenfant, says that an independent review group gave the project a high priority. The institute's governing council, however, said that the study was too costly and might not be able to prove or disprove the treatment's effectiveness.

Dr. Lenfant says, "If we had all the money we wanted, we certainly would fund the Type A experiment. We didn't have it at that time. Perhaps in the future we will."

Where does hostility come from? Experts agree that much of it is learned—from parents, siblings, and peers. We do live in a competitive society where, as baseball great Leo Durocher observed, "Nice guys finish last."

Dr. Friedman notes, however, that most executives will admit that they made their biggest mistakes when they were angry or impatient. Anger interferes with creative thinking. Being a "nice guy" often nets rewards that hostility doesn't.

Growing numbers of scientists maintain that you biologically inherit the tendency to Type A behavior from your parents. Something in your body chemistry makes you impatient and quick to anger. That may be the reason that so many people find it hard to change their behavior.

If you insist on being mistrustful and angry and showing your anger, remember: The scientific data suggest that, as a result, you are running risks with your life.

Do You Have a Hostile Heart?

It takes a long, probing examination to determine whether you are a hostile person (people do hide such truths, from others and themselves), but Dr. Redford Williams of Duke University has three questions that will raise a warning flag for you. In edited form, they are given here. Circle the word that best describes your behavior:

1. When anybody slows down or stops what I want to do, I think they are selfish, mean, and inconsiderate.

Never___ Sometimes___
Often___ Always___

2. When anybody does something that seems incompetent, messy, selfish, or inconsiderate to me, I quickly feel angry or enraged. At the same time, my heart races, my breath comes quickly, and my palms sweat.
Never___ Sometimes___
Often___ Always___

3. When I have such thoughts or feelings (statement 2), I let fly with words, gestures, a raised voice, and frowns.
Never___ Sometimes___
Often___ Always___

Dr. Williams says that if you answer "often" or "always" to two of these questions, you are in a high-risk group. You have a hostile heart.

How to Have a Trusting Heart

The key to reducing hostility may be a trusting heart, says Dr. Redford Williams.

Hostility begins when you mistrust others. In his book *The Trusting Heart,* Dr. Williams suggests these 12 steps for acquiring such feelings of trust:

1. Monitor your cynical thoughts by recognizing them.
2. Confess your hostility and seek support for change.
3. Stop cynical thought.
4. Reason with yourself.
5. Put yourself in the other person's shoes.
6. Laugh at yourself.
7. Practice relaxing.
8. Try trusting others.
9. Force yourself to listen more.
10. Substitute assertiveness (firmness) for aggression.
11. Pretend today is your last day.
12. Practice forgiveness.

If you cannot do it on your own, seek help from a psychologist, psychiatrist, or member of the clergy.

How You Might Help Turn Off Drug Abuse

WHEN YOU FIRST THINK ABOUT IT, IT LOOKS hopeless: 50 million Americans snorting, popping, smoking, and injecting powerful mind- and mood-changing drugs.

Many of them are your children. Many of them are hooked.

Until recently and for more than two decades, Americans—particularly young people—have "turned on" in increasing numbers to illegal substances. The drugs include marijuana, cocaine, heroin, amphetamines, barbiturates, tranquilizers, hallucinogens, and legal substances like alcohol and tobacco.

By any medical standard, this widespread abuse is an epidemic. And for a while it looked unstoppable as drug abuse spread from person to person. Friend turned on friend to drugs; brother turned on brother; and often, unwittingly, parents introduced their children to drugs.

We are still a nation deeply dependent on chemicals to make ourselves feel better emotionally (see the table). Among our young people between the ages of 12 and 17, about one in three plays around with

these substances in any month. One in three used alcohol, and one in eight has tried marijuana, or "pot." The use of both substances is illegal for this age group.

Illicit drug use is so widespread that it hits every American in unexpected ways. Two of my very best friends each have lost a son to drug overdose. The family was devastated, as were their circle of friends. For those of us touched in this way, we cannot imagine what "went wrong."

According to the National Institute on Drug Abuse, widespread drug use by Americans has exacted an annual cost of at least $100 billion in criminal activity, medical and legal services, and lost productivity. Officials at the Drug Enforcement Administration have estimated that

Percentage Who Have Ever Used the Drug

Drug	Youths (aged 12–17)			Young Adults (aged 18–25)			Older Adults (aged 26+)		
	1972	1982	1995	1972	1982	1995	1972	1982	1995
Marijuana	14	27	6	48	64	41	7	23	52
Hallucinogens	5	5	5	17*	21	14	1	6	15
Cocaine	2	7	2	9	28	10	2	9	22
Heroin	1	***	1	5	1	1	‡	1	2
Stimulants**	4	7	2	12	18	4	3	6	7
Sedatives**	3	6	1	10	19	2	2	5	4
Tranquilizers**	3	5	1	7	15	5	5	4	6
Alcohol	54*	65	41	82*	95	84	73*	88	90
Cigarettes	52*	50	38	69*	77	68	65*	79	76

SOURCE: The National Household Survey on Drug Abuse, courtesy of the National Institute on Drug Abuse. All figures are rounded to the nearest percentage.

*Figures are not available for 1972 and are from 1974.
**Nonmedical use.
***Less than one-half of 1 percent.

by 1980 we had spawned a $70 billion-a-year illegal industry with wads of cash to bribe and subvert local and state officials.

Recent Bad News about Drug Use

Twelve years ago, health officials saw some bright spots in this gloomy picture. The latest surveys from the National Institute on Drug Abuse showed modest but real declines since 1979 in puffing marijuana and popping hallucinogens and PCP, or "angel dust." The surveys also reveal a leveling off in cocaine use among the 18 to 25 age group.

In 1984, experts showed moderate optimism. Dr. Mitchell Rosenthal, director of New York City's Phoenix House, one of the nation's largest residential drug treatment programs said: "In our lifetime, you and I will probably see a significant decline in drug use. We will see high school kids dropping way back. We won't be in as dangerous a place as we are now."

It hasn't quite worked out that way. Over the period from 1992 to 1996 there was marked increase in the use of marijuana among high school teenagers. Parents met this with grim anticipation. Politicians used the statistic to batter their opponents. Experts had few solutions.

The Terror of the Addict

Health officials see a new and terrifying danger: young teenagers who regularly abuse and combine many different drugs.

They end up with shattered and impotent lives, out of school, unemployable, often in jail, and sometimes dead.

I talked to such a teen we'll call Ronny; I cannot give her real name. A pretty, brown-eyed high school junior of 16, she lives in a wealthy New Jersey suburb.

"I drank a lot," Ronny says, "dropped acid, smoked pot, did cocaine and everything else. I couldn't live without it." After months in treatment, Ronny freed herself from drugs.

George Beschner, chief of the treatment research branch at the National Institute on Drug Abuse, estimated then that multiple drug use had trapped as many as 1.2 million adolescents in America. Most of the multiple-drug abusers are youngsters who use marijuana every day.

"It cuts across all ethnic and income groups," he explains. "And we really don't know enough about how to treat them and prevent this problem."

Opening the Door to Hard Drugs

The worst consequence of marijuana use may be that it opens the door to harder drugs. Dr. Richard R. Clayton of the University of Kentucky in Lexington says flatly that marijuana "causes" heroin and cocaine use. He cites figures showing that the more marijuana a person smokes the more likely he or she is to use heroin or cocaine or both.

Dr. Denise Kandel of the New York State Psychiatric Institute in Manhattan says that "cause" is too strong a word because only a small fraction of marijuana smokers go on to use other drugs. But, she points out, her 1971 and 1980 studies of 8,000 public high school students in New York State reveal that nearly all cocaine and heroin users start with marijuana.

In the late 1970s a survey of 17,000 high seniors by the National Institute Drug Abuse, found young people understand that regular use of any drug carries a high risk. But, in a curious way, they don't feel at risk themselves. When they buy drugs on the street, they do not know the quality, cleanliness, dose, or the actual chemical they will be putting into their bodies.

The Reasons

Much research points to the family as the critical factor in determining whether children will use drugs. A strong family counteracts the influence of a child's drug-using peers. On the other hand, a weak family may actually encourage drug use. Parental leniency about marijuana, for example, may actually prompt young people to try pot (although strong rules against drugs in the home do not necessarily stop marijuana use).

Most important, psychologists say, the family provides the child with emotional support and models for correct behavior. If the child is unable to share his or her feelings, thoughts, and needs with the parents, the child is more likely to try marijuana and other drugs to feel better. Young people who get into deep trouble

with drugs are the ones who use drugs to cope with their environment.

Dr. George De Leon, then research director of Phoenix House, has studied the family's influence on drug use in detail. He compared the families of adolescents who use drugs and those who do not. He has come up with a formula for a good family that may immunize its sons and daughters against experimenting with drugs despite so-called "friends" who pressure them to do so.

"A good family," says Dr. De Leon, "provides good communication, closeness, and good role models. A good family shows no compulsive behavior: no gambling, drug use, or excessive alcohol intake."

In his study of drug abusers and drug abstainers, Dr. De Leon has found that, perhaps more than the mother, the father's behavior powerfully influences his children's drug-taking habits. A good father, Dr. De Leon says, shows his children that he is true to his ideals and does not lie to himself or others. In this sense, a good father shows his children strong, self-reliant behavior and honesty.

A Checklist for Fathers

Dr. De Leon suggests the following ways for a man to improve his "fatherhood."

• Review the amount of time you spend with your children. More is always better.

• Talk openly with your children about your behavior. Show them you are not afraid to confront your own weaknesses.

• Share with your children your real concerns about them, even if those fears are unfounded. For example, instead of curtly telling your son or daughter to check in with you by phone on a late-night date ("I'm your father, and you should call"), try a more honest explanation: "Look, I worry about you. It may sound silly, but it would make me feel better if you call."

• Emphasize personal satisfaction above material gains. Sons, particularly, admire fathers who work at a job for its psychological rewards.

• The good father does not generate in his children the feeling that they are at fault when something goes wrong at home or school. Such accusations generate guilt, the feeling that you have done something wrong even when you have not. It is a powerful emotion for a young person to handle.

"Often drugs are taken to relieve guilt," says Dr. De Leon. "We have a sign in Phoenix House: 'Guilt Kills.'"

What Parents Can Do

In the last seven years, more than 4,000 parent groups in the United States have organized to fight drugs, particularly marijuana, which they see as the key drug. They have banded together as the National Family Partnership. The federation shows mothers and fathers how to organize themselves to fight drug abuse, including the following advice:

• Learn about drugs and their dangers.
• Take a firm stand against drug use by your children.
• Share the information with the parents of your children's friends, school administrators, and communities.
• Fight commercial exploitation of drug use—for example, the "head shops" that sell drug paraphernalia.

Parents who want more information can write to the National Family Partnership, 11159 Suite B South Towne Square, St. Louis, MO 63123.

It's difficult for parents to notice whether a child is using drugs unless the doses are so high and frequent that the child staggers. But there are clues. A child who suddenly burns incense or uses air fresheners may be covering the smell of marijuana smoke. Look for a change in behavior, either to high activity or lethargy.

How to Find Help

Youngsters and adults who have a drug problem and want help can call a local hospital, mental health association, or drug outreach group. Doctors, ministers, and guidance counselors can also help. Cocaine users can phone a national 24-hour, toll-free help line for referrals to 300 drug abuse centers across the country. The telephone counselors, all former cocaine addicts, may be able to help with problems stemming from other drugs too. Dial 1-800-COCAINE.

Treating the Heroin Addict

Few proven treatment programs for heavy drug dependency are available, except these for heroin addiction:

- Methadone maintenance. Addicts take methadone, a heroin-like synthetic, which reduces craving for heroin.
- Residential community. Heroin users live together in a support-group setting and work toward freeing each other from heroin addiction.
- Drug-free outpatient. Addicts report regularly to a clinic for counseling.

An analysis of these treatments by researchers at Texas Christian University and Texas A&M University reveals that, in each of the programs, many addicts drop their habits, keep out of trouble, and find paying jobs.

Methadone does carry a risk. In 1 year, out of 95,000 methadone patients nationwide, 350 died. This figure is far lower than the risk of death from overdose and disease outside the program.

Few studies show that drug treatment programs can achieve similar results for cocaine and multiple-drug abusers, although residential treatment does seem to work the best.

John, 31, a heavy user of cocaine and heroin (with alcohol, LSD, amphetamines), entered Phoenix House. After a year of daily meetings with other drug abusers and learning how to build a positive self-image and curtail his destructive behavior, John is ready to leave Phoenix House, drug-free. The chances of his going back to drug abuse are high.

The Schools Lend a Hand

Out of the parents' movement have sprung school programs to help children in trouble overcome their drug habits and to prevent others from entering the drug arena. Almost every school district in Minnesota, for example, runs drug education programs. New Jersey sponsors similar projects.

In one New York City program, the board of education spends $3 million a year to deter 300,000 boys and girls in 100 high schools from drugs. In each school, a counselor tries to pick out the youngsters who are in trouble but not yet lost to heavy addiction.

Ron Austin, a counselor at Julia Richman High School in Manhattan, works with students who have serious problems. Clara, 15, became pregnant and tried to kill herself with drugs. James, 18, wanted to fit in with his friends, so he took drugs.

Like most counselors, Mr. Austin tries to help students rebuild their self-image and self-confidence. After a while, some of them realize that tending to school and future employment will truly solve their problems whereas drugs do not.

There are no simple solutions to America's drug problems. The Drug Enforcement Administration has believed that the fear of arrest and punishment will scare people away from the drug business. Cutting off the supply at the source by cracking down on illicit importers will keep supplies of drugs short and prices high. If drugs are costly, the DEA says, that can dissuade many potential users. After spending billions of dollars tracking and bringing down the big merchandisers of drugs, the effect on drug usage has been minimal. The DEA would disagree with this analysis.

Beyond that, parents and schools are making some progress in convincing our children that there are better ways to deal

with a harsh world than through dependence on drugs.

All experts agree that to loosen the grip of drugs on America we must:

- inform everyone—children, parents, schools, and law enforcement officials—about the real and widespread dangers of drugs to individuals, communities, and the nation;
- arouse parents to take a stronger stand against drugs and to be better parents;
- initiate more effective programs in schools to prevent drug experimentation and help children already in trouble with drugs, and
- finance more research to find better treatments for those already trapped by drug addiction.

Nobody is certain that this program will work. But there seems very little more that one can do to curb the use and abuse of drugs.

Are You a Gambler?

AMERICANS SEEM TO ADMIRE THE BIG-STAKES gambler-hero in movies, the guy who risks and wins thousands on the turn of a card. In real life, compulsive gamblers who risk all, despite the odds, are pitied. They are losers, not heroes. Because they cannot stop, they often are broke, in debt,

and "borrowing" or stealing money to gamble. Their families are desperate.

In 1991, *Parade* surveyed men and women chosen at random in the United States to learn how Americans view and use money. Two key questions we asked were these:

- Do you gamble with more money than you can afford to lose?
- Do you bet on something whenever you can?

Of the 900 respondents, 2 percent replied "almost always" to both. We identified them as being in trouble over gambling. Projected nationally, this would indicate that the United States has 3.5 million adult compulsive gamblers. In addition, say other estimates, 1 million high school students and 650,000 college students are also compulsive gamblers.

Of our respondents, 20 percent said they gamble recklessly "often." Projected nationally, this 20 percent represents the approximately 35 million adults who probably account for most of the $290 billion spent on gambling in the United States last year. (The 1991 portion of our national debt was about $300 billion: Could this be a way to clear our credit?). Gambling is legal in 48 states. In the more than 30 states with lotteries, $20.8 billion is being spent a year on tickets.

Preventing pathological gambling is difficult in the face of seductive ads promising untold wealth. Lottery posters and TV ads in New York, for example, tempt and urge bettors, saying, "It only takes a dollar and a dream."

Chances of winning are minuscule, even with casino odds, which take "only" 3 to 5 percent for the house. No system beats the house in the long run. Sure, someone hits the $10 million lottery or the $1 million slot-machine jackpot. But for the overwhelming majority who never win, the big win is a carefully nurtured fantasy.

By my projections, gamblers—legal and illegal—are $200 billion in debt. And gambling is growing. There are new casinos in Nevada, Maryland, Atlantic City, and on Indian reservations. As gambling becomes legal in more places, the number of problem gamblers rises proportionally. Americans in 1996 wager twice what they bet in 1982.

Dr. Sheila B. Blume of the South Oaks Hospital psychiatric treatment center in Amityville, New York, has studied compulsive gamblers. "Most are never recognized or treated," Dr. Blume says. "The sad fact is that we have elderly women playing bingo 7 days a week with money they cannot afford to lose." (Bingo is now legal in 44 states.)

Compulsive gamblers pile up huge debts, according to Valerie C. Lorenz, executive director of the private National Center for Pathological Gambling in Baltimore. She surveyed members of Gamblers Anonymous (GA), a program modeled after Alcoholics Anonymous. The study found that the average gambler owed $75,000. (One GA member said he had issued IOUs for $1 million.)

Ms. Lorenz also found that, in Maryland, gamblers' losses for 1990 totaled $4 billion. National gambling costs—for losses, wagering dollars "borrowed" or stolen, treatment and missed work—neared $80 billion a year.

Most people can gamble without becoming addicted. The problem is to identify those who can't gamble socially without falling into the pit of uncontrolled wagering. Next, it's even a bigger difficulty to get them to avoid gambling *before* it becomes an addiction. No one knows how—yet. But the experts agree: Giving money to a gambler is like giving alcohol to an alcoholic. If your gambler won't seek treatment, stand aside or you almost certainly will be drawn into a web of lies spun to support this habit. Of course, you can try to ease the way, but the gambler must want to help him- or herself.

How can you tell whether someone is a gambling addict? Look for clues: betting slips, casino chips, unexplained big credit card debts, absences from home or work. Here's how gambling grows into addiction:

• Phase 1: "Social" gambling. Gambling is done less to be social and more to fill a need. Men need gambling for excitement; women, for escape. Wagers—and wins and losses—will increase.
• Phase 2: The trigger. A very large win is heady stuff. The gambler feels Lady Luck will repeat the win. This leads to large losses of money and self-esteem.
• Phase 3: The chase. To pursue wins, the individual places more and more bets. Addiction has set in. Big borrowing begins.
• Phase 4: The gambler feels out of control and tries to stop, feeling he or she

has hit bottom. In debt, the family devastated, gambling stops, then resumes with greater frenzy.
• Phase 5: The gambler bottoms out and finally seeks treatment. It could take years to reach it, but there is yet another bottom, with family and assets gone, a huge debt, and possibly a criminal record. Now treatment is *wanted*. Few compulsives achieve long-term abstinence, but victory is all the sweeter for those who do.

Says Howard Shaffer, director of the Norman Zinberg Center for Addiction Studies at Harvard, "Gamblers don't get the sympathy drunks or drug addicts get. We blame alcohol or drugs, which aren't the *cause* but rather are the *expression* of these addictions. Gambling can't be blamed on a substance, but gambling too expresses an addiction, not an evil personality."

Compulsive gambling is destructive and costly, and we are doing too little to stop it. Medical and scientific research may yield a solution, some day. But our social attitudes about gambling also could yield a great deal through change, today.

Take This Quiz

The following is a modification of a test developed by Professor Henry Lesieur of St. John's University in Queens, New York, and Dr. Sheila B. Blume of South Oaks Hospital in Amityville, New York.

Also included are questions from *Parade's* national money survey.

1. Do you often gamble with more money than you can afford to lose? Yes___ No___
2. When you gamble, do you ever go back another day to recoup your losses? Yes___ No___
3. Have you ever borrowed from people and not paid them back as a result of your gambling? Yes___ No___
4. Do you bet on something whenever you can? Yes___ No___
5. Did you ever gamble more than you intended? Yes___ No___
6. Have people criticized your gambling? Yes___ No___
7. Have you lost time from school or work because of gambling? Yes___ No___
8. Have you ever felt guilty about the way you gamble or what happens when you gamble? Yes___ No___

Scoring: One yes answer: You may have a problem. Two or more yes answers: You may well be an addict or heading for addiction. Ask for help from your doctor or Gamblers Anonymous (see the listing in your local telephone directory), or call South Oaks Hospital Gambler's Help Line: 1-800-732-9808 in New York State, 516-264-4000 outside New York, and ask for the Gambler's Help Line.

The Great Progress against Mental Disease

MENTAL ILLNESS OFTEN STARTS EARLY IN LIFE and ends late, leaving shattered families in its wake. It is more frightening, more mysterious, and more costly than almost any other disease.

Or it used to be.

That dark picture is brightening very rapidly now, thanks largely to the development of at least 50 new drugs that help check, if not cure, the worst of the major mental illnesses. They are schizophrenia, bipolar mood disorder (manic-depressive psychosis), major depression, obsessive-compulsive disorder, anxiety disorder, and panic disorder.

Back in 1960, when the population of America's mental institutions totaled 630,000, most people with these afflictions were doomed to pass their lives in grim incarceration. Now, properly treated and medicated, up to 80 percent of patients with the worst cases of those six mental illnesses can and do live normal or nearly normal lives.

Dr. David Pickar heads the experimental therapeutics branch of the National Institute of Mental Health (NIMH) in Bethesda, Maryland. Speaking for his fellow researchers, Dr. Pickar says, "There is a generation of us who have spent 20 years or more of our lives hoping, looking and tracking a big jump. The next giant step is in the immediate future."

In 1964, Dr. Benjamin Pasamanick, a medical researcher, boldly forecast that one day 80 percent of serious cases of mental disease could be treated at home with drug therapy. Few believed him. When he died in 1996, his prediction had almost come true for those with the major mental diseases discussed here.

Schizophrenia

Dylan Abraham, 40, of Madison, Wisconsin, was diagnosed at age 18 as having schizophrenia. "My symptoms began when I was 16," Mr. Abraham recalls. "They started with a sense of anxiety and unease. By 18, I was having hallucinations: I saw a gold rim of light around people. I heard voices. God and Satan were talking to me, telling me that I was godlike. I thought the CIA, the FBI, and the Communists were after me. I had totally lost it. I was arrested for disorderly conduct. My mother came to get me at the jail. She hospitalized me. That was in 1974."

The voices he heard did not exist in reality, of course. But to Mr. Abraham, those voices were quite real.

"I was totally psychotic," he says. "It was very frightening—the most frightening thing I had ever experienced."

With all that going on inside his skull, Mr. Abraham could not work, study, make friends, or simply sit still. The disease crashed over him in waves.

"When I went to get Dylan from the police that time back in 1974," recalled his mother, Nancy Abraham, "had I not known that it was Dylan, I would not have recognized him. He was so ill. I had lost the son I knew."

Those terrible times are now part of the past for Mr. Abraham, and they probably will stay there, so long as he takes his medication. In 1990, he was given Clozaril, then a new drug.

"In the last 5 years," he says, "Clozaril has wiped out the schizophrenia in me. I study tai chi, play volleyball, go to the gym. I'm dating."

Mr. Abraham is active in his church and in the local National Alliance for the Mentally Ill chapter, cofounded by his mother. He works as an aide at a private mental health center. He has many public speaking engagements on the topic of mental illness and has been recognized by the Wisconsin State Assembly for his work on behalf of mental illness.

Manic-Depressive Psychosis

This disease is also called bipolar mood disorder because the patient's mood will swing between the depths of sadness and the peaks of mania. At the depressed pole of the disease, patients often sit and contemplate suicide. Tragically, 15 percent do take their own lives.

At the manic pole, victims reach frightening peaks of excitement and agitation, and they speak very rapidly. They also engage in such risky activities as impetuous spending, incautious sex, and reckless driving.

Dr. William Z. Potter heads the section on clinical pharmacology at NIMH. "The main advance in manic depression," he says, "is the recognition that therapy with lithium produces good control in 50 to 60 percent of patients. Fortunately, studies now show that drugs usually reserved for the treatment of epilepsy also are very effective for mania." These include Depakote and Tegretol.

Dee Mukherjee, 32, is an attorney in Bethesda, Maryland. In 1982 she had what was diagnosed as a depressive occurrence. "I believed I was completely normal," says Ms. Mukherjee. "In 1987, I graduated with all A's at the top of my college class. Then I failed the bar exam. I remember that I was crying, not eating, not sleeping. I thought I was Jesus Christ.

"I did not believe I was sick," she continues. "It took me years to see the truth. I would take psychiatric drugs, and when I felt better, I would stop taking them. Then I'd get manic."

Doctors at that time had prescribed Haldol and lithium for her. Now Ms. Mukherjee takes lithium, Depakote, Risperdal, and Klonopin. NIMH statistics show that by treating a patient with a variety of medications, doctors have controlled the symptoms of bipolar mood disorder 80 percent of the time.

Major Depression

Patients with major depression are alarmingly prone to suicide. Using many medicines, physicians have been able to lift the depression in up to 65 percent of these cases.

Kay Phillips, 49, of Birmingham, Alabama, teaches computer use to people with disabilities. After struggling for 5 years with many prescriptions, she says, she finally found Dr. Ed Logue in Birmingham. He was testing Organon, a new drug. Ms. Phillips recalls that other medications she had taken had interfered with her sleep so severely that she'd been unable to keep a job.

"I was tired for 5 years," she says. "But when you find the right medication, it is incredible. My energy level was restored. No more anxiety."

Eventually, Ms. Phillips no longer needed the medication. "I'm depression-free now," she says. But she stays in close touch with Dr. Logue, who reports, "Things in Kay's life are going well now, and she is off medication. Unfortunately, the drug did not work as well for most of the other patients in the study, so we discontinued it." But, he added, he would prescribe another medication for Ms. Phillips if needed.

Years ago, patients with major depression had no treatment available except electroconvulsive therapy (ECT). Because that therapy—which sends small electrical currents into the brain—used to be somewhat dangerous, people still fear it. But new techniques in the hands of well-trained scientists have removed the danger. In fact, despite what most people believe, ECT is safer than most of the drugs now being prescribed. It even has an advantage over medicine: it acts rapidly, within days or weeks; drugs take longer, leaving the depressed patient vulnerable to suicide.

Obsessive-Compulsive Disorder

Until now, OCD, as it is called, had defeated all efforts at treatment. The patient suffers first from obsessions— thoughts or feelings he or she knows are unreasonable but that can't be shed.

For example, a patient becomes obsessed with the thought that everything is covered with deadly germs. The obsession might drive him or her to remove all the germs, lest a fatal disease be contracted. To do so, the patient might persist in washing and rewashing his or her hands or, perhaps, scrubbing all the doorknobs.

Dr. Rudolf Hoehn-Saric, a professor of psychiatry at the Johns Hopkins Medical Center in Baltimore, has made a specialty of treating this disease.

"We now have a number of drugs with which to treat OCD," he says. "All are effective, yet none is 100 percent effective. The symptoms rarely go away completely."

They once had to make do without even one drug available for the treatment of obsessive-compulsive disorder, but psychiatrists now have several, including Luvox, Prozac, Zoloft, and Anafranil, which make the brain less sensitive to obsessions. These drugs combine well with therapy that trains the patient to avoid having unwanted behavior triggered by unpleasant events. National Institute of Mental Health reports show that the success rate for the treatment of this disorder is almost 60 percent.

Anxiety Disorder and Panic Disorder

Philip Bosco, 65, one of America's great character actors, has performed in everything from Shakespeare to modern farce and drama. He lives in suburban New Jersey. Much of his work is done across the river in the Manhattan theater district. That was fine, except for his panic attacks.

"I didn't know what caused them," Mr. Bosco relates. "Day after day, I would find myself parked alongside the highway, sweating, unable to move. I knew that if I didn't get to the rehearsals, my career would be over."

An emergency visit to a psychiatrist solved his problem. Medications were prescribed. "Almost as soon as I began taking them," Mr. Bosco says, "it was like the lifting of a great weight." Overall, drugs have raised the success rate for treatment of anxiety disorder to 80 percent.

Dr. Michael R. Liebowitz directs the anxiety disorders clinic at the 100-year-old New York State Psychiatric Institute in Manhattan. Much of the revolutionary research on medications and mental disease was done there.

"Between 6 percent and 8 percent of the population has had at least one panic attack," Dr. Liebowitz estimates. "More important is that 1.5 percent have had recurrent attacks. Fortunately, we now have the tools to handle it."

Psychiatrists classify panic attacks as one of the several kinds of anxiety disorders. For most people, anxiety refers to a sense of fear and doom. Sometimes there is a ready reason for such a feeling. The patient may have had a close brush with death, and the fear lingers. In many cases, though, no apparent reason exists for the oppressive sense of foreboding.

As with obsessive-compulsive disorder, says Dr. Liebowitz, various medications help treat anxiety disorder. And psychotherapy combined with drugs can lead patients to respond more healthily to the bad news or trauma that triggers their illnesses.

Most of the dramatic treatments for mental illnesses have come from new information about how the brain works. In particular, scientists have homed in on the natural chemicals (neurotransmitters) that pass between the endings of adjacent neurons to form the brain's great communication system.

For reasons not yet entirely clear, patients with severe or moderately severe symptoms of mental illnesses appear to be deficient in one or more neurotransmitters. Modern drugs help balance the deficiencies.

As research continues to progress, more drugs will involve more and different neurotransmitters, probably simultaneously. Unfortunately, drugs cannot cure or relieve every patient of the symptoms of serious mental disorders. Medication has helped considerably to control, if not totally to cure, the more serious and disabling behaviors and thoughts.

As a result, though many patients retain them, the crippling behaviors of their illnesses are of much weaker intensity. With help from community mental health agencies, many more of the patients who are discharged can live independently and hold down jobs.

Since the 1960s, NIMH reports, the number of Americans in mental institutions has fallen by 85 percent. The new drugs developed since then unquestionably have contributed to this. Still, many patients today desperately need hospitalization, at least intermittently, because they are not completely cured.

Though much more remains to be done to improve mental health nationwide, many experts look to the future with considerable optimism. Among them is Dr. Herbert Pardes, vice president for health sciences at Columbia University in New York City. He also has served as chief of the National Institute of Mental Health.

"I think," Dr. Pardes predicts, "that psychiatry will increasingly use high-tech methods to study brain systems, genes, and behavior. I also think that we will learn how to intervene in mental illness much earlier than we do now. That should translate into less suffering and better lives."

For more information on the symptoms and treatments of mental illness (but not requests for physician referrals), write to the National Alliance for the Mentally Ill (NAMI), 200 N. Glebe Road, Arlington, VA 22203-3754. You also may call 1-800-950-NAMI.

If You Have an Eating Disorder

IN FEBRUARY 1996, A BENEVOLENT THRONG OF psychiatrists, psychologists, and other health specialists trekked to 600 college campuses to help young people suffering from a potentially fatal condition.

In those few days, they reached 20,000 students (mostly women) with severe eating disorders. Using educational materials and their own skills, the experts helped the students assess the extent of their disorders. They also learned how to identify the health-threatening warning signs as well as how to prevent illness. Screening results were kept strictly confidential.

Videos dramatized the problem. A questionnaire (presented later in this section) helped individuals learn whether they are at risk. The colleges had mental health specialists on site.

Eating disorders can and do kill. Some have death rates of up to 5 percent—higher than most of the other diseases that affect those aged 12 to 24 (with the exception of cancer). The eating disorders come in three varieties:

• Anorexia. The individual scarcely eats anything; body weight falls to as low as 85 percent of his or her ideal weight.

• Bulimia. Weight can approach normal, though the individual binges on large amounts of food and is obsessed with preventing the calories from turning into body fat. So the bulimic purges with laxatives, vomiting, and water pills and exercises heavily and constantly.

• Binge only. With this disorder, large amounts of food are eaten in short periods, with no purging. Overweight often results, without other major symptoms. The binge-only person takes control, for a while, slowly diets to "normal" weight, then binges and gains again.

This new battle against eating disorders is being waged by the National

Eating Disorders Screening Program. It is an outgrowth of the National Mental Illness Screening Project, which began an annual program in 1991 to screen men and women for depression. The screenings, held each October and announced in *Parade,* may have saved thousands from suicide by identifying those with severe depression and helping them get treatment.

Dr. Douglas G. Jacobs, a professor of psychiatry at Harvard Medical School, is a director of the screening programs both for depression and eating disorders. He has calculated that, as a result of the 1995 screening, 37,400 individuals with depression were referred for examination. And more than 1,000 persons were found to be so deeply depressed that they were hospitalized on the very day they were screened. "Most will feel better in 6 to 12 weeks," Dr. Jacobs said, "thanks to good medical treatments. We hope to do as well with the eating disorders."

Starting with the idea that some symptoms of eating disorders resemble some symptoms of depression, researchers theorized that drugs known to reverse depression might help treat eating disorders as well. Tests indicate that the medications do decrease the urge to binge. Physicians also prescribe group and individual counseling to control eating and to cope with the pressures to be thin.

Medical literature shows that 30 to 40 percent of food disorder cases persist for years. Among the famous women who say they have conquered food disorders are the actress Jane Fonda; Ellen Hart Peña, the wife of secretary of Transportation Federico Peña; and Princess Diana of England.

Officials of the National Eating Disorders Screening Program lined up 21 organizations of students and medical professionals. They include the American Psychiatric Association, the National Panhellenic Conference (sororities), USA Gymnastics, the U.S. Public Health Service, the American College Health Association, and the American College of Sports Medicine.

Catherine Baker, coordinator of Eating Disorders Services at Duke University in Durham, North Carolina, is very sensitive to the subject. "At age 14," she explains, "I developed an eating disorder for a few years because I had been assaulted. Eating disorders help us survive pain. I went through a deep depression. I hope the screening program will help students see that these behaviors hurt their lives."

Becky Guiffre, a student at the University of Maryland at College Park, became bulimic at age 12. "I would not eat for a few days," she says. "Then I'd gorge, then vomit 10 to 12 times a day. A specialist looked at the lining of my stomach: No lining was left. I can't say I never mess up now. But, mostly, I am recovered."

The National Institute of Mental Health in Bethesda, Maryland, estimates that 5 million Americans (nine women for every man among them) have eating disorders. But there are hints of improvement, probably as a result of changes in diet and self-image. The psychologist Todd F. Heatherton and his colleagues from Dartmouth College in Hanover, New Hampshire, report a drop of almost 10 percent in eating disorders at Harvard/Radcliffe, where students were surveyed in 1982 and again in 1992. Still, they found that one woman in 10 reported symptoms of serious eating problems. Their findings appeared in the November 1995 issue of the *American Journal of Psychiatry*.

Dr. David Herzog, a professor of psychiatry at Harvard Medical School and head of the Harvard Eating Disorders Center, is scientific director of the screening program. "Our culture demands thinness," he says, "especially among women. If the screenings help us identify symptoms before conditions become full-blown, we can help people back to health much earlier."

Do You Have an Eating Disorder?

Ask yourself these questions:

1. Do you restrict your intake to under 500 calories a day? Do you skip two or more meals a day?
2. Do you eat a lot of food within 2 hours, while feeling out of control?
3. To lose or control weight, do you use laxatives or water pills? Do you vomit or exercise excessively?
4. Do you avoid social functions or stay home from school or work to keep to an eating or exercise schedule?

"Yes" to any question indicates that you could be suffering from an eating disorder. Seek evaluation from a psychiatrist, psychologist, your physician, or a social worker.

For more information on eating disorders, write to Eating Disorders Awareness and Prevention, P.O. Box 14469, Seattle, WA 98114.

When Baby Needs a Therapist

TO THE OUTSIDER, THE SETTING RESEMBLES AN ordinary nursery school, except that there are far more "teachers" than usual, and some of the children are so young that they are still crawling.

Also on her hands and knees, one of the adults "plays" with Johnny, 2.5 years old. Dr. Eleanor Galenson, a psychiatrist, has just handed him a huge yellow-and-gray hammer made of sponge. He takes it and begins whacking away with all his might on a large red sponge block.

With each blow, Dr. Galenson says to Johnny, "Gee, you must be really angry. You really want to hit that block." Up to now, Johnny had pounded away with his fists—on other children, including his brothers. Johnny is one of a set of triplets. The psychiatrist is teaching him two things: First, it's OK to hit *nonliving* things. Second, he's putting a name on his feelings—anger.

"A healthy angry adult might work out his anger by talking or painting an angry picture or going for a run," says Dr. Galenson. "Sometimes, an unhealthy angry adult shoots somebody. Generally, that's a person who never learned to put a name on his feelings."

Dr. Galenson wants to intervene with Johnny before he grows up with twisted feelings. She wants him to experience the sort of babyhood that his mother, overwhelmed by having to care simultaneously for three infants, simply couldn't give him.

We are visiting a therapeutic nursery for disturbed children at Mount Sinai Medical Center in New York. Dr. Galenson and her partner, Dr. Herman Roiphe, with a squad of psychiatrists, psychologists, and volunteers, teach healthy babyhood to children between the ages of a few weeks and 3 years. These babies feel bad but cannot say how they feel.

Statistics are hard to come by, but one study suggests that three out of 100 children under the age of 3 have grave emotional problems and need help. With 9 million American children in that age group, that could mean that 270,000 babies are troubled. And such troubles could trigger personality problems that follow them into adulthood.

"These children are the ones who are most at risk for committing crimes and taking drugs, especially the boys," warns Dr. Galenson. (Since I visited Dr. Galenson, the nursery has been dismanteled because of a lack of funds.)

Dr. Jerry Wiener, of the American Academy of Child and Adolescent Psychiatry, says that the field of infant psychiatry has blossomed in the last 10 years.

"The most exciting change," says Dr. Wiener, "is this: We used to view the infant as a blank slate, molded and shaped by the home environment. But now we know that babies are much more active participants than we used to think."

For example, scientists now know for sure what parents had only suspected: each baby is born with a temperament unlike that of any other. Johnny is one of triplets, yet only he gives his mother difficulty; only he bites and hits. His two brothers are quiet and friendly.

Some children, from birth onward, do not like to be touched. Others may find high noise levels to be irritating. In fact, a baby comes into the world with a distinct personality, ready to respond in his or her individual way to parents and the environment. Each child is different.

Through his research, Dr. Jerome Kagan, a psychologist at Harvard University, found two types of children: One, by the middle of the second year, is timid and shy, fearful and wary. The other is outgoing, sociable, and not easily frightened. Both types can come from similar families.

By school age, half the fearful children Dr. Kagan had studied had lost their timidity; 10 percent of the fearless had become fearful. This, Dr. Kagan says, shows that although biology may produce a child who tends to be vulnerable (fearful), environment can push him or her into the other column. In short, if parents knew what to do, they could overcome biology.

Dr. Paul V. Trad, assistant professor of psychiatry and director of the Child and Adolescent Outpatient Department at Cornell University Medical Center in White Plains, New York, teaches the parents of his difficult infant patients how to deal with them. One, a 32-year-old mother who works outside the home, had given birth to a baby daughter who cried all the time. We'll call them Diane and Maggie.

"Every time Maggie cried, I'd think she needed feeding," Diane says. "I'd try to feed her, and she'd cry more. I'd try to play with her, and she would cry more. Then I'd get anxious, and it would get worse."

Diane and Maggie had what psychiatrists call a poor mother-child fit. Just because you're the parent doesn't mean you and your baby are guaranteed to like each other from the start. Some parents have to *learn* how to play with and love their babies.

Dr. Trad took videotapes of Diane playing with and feeding Maggie and then played them back. "It became clear that I was overanxious," Diane says. "I wasn't watching her. I didn't wait for her signal. I was doing too much. Watching the tape, you can see her turn away—that's a signal telling you, 'Don't press it.'"

Dr. Trad took Maggie on his lap and played with her to demonstrate how to watch for a baby's signals. "It's an adventure, learning about your own child," Diane says. "Now I am able to respond to her, and she has become a relatively easy baby."

But the adjustment is harder for babies born into what Dr. Stanley Greenspan calls multirisk families. Dr. Greenspan is clinical professor of psychiatry at George Washington University Medical School in Washington, D.C. In one study, he and Dr. Arnold Sameroff observed families without "difficult conditions" and others with problems that included one or more of the following:

- The father was absent.
- The mother had suffered from mental illness at least twice in her life.
- The mother was not spontaneous (i.e., didn't smile at or touch the child).
- The mother was highly anxious.

- The head of the household was unemployed or unskilled.
- There already were four or more children in the family.

If a family had none of these "risks," the average IQ for the child was 118. If more and more risks existed, the child's IQ dropped steadily, reaching 85 with seven or eight family problems. Generally, the high-risk families produced children with emotional problems.

Dr. Greenspan videotapes mother and child to find out how they get along. One 21-year-old unmarried mother with two children was videotaped with her infant son, Albert, when he was 4, 8, and 12 months old.

At the first taping, she played rough-and-tumble with Albert, then 4 months. She rocked him in her arms and held him affectionately—all good mothering techniques. At this age, Albert reacted far more often with pleasure than distress.

But by the next two tapings, Albert's mother had turned on him. She would take toys away from him and tease him by pretending to play with them herself. She slapped him on the wrist for no reason or threatened him with an upraised hand. Albert responded by avoiding his mother; he showed few signs of pleasure and gave many exclamations of distress. His behavior became aggressive. Mother and son were locked in battle.

How, as a parent, can you learn what to do? First, find out what behavior can be expected of your child at different ages. Dr. Greenspan gives the following timetable:

- 0–2 months: responds to sights and sounds; can calm self down
- 3–7 months: shows signs of pleasure and joy
- 4–9 months: communicates wishes by showing various feelings with gestures, facial expressions, and sounds
- 10–18 months: expresses complex feelings and demands with gestures, words
- 24–36 months: uses language and pretend-play to work out fears and emotional needs (e.g., may hug a doll when Mom is away)
- 30–48 months: employs logical thinking and demonstrates knowledge of the difference between reality and fantasy

Parents should seek help if a child does not show these coping skills roughly on this time schedule. Parents also should seek help if the child is constantly irritable, inattentive, withdrawn, won't eat, can't sleep, bites or hits other children, or doesn't talk by 18 months.

With help, parents can overcome some of these problems by learning to understand the baby's behavior and to respond to it by adjusting their own behavior accordingly. The first step, says Dr. Greenspan, is to establish a connection. You do this by playing on the floor with the baby. You learn to read the child's signals. With a passive infant—one who doesn't do or say much—you exaggerate: "Oh, what is this? Do you want to see that?" Then you follow up by engaging the baby's interest by pointing out details. With an active child, you try slowing and focusing techniques. If he or she stops at a toy, for example, engage the baby in talk about the object.

"One child we had in treatment," Dr. Greenspan relates, "would stop at a toy for only 2 seconds. We extended the stop to 6 seconds, eventually to 30 seconds."

He cites the following as problems likely to begin in infancy:

- Autism—The child doesn't communicate with any other human being.
- Depression—The child is sad, weepy, cannot sleep, cannot eat.
- Attention disorder—The child seems unable to focus on anything—toys or humans—for more than a few seconds.

Dr. Phillip Strain, an associate professor of psychiatry at the University of Pittsburgh, has a new way to deal with autistic children. In LEAP (Learning Experiences, An Alternative Program for Preschoolers and Parents), at the Mifflin School in Pittsburgh, he places normal children with the autistic children to serve as role models for behavior and communication.

"We get many to go on to kindergarten," Dr. Strain says. "And if we get the autistic child by 2.5 years, we usually can prevent the self-injury so common in these children." (Some of their self-destructive acts are head banging, eye gouging, hair pulling, and hand biting.)

Autism remains a mystery. Doctors theorize that some autistic children have a chromosome deficiency that may have caused the illness, while others may have got it from a virus. Under the best programs, some autistic children develop to their maximum potential.

Patty Caito placed her two normal children in Dr. Phillip Strain's autism program when they reached age 3. The experience of helping other children, says Mrs. Caito, enriched her children, too.

"There was an autistic child named David who never said a word," she relates. "He just screamed. After a few months, he was saying words. My kids would come home and say, 'Dave said this and Dave said that.' They loved seeing his progress."

Infant psychiatry itself is still in its infancy, but Dr. Stanley Greenspan asserts, "If we can provide them with the right emotional environment early enough, most of these troubled babies can be won."

For more information or for locations of the nearest therapy centers for children, write to the American Academy of Child and Adolescent Psychiatry, 3615 Wisconsin Ave., NW, Washington, D.C. 20016, or call (800) 333-7636.

Is That Child Bad—or Depressed?

AT FIRST, THE CHANGES IN JIM, 16, WERE MORE bothersome than frightening. A good student, he slowly dropped his studies. He wore his hair long and uncombed. He stayed up all hours of the night, keeping to his room, avoiding his family. Once a healthy eater, he turned to junk food. His table manners became messy.

Jim's parents reacted predictably. They nagged him to shape up. Despite a 10 P.M. curfew, Jim would stay out all night. Asked by his mother if anything was bothering him, he'd say, "Every thing is fine. Stay out of my life."

The story of Jerry, a high school senior, mirrored Jim's—until he tried to hang himself. He changed his mind at the last minute. "I didn't want to die," explains Jerry. "I was just frustrated." Jerry's attempted suicide so frightened his dad that he had his son hospitalized.

Parents of depressed teenagers say they feel "trapped," as if they are holding a hand grenade about to explode. They know something awful is happening to their child, but they don't know what.

Psychiatrists now say that teenagers like Jim and Jerry suffer from what once was seen as an "adult's disease": depression.

Dr. Mark Gold, former research director of Fair Oaks Hospital in Summit, New Jersey, says that depression seems different in teens because they are not fully developed. "An adult can tell you about his sense of foreboding, of unremitting sadness," says Dr. Gold. "He will tell of his problems with clear thinking. He will withdraw socially. He will use the words 'I'm depressed.' A teenager can't. His actions tell the story. A patient like Jim—with his food, behavior, and study problems—shows all the signs of a full-blown depression. He's sick. But to his parents, teachers, and friends, he seems to be a bad kid."

An estimated 10 percent of teenage boys and girls suffer bouts of depression. With teenagers numbering 20 million in the United States, that makes it a major problem. The annual suicide rate for ages 15 to 19 per 100,000 rose from 5.9 in 1970, to 8.5 in 1980, to 11.1 in 1990 (est.)

Doctors estimate that depression afflicts 40 percent of all teenagers who attempt suicide. Among them, the boys more often die than the girls, because boys generally choose more violent and lethal methods.

The victim of depression feels extremely sad for long periods, during which there is a loss of interest in life and an inability to manage well in everyday situations. In another form, manic depression, moods swing between depression (ranging from irritability to hopelessness) and mania (high elation, in which the patient feels like a superhero, with high levels of sensuality and talkativeness). Tragic events—a death, a traumatic accident—trigger some depressions; others seem spontaneous.

The illness need not end in suicide, life failure, or deep unhappiness. Doctors now prescribe mood-elevating drugs that reverse the symptoms in four of five patients. And new psychological techniques often work as well as drugs in lifting depression's dark cloud.

Jim, who doesn't want his real name used here, worked through his emotional problem with the help of a new psychological method. It's called cognitive therapy, because psychologists help patients change the way they think about things.

For example, at the hospital near San Diego where he began his treatment, Jim felt that the doctors and nurses judged him a failure. Craig Wiese, a psychologist, guided him in learning the truth. He had Jim interview the staff members and ask each, "How do you see me? Am I acting out of line?" To Jim's surprise, most said they thought he was a nice guy and his condition was improving. Once Jim confronted reality, he found that if he asked for help, he got it.

Step by step over several months, Dr. Wiese worked on Jim's distorted thoughts, especially his low self-esteem and his belief that anything he tried would end in failure. Jim went back in school, studying computers and electronics. He showed no signs of depression.

Another psychological approach is interpersonal therapy, based on the premise that the patient's depression is rooted in relating with others. It aims at improving social functioning.

Many psychiatrists, faced with treating acute cases (e.g., a potential suicide), turn to powerful drugs to lift the young person out of depression. Dr. Gold says, however, that the physician first must have the patient thoroughly tested to rule out a physical disease. "We found one youngster complaining of leg pains that his psychiatrist thought might be another symptom of depression," he notes. "It turned out that the boy had cancer of the bone."

First comes the diagnosis, then the treatment, which may include drugs. The drug imipramine works very well for young people, says Dr. Gold. A new method measures the amount of the drug in the blood to determine whether the patient is taking the right dosage. Such measurements have revolutionized drug treatment for depression and made it successful in up to 80 percent of teenage cases. Lithium salts also help young people, but they are mainly prescribed for manic-depressives.

Jerry, whose attempted hanging had led to hospitalization, eventually was cared for by Dr. Russell Marx of Regent Hospital in Manhattan. Dr. Marx prescribed desipramine, a chemical cousin of imipramine. Within 2 months, the depression lifted. Jerry was able to concentrate on his studies.

As do other physicians, Dr. Gold cautions that "you cannot just throw medication at a child." Psychological treatment helps the child develop socially and emotionally while fighting the depression. Without such help, Dr. Gold adds, the young person falls behind peers in learning how to deal with others and problems.

Family history plays a big role in teen depression. If depression afflicts one of the parents, chances are two in five that the children will suffer the same disease. Bad life circumstances also can trigger or prolong depression. Physically or mentally abused children tend to be depressed. Children in families with marital discord also suffer from depression.

It is extremely important that the family participates in treatment; otherwise, the teen whose depression has been lifted by drugs or therapy or both might return to a family situation that could trigger the illness all over again.

"Depression is a disease," says Dr. Gold. "It's treatable. Untreated, it's deadly."

A Father's Story

A father who first denied the truth, then dealt with it, tells of his experience to help other parents who might be baffled as to what to do to help their own depressed teenagers.

"At first, you tell yourself, 'He's a teenager and is just going through a phase.' So you reassure yourself: 'This will pass.' But, little by little, the behavior becomes more aberrant. Initially, your child does attention-getting things that are out of line but fall just short of crossing that socially acceptable line— they are not quite 'abnormal.'

"Then the phone calls start coming from his friends, from their parents, from his teachers, his coach, his principal, from neighbors, from the preacher. They tell you they've seen him do reckless things—diving from a cliff into lakes he has never swum before, taking ski jumps when he's never been trained to do them. I got to hoping he might break a leg and be hospitalized for 6 weeks or so. It would keep him from killing himself and give us all a rest.

"Next came the flamboyant dressing—necklaces, eyeliner, punk clothing. He's determined to shock.

"He objects strenuously even to the mildest household rules—a 10 P.M. curfew on school nights, for example. He begins to make sexually suggestive comments about girls. And he starts dating a string of girls from school—six or seven—regularly. All of this is uncharacteristic. We had a stranger in our house who looked like our son but acted like no one we knew.

"Anger or scolding produced violent reactions in him. We found a psychiatrist who was helpful, but still we weren't fully satisfied.

"Then our son changed again. He started to make frequent references to deep unhappiness. He couldn't concentrate on his studies. Passively suicidal feelings began to emerge. He'd say things like, 'I wish I were dead.'

"That, we came to learn, was the downside of his illness—the depressed phase of manic depression. In the up side—the manic phase—you don't feel effective as a parent, and you aren't, but you sometimes do have some impact on him. In the depressed phase, you can't get through at all. For instance, he'd play basketball and blame himself mercilessly for imagined blunders. He confided how he'd be in the middle of a game and find himself observing his actions as though he'd stepped out of his body. In a very real sense, he was disconnected from himself, from others, from life.

"We could see he was on the borderline of crossing from normal to something terrible. We found another psychiatrist. We had him institutionalized for about 6 weeks. Probably he'll never forgive me for this. But it did help.

"The doctors finally diagnosed him: manic-depressive. Now, at least, what was wrong with him had a name—and a course of treatment.

"Once word got around about his illness, confidences came pouring in. People who never would have told you such things before came out with confessions and reassurances. They were manic-depressive. Or their son or husband or sister was, and lithium helped them.

"Knowing what I know now, having learned the hard way, I can see that this illness, manic depression, was as readily observable as mumps.

"He has made great progress, thanks to lithium treatments the doctor prescribes. But it's a rough go, and the parents and the siblings of manic-depressives need help to cope. If there were a group of people who have lived through similar experiences or who are living through them now, I'd certainly welcome the chance to join them."

There is such a group. For information about how to join, write to the National Depressive and Manic-Depressive Association, 730 North Franklin, Chicago, IL 60610.

What Parents Can Do

Parents can get help before depression overcomes their child and before suicide looms. Here are some pointers:

- Be ready to accept the idea that your child may be depressed; denying it may blind you to the facts.
- Make room for the adolescent's thoughts and concerns; concentrating on yourself shuts out your child.
- *Really* listen to what your child is saying; allow for differences of opinion.
- Be aware: Are you pressing your child to live out your fantasy—to be the baseball player you were not, perhaps?
- Keep communicating; if you stop, you're walking away.

- Listen to your child's teacher; don't blame the teacher for having noticed signs of the disease.
- Be ready to accept outside guidance—first, perhaps, from your family doctor, later from a psychiatrist or psychologist.

Warning Signs

You can spot early warnings of the onset of depression, such as these:

- Changes for the worse in personal habits—dirty clothes, messy room
- Decline in school achievement
- Loss of interest in activities that once gave pleasure—participating in sports or going to the movies, for example
- Quick to tears; increase in sadness, moodiness
- Changes in sleep behavior; too much sleeping or too little, including fitful sleep or rising too early
- Loss of appetite
- Use of alcohol, marijuana, or other drugs
- Talk of death and dying, even in a "joking" fashion
- Sudden withdrawal from friends, family; moping around the house

If these symptoms persist for more than 10 days, seek professional help.

Should You Spare the Rod?

WE ALL KNOW THAT PRAISE WORKS BETTER than punishment in helping a child learn or behave. Or do we? Scientific observations reveal that parents and teachers alike tend to scold, mock, deprive, and strike children more often than they offer a few kind words.

Walk into any classroom. Count the number of times the teacher praises his or her pupils; also count the condemnations, insults, and threats. Negative words, as scientific research shows, outnumber helpful words by three to one (or more) in most classrooms. Ironically, punishment works only to control the worst behavior—fighting, lying, cheating, stealing.

The National Institute of Education estimates that school vandalism costs this country almost $500 million a year. In one California school system, a praise-and-reward program paid off by cutting school vandalism by 78.5 percent, and one school saved $25,000 over the previous year. Other schools have reduced absenteeism from 33 percent to a scant 2 percent with free pizza and other rewards for perfect attendance.

The Los Angeles County Office of Education developed a "constructive discipline" program for students. Its chief architects were G. Roy Mayer, a professor of education at California State University at Los Angeles, and Thomas W. Butterworth, now a retired consultant. The program cut vandalism and absenteeism in Los Angeles schools. Parents easily can adapt it at home. The technique has three parts:

1. Reward good behavior with praise, recognition, prizes, and privileges.
2. Ignore minor infractions or work out deals to reward children for reducing minor misbehavior.
3. Punish only major misbehavior—vandalism, truancy, disruption, fighting, resisting authority, drug use. (The punishments in schools range from a conference called with student and parents to suspension, expulsion, and even a call to the police.) Constant punishment actually induces students to escape through being tardy, skipping class, or dropping out of school. Children punished for every little thing also become more violent and destructive. It was found that vandalism was highest in schools where teachers abused their students the most. After a special teachers' training program on how to be more positive, the incidence of vandalism in those schools plummeted.

Corporal punishment—spanking, paddling, whipping—actually may teach children to be physically aggressive toward those less able to defend themselves. (Physically abused children often grow up to be abusive parents.)

The absenteeism program at San Gabriel High School in California uses constructive discipline this way: Marisela Adams, the attendance counselor, sets up clear rules for unexcused tardiness or absences. The first incident results in a talk with a teacher; the second causes a postcard to be sent to the youngster's home. At the ninth incident, the student comes in for a 4-hour Saturday work/study program. The 12th truancy or tardiness results in suspension.

On the positive side, students with perfect attendance are eligible for free pizzas, hamburgers, football game tickets, and buttons saying, "I am perfect."

Dr. Beth Sulzer-Azaroff, a professor of psychology at the University of Massachusetts at Amherst, says, "With positive techniques, children learn better and retain their lessons longer. What's more, the positive approach to learning is fun."

She cautions to be careful with praise, however, and gives these hints: Praise the deed, not the child. You might say, for example, "That's a well-drawn picture, Lilly." Not, "You're a good artist, Lilly." And your facial expression must say, "I mean it."

For children who have been starved for praise, words alone may not work, so tangible rewards are given. Some teachers give out points for good behavior, and children trade the points later for prizes. Such a scheme is called a *contract*. And parents can adapt it to reward a child for any desired behavior—washing dishes, taking out the trash, studying, using good table manners. Parents and child agree on what kind of behavior wins points, how many points get the prize, and what the prize is. Parents must never fail to honor a commitment.

Once the behavior is learned, set up a new contract for a new behavior. Phase out the rewards for learned behavior, so that it becomes important for its own sake. Also, to keep the contract intact, if a child fails to win points for some days, ignore this failure.

Many teachers and parents argue that children should not be rewarded for things they ought to do anyway. They call that bribery. Professors Sulzer-Azaroff and Mayer point out that bribery induces illegal or immoral acts. By re-

warding good behavior, they note, you are not inducing something illegal or immoral. The reward is to the child's advantage, not to the advantage of the reward giver.

While most psychologists agree that praise works better than punishment as do tangible rewards, teachers and parents must be wary of killing a child's curiosity and innate eagerness to learn. If a child learns to work only for rewards, they soon lose interest in studying or practicing for their own sakes. However, praise and tangible rewards can jumpstart a change of miscreant behavior.

Dr. Mayer adds that most adults are paid for their work and says there is nothing wrong with paying children for *their* "work." So give children their "paycheck": smile!

Relax—It Can Be Good for What Ails You

RELAXATION, SCIENTISTS ARE FINDING, DOES much more than reduce stress. It also can relieve pain and help control sickness. More and more is being learned about how tension—emotional stress—is bad for both your mind and body. Doctors are now prescribing relaxation training as part of the treatment not merely for

minor ills but also for infertility, heart disease, and, sometimes, even cancer.

The concept of relaxation as good medicine, once totally dismissed by scientists, is accepted now, thanks largely to Dr. Herbert Benson, an associate professor at Harvard Medical School and the founder of the Mind/Body Medical Institute at New England Deaconess Hospital in Boston.

When the mind is stressed—by anxiety or anger, for example—the body responds. Metabolism, heart rate, blood pressure, breathing, and muscle tension rise. These reactions date to prehistoric humans, who, if faced with danger, chose either to fight or to take flight. Hormones pour out to ready you for action. One hormone, epinephrine, speeds up the heart. But if your heart is weak and the small arteries feeding blood to it are blocked with fats, epinephrine might overload your heart. It is in just such a case that relaxing could help save your life.

Through effort and training, Dr. Benson says, you can learn how to quiet yourself down and summon at will the healing changes in body chemistry called "the relaxation response." For 20 years, Dr. Benson tested and ultimately proved the healthful effects of relaxation. He recorded changes in the bodies of his subjects and their diseases after treatments combining medication, relaxation therapy, nutrition, exercise, and stress management. He compared them with control groups of similarly ill but untreated subjects. In *The Wellness Book,* Dr. Benson and Eileen M. Stuart, R.N., tell how to elicit the relaxation response and gives details on many routes to reach it.

Dr. Redford Williams, professor of psychology and director of the Behavioral Medical Research Center at Duke University in Durham, North Carolina, terms relaxation "a critical element" in stopping or slowing disease when combined with a variety of psychological methods. "Studies published recently have shown these interventions improve prognoses in cancer and heart disease," says Dr. Williams. Today, data support relaxation as being able to, among other things:

- cure some cases of infertility,
- lower high blood pressure,
- help control glucose and insulin levels in those with diabetes, and
- slow the progress of heart disease.

Amazingly, relaxation has also been proved to cure cases of infertility that have no obvious biological cause. (Good news for those enduring costly, sometimes painful infertility tests and treatments.)

Dr. Reed C. Moskowitz of New York City and his wife, Debra, had taken every test known to medical infertility experts. Nothing worked. At New York University Medical Center, he is director of Stress Disorders Medical Services and a clinical assistant professor of psychiatry. Debra Moskowitz is an attorney. In 1989, she complained of stress at work. Dr. Moskowitz knew of a study led by Dr. Benson. In it, childless couples with no known physical cause for infertility showed good results after relaxation therapy: 18 pregnancies of 54—a success rate of 33 percent, compared with 25 percent at fertility clinics. Dr. Moskowitz reasoned that stress-induced hormones were pouring into his wife's system, perhaps impeding conception. He'd helped patients overcome stress; now he'd help his wife.

They practiced breathing and muscle relaxation, visualizing a healthy, growing baby. In days, Mrs. Moskowitz mastered the relaxation technique. In months, she was pregnant. On October 10, 1990, their daughter, Marissa, was born; their son, Craig, arrived on January 25, 1995.

Relaxation helped Don Wood, too. "I had borderline high blood pressure but didn't want to take drugs," says Mr. Wood, 48, a computer technician at New England Deaconess Hospital. He also had tension headaches and neck pains. In early 1992, he entered a cardiac risk reduction program at Deaconess emphasizing diet, exercise, and relaxation. His pain eased, and he had 75 percent fewer headaches. "I was amazed," Mr. Wood says.

The American Diabetes Association reports that research shows relaxing can help some diabetics to control blood glucose levels, which can be harmed by stress. Stress also can raise the need for insulin while blocking its release.

The relaxation response can be induced in several ways. I learned how with a method introduced back in the 1920s by Dr. Edmund Jacobson of the University of Chicago. He taught patients to unwind by progressively relaxing muscle groups, from their soles to their scalps. "Curl your toes," he would say. "*Hold* them in that position. Feel the tension in the muscles of your feet [soles, toes, arches, heels, ankles]. Now, slowly release the muscles; let the tension drain away. Think of something pleasant."

Later, listening to his tape-recorded instructions, I soon felt the relaxation response of floating above my bed.

Here are some other tools to help you induce a relaxation response:

• Biofeedback. By recording biological changes in your pulse rates, temperature, muscle tension, and sweat, machines can show your body's feedback. A TV monitor shows your heart speed up or slow down in response to your thoughts, to see which relax you.

• Hypnosis. A hypnotist might put you into a quiet state. By self-hypnosis, some can learn to do this for themselves.

• Imagery. Imagining quiet scenes often seems to trigger the relaxation response. Some researchers contend that imagery can help patients to slow their cancer, but doubt persists.

• Breathing. Most of us don't breathe deeply enough. Shallow breathing will lead to shortness of breath and chest tightness—symptoms of stress. Focus on deep breathing for relaxation.

The World Health Organization has approved the relaxation response as part of the treatment for high blood pressure. Combined with nutrition and exercise, doctors see it easing depression, painful AIDS symptoms, headaches, back pain, and other ills.

Dr. Williams, of Duke, in his study of the impact of hostile feelings on the heart, found that angry people suffered more heart disease than calm ones. "These studies of relaxation and other stress management techniques," he says, "suggest stress management is ready for more extensive clinical trials."

The wide range of research on relaxation, and the role the mind plays in healing the body, offer hope for controlling an ever-widening range of diseases.

For more information, write to Division of Behavioral Medicine, Mind/Body Medical Institute, Deaconess Hospital, 1 Deaconess Road, Boston, MA 02215.

Is Your Job Killing You?

IF NEWS REPORTS TOLD OF JET PLANES CRASHING everyday, killing 243 passengers and crew each time, neither the public nor government authorities—including the President—would stand idly by for long. Things would begin to happen quickly either to improve the safety of the planes or to put them out of business.

But according to studies by the National Safe Workplace Institute in Chicago, an estimated 240 people die every workday in this country as a result of on-the-job accidents or protracted job-related illnesses. And not much—certainly not nearly enough—is being done about it.

Add it up: 243 deaths every workday equals 60,000 deaths a year, and the figure might be as high as 70,000. Each year, 6,000 individuals die in this country from *injuries* sustained on the job, according to 1985 figures compiled for Congress by the Office of Technology Assessment. Others suffer illnesses brought on by exposure at work to chemicals, dust, and other noxious materials, which cause their deaths many years later. Most workers in dangerous jobs aren't even aware of the risks they run simply by working at them. (Most of the figures in this section have increased since 1990; exact totals are not known.)

And, except in California, where employers convicted of operating unsafe workplaces are sometimes sent to prison, most public agencies seem to make light of the situation. In the last 8 years, the federal government has won only two criminal cases against employers who defied safety rules. In that same period, California won 112 cases against employers.

Joseph A. Kinney, an ex-marine and Vietnam vet, got mad enough to fight for safe workplaces. His youngest brother, Paul, died in 1986 at age 27 when a building scaffold collapsed in Denver. His brother's death tore him up. "The fire captain who supervised the rescue called my brother's death a travesty," Mr.

Kinney recalls. "He could see that the scaffold was not properly erected." In May 1987, he started the National Safe Workplace Institute to research job safety and prod lax government agencies.

Not only construction work holds dangers. Shockingly, for women at work, murder is the greatest risk, according to J. Paul Leigh of San Jose State University in California. He studied the risk of death in 347 occupations, using 1970 Census Bureau job categories. Nothing has changed much since then.

"Women are not taking a lot of blue-collar jobs that involve a lot of danger," Mr. Leigh says. "They take service jobs at an all-night grocery or a liquor store or a photo development booth. They get robbed and they get killed."

Kathy Fisler, 28, works in a convenience store near her home in San Jose. She has been robbed once, and an 18-year-old girl was killed while working nearby in a photo development booth.

"It got me a little leery," she recalls. "But if you're paranoid, you shouldn't work here. I had a cop tell me he would not want my job."

Mr. Kinney says that of an estimated 7,000 people who die on the job each year, he has seen research indicating that 350 are women and that murder accounts for 42 percent of their deaths.

One expert suggests that taking easy measures could reduce the number of attacks on women clerks in stores: Keep the cash register in view from the street. Use a drop safe to deposit bills larger than $1. Greet each person who enters.

In Mr. Leigh's analysis, all but one of the 30 occupations ranked as having the highest risk of death in the United States are in the blue-collar or service trades. The exception is airplane pilots, who are second only to loggers overall. Among white-collar workers, messengers and office helpers follow pilots in risk of death. Managers and department heads of retail stores are third. Unexpectedly, astronomers and physicists are seventh, coaches and gym teachers 14th, and athletes 18th. Editors and reporters ranked 35th. Mr. Leigh ranks job risks for embalmers and librarians at zero.

By industry, farming placed first for 1987, passing mining as most dangerous, according to the National Safety Council. Building construction was next, followed by transportation and public utilities. Even though in 1987 the manufacturing industry had fewer on-the-job deaths and was ranked as four times safer than transportation, it still accounted for 1,100 deaths and 300,000 disabling injuries. Exposure to toxic materials may make manufacturing the most risky segment in the long run. Overall, 1.8 million Americans suffered crippling injuries on the job in 1987.

On the farm in 1987, tractor rollovers, accidents involving machine gears, and dozens of miscellaneous mishaps took 1,600 lives and caused 160,000 others to be incapacitated. Some studies indicate that a quarter of the farm casualties were children under the age of 15.

Two years ago, Darrell and Marilyn Adams, who own a 500-acre farm in Earlham, Iowa, lost their son, Keith, 11. He was sucked into a grain-filled wagon and suffocated.

Family-owned farms are not under government safety supervision, and they often lack the money needed to update and improve the safety of their equipment. Children frequently do farm chores that exceed their abilities. Farming illustrates the main causes of the safety malaise that afflicts the American workplace: little or weak government regulation, lack of safety features on equipment, and inadequate training.

Until recently, the burden of safety was put on the worker, with urgings to be careful. Most experts now say that, in a dangerous occupation, even the most cautious operator runs too high a risk. Many bosses ignore safety problems because they see the costs of workers' protection cutting into profits.

In Los Angeles, former District Attorney Ira Reiner gave bosses of unsafe operations a new motivation to make their places safe: he arranged for their prosecution and trial; some even were sent to prison. Twenty-four hours a day, 7 days a week, Mr. Reiner had a lawyer and an investigator standing by, ready to respond to the report of a death on the job.

"When a worker is killed, fellow workers are appalled and upset and will speak candidly to investigators immedi-

ately after the accident," Mr. Reiner explained. "But if you wait a few days, things change. The employer talks to the other workers, who see their jobs at stake.

"By then, an entirely different attitude has set in. If there is a deliberate violation of the law, the highest company official who had guilty knowledge will be personally charged. We are now getting phone calls from lawyers at corporations, asking our advice on how to set up safety programs."

In July 1987, California Governor George Deukmejian killed the state's office of the Occupational Safety and Health Administration (CAL-OSHA). He turned inspection and regulation over to the Federal OSHA. Last November, voters restored the state's jurisdiction to inspect private-sector workplaces.

John Lynch, who once headed Ira Reiner's occupational crimes unit says, "I have seen a dramatic increase in fatalities since the feds took over." The federal agency rarely refers cases for prosecution. Instead, the agency relies on "megafines," penalties that can total more than $1 million.

John Pendergrass, of OSHA, says that his is a civil, not a criminal agency. "We want the employer to make the workplace safe in a timely manner," he says. So OSHA imposes the heavy fines, which can increase as time elapses, to motivate employers to act promptly.

Joseph Kinney of the National Safe Workplace Institute says that OSHA often ends up cutting its fines by 50 percent or more, taking the bite out of them. Mr. Pendergrass says OSHA's approach obviously works because the on-the-job death rate is dropping. This, counters Mr. Kinney, is a mirage due in part to a shift in employment—from risky manufacturing, mining, and farming jobs to jobs in the far less hazardous service in-

dustries, including retail trades, repairs, and offices.

Moreover, Mr. Kinney says, in the last 8 years, owing mainly to OSHA's weak approach to job safety, the decline in the death rate has slowed from 2.2 percent annually to only 0.7 percent. If the reduction had continued at the old

A Listing of Occupations Ranked in Order of Risk

Blue-Collar Jobs		White-Collar Jobs	
Rank/Job	Deaths per 100,000	Rank/Job	Deaths per 100,000
1. Timber cutters and loggers	129.0	1. Airplane pilots	97.0
2. Asbestos and insulation workers	78.7	2. Office helpers and messengers	14.5
3. Structural metal workers	72.0	3. Retail sales managers and department heads	12.3
4. Electric power-line and cable installers and repairers	50.7	4. Geologists	9.5
5. Firefighters	48.8	5. Agricultural scientists	9.0
6. Garbage collectors	40.0	6. Vehicle dispatchers and starters	8.3
7. Truck drivers	39.6	7. Physicists and astronomers	7.6
8. Bulldozer operators	39.3	8. Construction inspectors (public administration)	7.6
9. Earth drillers	38.8	9. Meter readers, office machine operators	7.4
10. Craft apprentices	37.5	10. Engineers	7.3
11. Miners	37.5	11. Public administrators and officials	7.2
12. Boilermakers	35.0	12. Weighers	7.1
13. Taxicab drivers and chauffeurs	34.0	13. Science technicians	6.7
14. Construction workers, carpenters' helpers	33.5	14. Coaches and physical education teachers	6.6

(continues)

2.2 percent rate, Mr. Kinney says, nearly 4,000 fewer deaths would have occurred in the last 4 years. Pendergrass calls this "statistical manipulation."

The records show that OSHA issued 1,238 citations for "willful" violations (the gravest of its offense categories) in 1980 but only 523 in 1981, the first year of the Reagan Administration. Last year's total was 1,159. In addition, OSHA cut its inspectors from 1,350 in 1980 to 1,150 in 1981.

Mr. Pendergrass says OSHA is doing better with fewer inspectors and fewer citations. But the experts we talked with say they doubt this. They also criticize

A Listing of Occupations Ranked in Order of Risk (continued)

Blue-Collar Jobs Rank/Job	Deaths per 100,000	White-Collar Jobs Rank/Job	Deaths per 100,000
15. Millers	33.3	15. Private administrators and managers	6.6
16. Surveyors' helpers	33.3	16. Real estate agents	6.6
17. Sheriffs and bailiffs	32.4	17. Pharmacists	6.5
18. Roofers and slaters	31.9	18. Athletes, kindred workers	6.5
19. Metal molders	26.6	19. Surveyors	6.1
20. Flight attendants	23.0	20. Building superintendents	5.8
21. Oilers and greasers	22.5	21. Veterinarians	5.2
22. Excavating, grating, and road machine operators	20.9	22. Assessors	5.2
23. Crane operators	19.3	23. Restaurant managers	5.1
24. Police and detectives	17.5	24. Computer specialists	5.0
25. Bakers	16.9	25. Insurance adjusters	4.9
26. Engravers	16.6	26. Sales managers	4.7
27. Millwrights	15.5	27. Union officials	4.6
28. Sawyers	15.4	28. Funeral directors	4.5
29. Tailors	15.0	29. Architects	4.3
30. Forge and hammer operators	14.2	30. School administrators	4.2
31. Farm machine operators	14.2	31. Chemists	4.0
32. Plasterers	14.2	32. Inspectors	3.9
33. Ship fitters	14.2	33. Ticket agents	3.7
34. Butchers	13.8	34. Advertising agents	3.6
35. Loom operators	12.5	35. Editors and reporters	3.6

him for not setting priorities to go after dangerous industries, and they say he has not established safety standards in a timely way. It takes 2 to 6 years for a regulation to get on the books. And hundreds of industrial chemicals are so new that no rules have been formulated yet to regulate their use or storage.

Has OSHA been effective?

Says Stephen Bokat, vice president and general counsel of the U.S. Chamber of Commerce, an organization of businesses, "On the whole, yes. But there are failings. The standard-setting process is ludicrous. They don't set priorities and they don't help employers—especially the small ones—to comply with the rules."

Asked the same question, John Moran says he has reason to doubt that OSHA and the federal government have a serious interest in preventing on-the-job injury and death. For 4 years, Mr. Moran headed the safety division of the government's National Institute for Occupational Safety and Health. He created the first national census of occupational deaths, a study that revealed 7,000 job fatalities a year. He resigned soon after the study's completion, in February 1988.

"After this report was issued, we were not able to publish anything else," Mr. Moran says.

Many experts worry about the unseen chemical "time bombs" that lurk in many workplaces. Asbestos is the most notorious example. Dr. Philip Landrigan, director of the Division of Environmental and Occupational Medicine at Mount Sinai School of Medicine in Manhattan, says we are beginning our third wave of asbestos illness.

The first came in World War II, when thousands of shipyard workers breathed in the asbestos fibers that lined ships' walls and hot pipes. Three decades later, these same workers came down with lung cancer and other diseases. In the 1950s and 1960s (second wave), construction workers sprayed asbestos on steel beams. We are seeing their illnesses now.

In the 1980s (third wave), the workers removing the asbestos were inhaling its microscopic fibers; they will be sick by the year 2000.

For years, tannery workers have breathed and touched powerful chemicals used to cure leather. Some of these chemicals, new research indicates, may trigger cancer.

In a tannery in Johnstown, New York, three coworkers on the same shift on the finishing line developed cancer of the testicles. All had been exposed to DMF—dimethyl formamide—a chemical used widely in the tanning industry. Dr. Stephen Levin of Mount Sinai's Department of Environmental Medicine says a New York State Department of Health study found that the case histories of those with testicular cancer frequently show them to be tannery workers who possibly were exposed to DMF. "The relationship between DMF and testicular cancer has not yet been directly proven," says Dr. Levin, "but this is of concern to the scientific community."

Do you believe your job threatens your health or safety? You can report bad working conditions to OSHA by filing a complaint under Section 11(c) of the Job Safety Act. The system is *supposed* to help and protect workers against discrimination by the boss.

But some workers say they complained to OSHA and later learned that they had been named as informers to their bosses. They suspect OSHA of the leak. Joseph Kinney says it must be noted that the OSHA inspector's job is not problem-free. "Sometimes," he explains, "workers

who are angry will take revenge by phoning in a false safety violation."

Now a new approach is being tried. In 1987, the New York State Legislature set aside $1 million for a network of clinics to diagnose and treat job-related illness.

"With this program," says Dr. Landrigan, "we can go to the workplace, speak to the manager or union bosses, and screen other workers who might be exposed to similar hazards. This is a way to prevent disease, which you cannot do under workers' compensation." He adds that New Jersey and Massachusetts may start similar programs.

Is Your Job Good for You?

NEARLY ANYONE WHO HAS WORKED FOR SOMEone else has run into a manager who was cruel or incompetent or both. That manager's qualities kill your desire to work. New research shows that they could kill you, too—by eliciting from you feelings of being trapped, helpless, and inefficient in a bad job. This can become unhealthy for you and the business too, harming both job performance and product quality.

Evidence is mounting that a bad job can raise your blood pressure during working hours and keep it elevated long after quitting time. Doctors are accumu-

lating biological data that support this observation. And other bad-job studies show they can boost the risk of hospitalization for suicide attempts, alcohol-based illnesses, digestive diseases, mental problems, and traffic accidents. Bad jobs also are linked with higher rates of heart disease.

What are the markings of a "bad job"? Yours is bad if *both* of the following hold true:

• You have no or low control over what you do and how you do it. (Your boss

insists on making and enforcing decisions.)
• You have a job with high psychological
demand. (You must do too much work
in too little time.)

A low-control/high-demand job lands
a one-two punch to your psyche, brain,
heart, and body. You're locked into using
work methods that don't suit you, and
you're pushed to work too quickly.

There's a third job element: social
support. Without it, a bad job becomes a
horror. With it, a bad job is less bad. You
get social support when your coworkers
and supervisor reach out to help when
you need it.

Lisa Webster, 21, says she loves her
customer service job at Smalley Transportation Company, a trucking outfit in
Tampa, Florida. She says she quit a "very
stressful" job as an airline reservations
agent, taking hundreds of calls from
irate customers with no chance to respond creatively or discuss problems or
ideas. "Now," says Lisa, "I can share a
problem with a coworker. My supervisor
wants to hear my suggestions. The big
boss listens too."

Robert A. Karasek, professor of work
environment at the University of Massachusetts at Lowell, says about 20 percent
of American men hold bad jobs. He began
researching job strain and heart disease in
1980. Dr. Karasek says holders of low-in-
come jobs—clerks, laborers, waitresses—
are more likely to face job strain than are
bosses or various professionals, such as
engineers. More research may prove that
workers in high-strain jobs also are more
at risk for heart disease.

A study of 215 men by Dr. Peter L.
Schnall, a cardiologist at New York Hospital in Manhattan, revealed that those
who complained of job strain were more
likely to have high blood pressure. Pictures of the heart made by high-frequency
sound waves—sonograms—revealed that
the muscled walls of their hearts were
thicker. Such pictures predict a high risk
of heart attack.

"We identified a risk factor that
links job strain and hypertension," says
Dr. Schnall, "but more research must be
done."

The stress culprits, Dr. Karasek says,
are bosses and supervisors who, in the
name of short-term efficiency and profits,
dehumanize work and tell people how
to do their jobs, allowing employees no
input.

Robert Hogan, chairman of the psychology department at the University of
Tulsa, asserts that "60 percent to 75 percent of American managers are incompetent." He says bad managerial styles
include these:

• The arrogant manager. Know-it-
all; beats up on workers; makes a sudden
impact, then moves on
• The charmer. Highly likable, lazy;
has no agenda; does no work; can't be
fired; has no enemies

- The passive aggressive. Very smart, with lots of social skills; seems non-hostile but strikes back sneakily when criticized

A *good* manager, says Dr. Hogan, is considerate, provides structure for the workers, tells them what needs to be done, when it is due, how a good job should look, and gives them frequent feedback. He wants subordinates to evaluate their managers—anonymously—so bad managers can learn quickly that they are not liked, not leading, and not obeyed.

"Bad management is a principal cause of stress in the workplace," Dr. Hogan says. "It also is costly: employees get ill, complain, and don't perform."

Professor Karasek notes that since 1911, American business has been ruled by the theories of the "efficiency expert" Frederick Taylor. Mr. Taylor broke down industrial production into elemental skills. Result: specialization and isolation of workers from each other. This, Dr. Karasek says, has led to jobs that "destroy both mental and physical health and harm the worker's productivity skills."

Fortunately, more employers today are inviting workers' input—and *using* it. For example, at the Newcastle Machining and Forge Division of Chrysler in Newcastle, Indiana, workers now manage work flow and act in teams. Mike Atkins, a plant worker, says, "Before, we drove to work and left our brains in the parking lot. Now, like people—not machines—we use our brains."

What to do if you hate your job?

Dr. Hogan: "You just have to take it. Sooner or later, bad managers derail, but before they do, they take everybody down with them. Whistle-blowers always lose. It's a terribly grim picture."

Dr. Karasek: "Try to develop a strong support system among coworkers. Talk to one another and identify bad spots. Set up a plan for steps to take to help one another when needed. And—hardest of all—keep trying to find a way to get management and labor at *all* levels to discuss how to improve communication and work methods."

Manage some of these, and you'll have made your bad job better—and, perhaps, you'll have saved your life.

Are You in a Bad Job?

This condensed questionnaire was extracted from the book *Healthy Work*, by Robert A. Karasek and Töres Theorell of the Karolinska Institute, Stockholm.

Control (score 1 for each no answer):

1. Do you learn new things on your job? Yes___ No___
2. Does your job require a lot of skill? Yes___ No___
3. Are you free to make a decision on your job?   Yes___ No___
4. Do you have a lot to say about how to do your job?   Yes___ No___

Total:

Score: Three or more indicates *low control* over your job

Demand (score 1 for each yes answer):

1. Do you have more work than you can easily handle?   Yes___ No___
2. Do you get conflicting orders?
Yes___ No___

3. Are you required to work fast?
Yes___ No___
4. Do you work hard?
Yes___ No___

Total:

Score: Three or more indicates a *high-demand* job.

How to Think Clearly

SALLY: "JUDY IS 5 MINUTES LATE."
Jean: "Yeah. Judy is always late."

Bill: "That's a pretty nice tie, Harry."
Harry thinks: "Bill has no taste. This tie must be terrible. I'll throw it away."

Jean and Harry are thinking illogically. Just because Judy may have been late once or twice, Jean jumps to the conclusion that Judy is *always* late. And Harry does not know how to accept a compliment; he sees only the negative side.

Jean's and Harry's twisted logic are but two examples of a dozen kinds of distorted thoughts that hold us in their grip, producing depression, anxiety, and frustration, ruining our relationships with others, and making it difficult for us to think, to work, to love.

I call them the "dirty dozen of distorted thinking." Psychologists call them *cognitive distortions.* The word *cognitive* comes from the Latin *cognoscere,* which means "to know." Cognitive refers to what you know and believe rather than how you feel, your emotions.

Psychologists say that almost no one escapes cognitive distortions. If twisted logic is giving you trouble with your spouse, children, friends, or boss, or if you are ever anxious, depressed or puzzled over emotional problems, you too may be a victim of one or more of these "dirty dozen."

1. "Every." Although psychologists call the first distortion "overgeneralization," I call it the "every" distortion. After only one or two instances of an event, you leap to the conclusion that it happens every time, or to everybody, or everywhere. A prime example of the every distortion is Jean's twisted thinking. Jean thinks her friend is always late even though Judy may have been late only once before.

2. The shoulds. You set up impossible standards of behavior for yourself or others, telling yourself and others what *should* or *must* be done. It's easy to fail this way. Reasonable people make suggestions more tentatively. "Such and such *might* be better," they say.

3. All or nothing. Some of us see everything in terms of one extreme or the other; there is no in-between. For example, we either love or hate something, or we think everybody is either good or bad. We view everything in stringent black-and-white terms when, figuratively speaking, real life is shades of gray.

4. No! No! No! If something is even remotely negative in another person's actions or words, you will find it and harp on it.

5. Mind reading. You really believe that you know what another person is thinking. ("I know my boss likes long memos, even though he says he doesn't.") Then when you act on your beliefs, you get into trouble. The success rate of all mind reading is low, no matter what you've seen in the movies or on television. Even trained psychologists fall into the trap. An actual test shows that psychologists could guess correctly only 50 percent of the time what their patients were thinking.

6. Catastrophizing. If you suffer from this distortion, you view everything as a catastrophe. One gray hair on your head means that you are old. One lost sale signals the end of your job. Catastrophizing paralyzes action; if you fear the worst, you won't make a move.

7. I! I! I! You think that everything happens because of you or to you. If your best friend gets the flu, you think it's because you served her iced tea on the rainy afternoon that she visited, and then you fret that you're sure to catch an even worse case. Most such occurrences have more than one cause, the least of which is probably your contribution.

8. Mislabeling. With mislabeling, you tend to paint a picture of reality that you want or fear rather than what exists. You may say, "I'm a failure" and think that you really are, when all you actually did was make a mistake.

9. Poisoning the positive. Like Harry, you find reasons to distrust and dismiss compliments or friendly moves. Such poisoned thinking discourages friendships and undermines intimacy.

10. Thoughts as things. You take something that exists only in your head and you make it real. This, in turn, leads to a form of mislabeling. You *think* you're being given all the bad jobs in the office when in fact you are not.

11. Emotional reasoning. Essentially, you think, "I feel it; therefore, it must be true." For example, you feel anxious, so you conclude that something terrible will happen to you.

12. Magnify/minimize. You either exaggerate or downplay a situation, depending on your needs rather than the reality. If you have a pimple, you may say it's skin cancer. Or, you insult someone and minimize the effect by saying, "I was only joking."

As you read the 12 types of warped thoughts, did you recognize some of your own? If so, you may be a victim of cognitive distortions. As a result, you may be anxious, depressed, or puzzled over your emotional problems.

Dr. Aaron T. Beck, professor of psychiatry at the University of Pennsylvania, identified many of these cognitive distortions. He says that unless cognitive distortions are caught early, they can mushroom.

"They are particularly deadly in marriage," Dr. Beck says. "You get a couple who has a controversy about a minor point. Instead of seeking a common ground, they begin to look at each other as adversaries and look at their differences. The husband thinks the wife is just being 'hysterical': the wife sees the husband as 'tyrannical.'"

Then one or more of the dirty dozen takes over. First, the "every" distortion. The wife, after one or two battles, thinks the husband is *always* tyrannical; the husband sees the wife as *always* hysterical. From then on, the relationship spirals downward.

Enter the second distortion: "poisoning the positive." When the wife cozies up to the husband in an attempt to make up, the husband thinks, "She's manipulating me." And when he rejects her overture, she thinks, "He's trying to control me." And then they are trapped.

People troubled by illogical thinking often need the help of a psychologist or psychiatrist who is trained in recognizing cognitive distortions. The expert can point out illogical thinking and actually train a couple to think clearly.

You also can train yourself. The primary rule for clear thinking is to confront your belief with *reality,* that is, with real evidence. For example, what are the real chances of something you do ending in catastrophe? How many catastrophes have you actually had? Are you really ugly? Or do you have nice features, such as eyes or hair?

Therapists often ask their clients to make lists of good or bad things about themselves. This exercise shows patients that reality is different from their negative ideas. (Likewise, if you believe that nobody likes you, try writing down the names of people with whom you are friendly.)

Dr. Beck has shown that many depressed individuals owe their conditions to cognitive distortions. By removing the distortions, Dr. Beck and his colleagues say, they have been able to clear up depressive symptoms as effectively as drugs do.

In depressed patients, cognitive distortions foster a sense of worthlessness. For example, the patient thinks, "If *everybody* hates me" (or "If I am ugly," or "if *everything* I do is a catastrophe"), "then I must be worthless." A feeling of worthlessness often attacks nondepressed people who think this way, too.

Dr. Albert Ellis of the Institute for Rational Emotive Therapy in New York City thinks the tendency to distort is built into the human brain.

"When the human race was running through the jungle, thinking that a lion was around the corner was not unreasonable," Dr. Ellis says lightheartedly. "Even if your perception was distorted—that is, there was no lion—you could live to run another day. Today, perceiving danger where there is none can be crippling."

Much illogical thinking, he says, also comes from copying the thinking style of one's parents, teachers, and peers, many of whom may have been trapped by their own distortions.

Dr. Beck reports that, once your thinking is crooked, you will distort what you see and hear and not know you've done so. As evidence, he videotaped confrontations between spouses. Later, he asked them to list the good things said. Couples in trouble could not list any. Yet, when the videotape revealed otherwise, neither the husbands nor the wives could remember having heard anything positive. Such distorted perceptions reinforce our mental distortions.

Dr. Ellis says many of the distortions come from unrealistic needs to be totally loved by everyone. Other unrealistic needs include these: "I must be 100 percent right all the time." "I must have adoring, well-behaved children." "I must be fashionably dressed all the time." "Nobody matters but me."

The bottom line is that the outside world cannot *make* you feel bad. Unbelievable as it sounds, it isn't the actual loss of money, fame, or loved ones that affects your feelings. It is what you believe that counts.

Dr. Ellis cites the Roman philosopher Epictetus, who said, "What disturbs men's minds is not events but their judgments on events."

Sex

AMERICANS TODAY BEHAVE SEXUALLY WITH astonishing variety. In an unprecedented national survey that asked people about their sexual attitudes, preferences, and practices, *Parade* has discovered eight styles of sexual behavior in America.

These eight styles show the nature of the sexual revolution that, experts say, America has been undergoing for a generation. Old values now face new challenges; traditional ideas of what constitutes normal and abnormal sexual behavior are no longer universally accepted.

Likewise, in addition to identifying the eight sexual styles, our survey found that no single style predominates—that is, there is no typical way to have sex. Americans have, in approximately equal numbers, settled on one of the eight styles for themselves.

Nor is a sexual style exclusively male or female. Men's and women's patterns of sexual activity are, in fact, remarkably similar. Although percentages can vary considerably in individual categories, substantial numbers of both men and women show up in each sexual style.

What Is Sexual Style?

It consists of your thoughts and feelings about sex, what arouses you and what doesn't, and your actual sex activity. Although each person's sex life is uniquely shaped by family, social, religious, and other influences, much of what we think, feel, and do sexually is not unique—other men and women share the same pattern. Each sexual style is the sum of those common attitudes and behaviors.

We discovered, for example, one sexual style we call *The Pansexual*. The men and women in this group are generally happy and take sex in many forms. One American in five is pansexual.

At the other end of the sexual spectrum, there's *The Nonsexual*. This is the style of one person in seven. They are unhappy in most aspects of their lives, and they dislike their bodies. No sort of sexual stimulation arouses them; they have a low sex drive.

For a description of each, see "The Eight Sexual Styles in America" later in this chapter.

Parade's survey revealed other surprising findings:

• Men and women are more alike sexually than they are different. Up to now, most sex researchers treated men and women almost as two distinct species.

• Age does not dictate sexual style. In fact, once you adopt a certain sexual behavior, you may respond to sex that way for the rest of your life.

• Neither religious devotion, nor marital status, nor political leaning powerfully influences how you take your sex, although each factor may exert some influence.

• Homosexuals may not be as aroused by traditional foreplay (such as kissing, hugging, and touching) as heterosexuals are. Homosexuals are more likely to be aroused by extremely erotic behavior. Eleven percent of the men and women in our sample had had some homosexual experience.

The Survey: Who? How? Why?

Parade queried 1,100 men and women who were randomly selected nationwide from all walks of life. Mark Clements, president of Mark Clements Research, Inc., supervised the data collection.

"The *Parade* survey is the first study of American sexual behavior and attitudes ever conducted with a national probability sample," Mr. Clements says. "This means that the respondents are a cross-section of the United States population."

Ranging in age from 18 to 60, they included married, single, and divorced people.

The questions were designed by Dr. Carol C. Flax, a sex researcher and therapist and adjunct associate professor of biology at New York University, and me. The data were then computer analyzed by Dr. Philip Merrifield, professor of educational psychology at New York University, and Deborah Hecht, his student.

Dr. Flax says that the concept of sexual styles could help in treating sex problems. "If we can get troubled couples to understand each other's sex styles," she says, "we can draw partners closer together."

And sex problems do abound: one person in seven reported trouble. The rate was about equal for men and women. However, women most often complained about sexual incompatibility with their partner (18 percent), difficulty reaching orgasm (17 percent), and low sex drive (17 percent). Men were mostly troubled by impotence (18 percent), feelings of sexual inadequacy (13 percent), and low sex drive (11 percent).

The Three Components of Sexual Style

We discovered that people's sexual behavior—both men's and women's—could be described in terms of three distinct traits. We call them *life satisfaction, sensuality,* and *eroticism.*

To see how much life satisfaction a person had, we asked such questions as, Are you happy or unhappy about your sex life? About your life in general? Your state of being single or married? The way your body looks? How easy is it for you to talk to your partner about sex? How good are you as a lover? How often do you have intercourse?

We then discovered that if you answer that you are happy about your life in general, you are most likely to answer that you are happy with your sex life, your marital status, and the way your body looks. You are also more likely to be at ease with sex talk, be proud of your lovemaking, and say that you have intercourse frequently. You are essentially a happy, satisfied person. You therefore have a high life satisfaction trait.

If you say you are unhappy with life in general, then all of your answers to these questions will likely be negative. Unhappy and unsatisfied, you have a low life satisfaction trait.

To measure the trait called sensuality, we asked questions such as, Are you aroused or repulsed by kissing? Hands on breasts? Mouth to breasts? Hugging? Tongue kissing? Genital touching?

Again, people who are aroused by one of these activities are likely to be aroused by the rest. They like cuddling, fondling, nestling. Many people were not aroused by such sensual behavior, which

we usually call foreplay. They scored low on sensuality.

The eroticism trait comes from answers to such questions as, Are you aroused by pornography? By erotic fantasy? By mouth to genital contact? By anal sex? Do you have a strong sex drive? Is sex important to you? Do you frequently masturbate?

If you answer yes to such questions, you have a high degree of the erotic trait; answer no and you have low eroticism.

Here's an important point: You may score high on one trait, low on the other two; or high on two, low on the third, and so on. In fact, eight different combinations of the three traits are possible; hence, the eight sexual styles.

What the Experts Say

Dr. Wardell Pomeroy, an author of the famed Kinsey reports on sex (published in 1948 and 1953) with whom we shared our findings, comments, "The sexual styles identified in the *Parade* survey give us a new and interesting classification and a way of looking at human sexual behavior that we have not really had before. And, in essence, the discovery of such styles emphasizes once again that there is no 'normal' way of sex, just different ways."

Dr. William H. Masters, who developed the Masters-Johnson technique of sex therapy, called *Parade*'s findings an "original presentation that opens a new door to the understanding of sexuality."

"I have said repeatedly," Dr. Masters says, "that there is very little difference in the response patterns between male and female, other than the female's greater capacity to respond."

The sex survey has increased our understanding of sexuality. This is just the first glimpse of the findings.

The Eight Sexual Styles in America

The Pansexual

Life satisfaction: High

Sensuality: High

Eroticism: High

198 persons per 1,000

45 percent women, 55 percent men

These people take life at the crest. They are happy with all aspects of their lives. They like themselves and the way their bodies look. They have sex frequently with a partner, and they are happy, whether single or married. They believe they are great lovers and find it easy to talk to their partners about sex.

We call them pansexual because they take sex in all forms. Very sensual, they are aroused by traditional foreplay. But they enjoy more erotic activities as well, such as pornography, erotic fantasy, and oral sex. In addition to frequent sex with a partner, they often masturbate. To them, sex is very important.

The Satisfied Erotic

Life satisfaction: High

Sensuality: Low

Eroticism: High

117 persons per 1,000

30 percent women, 70 percent men

To be aroused, these people need special stimulation. They are intense about their sexual experimentation; they like fantasy and pornography and other erotic activities. They are particular about what they need to complete the sex act.

Kissing, hugging, and other sensual activities do little for them. But they are very happy with themselves and their lives, whether married or single. They have sex often, both with a partner and by themselves. One of five Satisfied Erotics has had some homosexual experience. (Only the Lonely Erotics had as much homosexual experience.) Although men predominate by a larger than two-to-one margin, one Satisfied Erotic of three is a woman.

The Unsatisfied Erotic

Life satisfaction: Low

Sensuality: High

Eroticism: High

127 persons per 1,000

51 percent women, 49 percent men

The men and women of this group take sex wherever they can get it. For them, sex is very important, yet they are unhappy with their sex lives and with their lives in general, including the way they look. They are aroused by both sensual behavior and erotic activities. For all their arousability, however, they are more likely to masturbate than to have sex with others. Frustrated and seeking arousal by any means, they want sex frequently but cannot get it.

A 47-year-old divorced man wrote on his questionnaire, "I like a variety of experimentation and adventures. I find difficulty in finding someone of quality who has similar sexual tastes." In his lifetime, this Unsatisfied Erotic has had 45 sex partners.

The Lonely Erotic

Life satisfaction: Low

Sensuality: Low

Eroticism: High

121 persons per 1,000

27 percent women, 73 percent men

These are lonesome people who respond more to sexual imagery, depictions (i.e., pornography), and certain sexual activities than to their sexual partner per se. They have difficulty forming relationships, and their main sexual outlet is masturbation. They get nothing out of foreplay and are unhappy in most aspects of their lives, including sex. They dislike their bodies.

Although a significant number of women are Lonely Erotics, men outnumber them by more than two to one. People who have had homosexual experience also congregate in this style.

The Satisfied Sensualist

Life satisfaction: High

Sensuality: High

Eroticism: Low

109 persons per 1,000

54 percent women, 46 percent men

These people are happy with their sex lives, their partners, and themselves. Most are married. They love to snuggle up to their partner, kiss, fondle, and hug. Such foreplay is sufficiently arousing for intercourse. Most of the more erotic sexual activities—such as pornography, fantasy, oral sex—turn them off, however. They have sex with partners frequently but not often by themselves.

Says one typical Satisfied Sensualist, a 50-year-old man who has been married for 25 years with only one sex partner in his entire life, "It's important for me to be in love with the person I am making love to."

The Unsatisfied Sensualist

Life satisfaction: Low

Sensuality: High

Eroticism: Low

85 persons per 1,000

67 percent women, 33 percent men

Very unhappy in many aspects of their lives—their looks, feelings, and sexuality—these people seek human contact. For them, sensual behaviors such as kissing and fondling are arousing, so there is some spark of sex. But their sex lives are unsatisfactory. Many Unsatisfied Sensualists lack partners, because they never married or are no longer married. In fact, many are older women alone. They are lonely people with a low sex drive who infrequently have sex, even by themselves. Generally, sex is not important to them.

The Sexually Conservative

Life satisfaction: High

Sensuality: Low

Eroticism: Low

111 persons per 1,000

67 percent women, 33 person men

Sex may not be central to the lives of these people, who are otherwise happy and who like themselves. They do not find most foreplay arousing. In fact, they may be turned off by it. Yet, with frequent intercourse, they are satisfied with what they are getting. Six of seven are married. A 37-year-old woman, typical of the Sexually Conservative, wrote on her questionnaire, "I think that a couple's ability to work together so that they are both happy far outweighs location, 'climate,' sexual frequency, or technique."

The Nonsexual

Life satisfaction: Low

Sensuality: Low

Eroticism: Low

132 persons per 1,000

68 percent women, 32 percent men

Very unhappy with their lives and bodies, without frequent sex, and unaroused by any sexual stimulation—even the most erotic—these people have no interest in sex. A 40-year-old woman reflected this by writing, "I am too uptight."

What Is Your Sexual Style?

To help you identify your own sexual style, here is an abridged version of the *Parade* sex survey. Check the box that most closely describes how you feel about each statement.

Part I. Life Satisfaction

Do you agree or disagree?

	AGREE	DISAGREE
I am happy with my life generally.	☐ 7	☐ 1
I am happy with my marital status.	☐ 6	☐ 2
My sex life is happy	☐ 6	☐ 2
Talking sex with my partner is easy.	☐ 6	☐ 2
I am happy with how my body looks.	☐ 5	☐ 3

Total Life Satisfaction score _____

Part II. Sensuality

Do you agree or disagree?

	AGREE	DISAGREE
I am aroused by kissing.	☐ 7	☐ 1
I am aroused by hugging.	☐ 6	☐ 2

	AGREE	DISAGREE
I am aroused by tongue kissing.	☐ 6	☐ 2
I am aroused by hands on breasts.	☐ 6	☐ 2
I am aroused by mouth to breasts.	☐ 5	☐ 3

Total Sensuality score _____

Part III. Eroticism

Do you agree or disagree?

	AGREE	DISAGREE
I am aroused by oral sex.	☐ 7	☐ 1
I am aroused by body kissing.	☐ 6	☐ 2
I am aroused by pornography.	☐ 6	☐ 2
I am aroused by erotic fantasy.	☐ 6	☐ 2
My sex drive is strong.	☐ 5	☐ 3

Total Eroticism score _____

To score each trait, add up the numbers next to each box that you have checked. If you total 20 points ore more, you score high on the trait; less than 20 points scores low. Then, look at "The Eight Sexual Styles in America" and find the combination of highs and lows that matches yours. That is your sexual style.

Sex Education Programs That Work— and Some That Don't

FOR 25 YEARS OR SO, MOST PUBLIC SCHOOLS have taught a brand of sex education that supplies students with information about the body's sexual system. They also have taught that sex is healthy, not "dirty," but that waiting until marriage to have intercourse is a wise thing to do.

Many teachers and public health officials felt that this approach would reduce the terrible toll of teenage sex:

unwanted babies and sexually transmitted diseases. They were wrong. Mostly, these programs have failed.

But over the last 10 years, a new approach has been developed. Tightly focused on teaching methods that help teenagers change their behavior, this new method is showing signs of success. Instead of relying mainly on conveying information about sex or moral precepts, the new approach focuses on discovering and actually using behavior that will prevent pregnancy or disease.

Teachers of the new sex education approach are like coaches who help players perfect and apply what they learn at practice sessions. The goal is to win in an actual game. Through role-playing practice, for example, students anticipate some of the moves of their "opponents," whose goal would be sexual intercourse or sex without protection. The strategy is to know what moves to expect and to achieve one's own desired outcome: having fun without an unwanted pregnancy or a disease. Using games and interesting exercises that strengthen social skills, youngsters learn to say no effectively and confidently.

Acknowledging that many teens are sexually active, the new sex education pinpoints real-life results of irresponsible sex and urges self-protection. Pragmatic, not preachy, it combines learning theory with a hard look at the realities:

• Since the early 1970s, the teenage birthrate has been rising. Yearly, more than a million girls become pregnant, and about half of them give birth.

• In some inner cities, 80 percent of teenagers' babies are born out of wedlock. Nationally, the figure is closer to 50 percent.

• More than $25 billion a year in federal taxes support teenagers and their babies.

• Most children who are parents before they leave high school—and before marriage—face a harsh future: less education, less chance of getting a job, dismal prospects for a happy marriage. Most of the hardship falls on the female.

• Females more easily catch sexually transmitted diseases, including AIDS, one of the leading causes of death for Americans aged 25 to 44 (number 1 for men, number 4 for women). AIDS can be dormant for up to 10 years, so it would seem that many were infected as teenagers.

• Teenage girls get gonorrhea at a rate 22 times greater than older women. And despite antibiotics, sterility can result.

The newer sex education programs, which require student interaction, can help teenagers change their sexual behavior for the better, social scientists say. Early studies of two new programs show that junior and senior high school students in the programs delayed first sexual intercourse by at least 2 years longer than their untaught peers. Also, unprotected sex among older students already sexually active fell by 40 percent. Research on other, similar programs showed that many students had even reduced the number of sexual partners.

Finding Out What Works

Ideally, the best protection against pregnancy and infection is no sex at all.

Social scientists, finding no sexual abstinence program that could prove all participants had achieved that goal, fostered this approach: Give teenagers strong behavioral training aimed either at delaying first sexual intercourse or at turning aside unprotected sex.

By the 1990s, many such programs were available. To evaluate them scientifically, the projects were cast as experiments and written up as studies. Eleven were checked by a team of scientists and statisticians from the Centers for Disease Control and Prevention in Atlanta. Their leader was Douglas Kirby, director of research at ETR, a nonprofit health education group in Scotts Valley, California.

"We were looking for common characteristics of programs that worked," Mr. Kirby says. He adds that in half the sex ed courses studied, students had changed their behavior (reduced sexual risk taking), and in half they had not. "For the first time in history," he says, "we can pinpoint programs that delay sexual intercourse and/or inspire using safety devices, ultimately reducing the teenage pregnancies and sexually transmitted diseases."

This is a major advance. Educators now believe they know how to help students change their sexual behavior.

What They Teach

Grounded in modern learning theory, the new programs teach that actions have consequences and that students can change their behavior to get the results they want. Before classes begin, parents are sent a letter detailing the approaches to be taken. Efforts are made to keep lessons age-appropriate. Students learn these points:

- That they will benefit—socially, physically, economically—from avoiding unwanted pregnancy and disease
- How to delay starting intercourse (The student learns and practices, through role-playing with classmates, how to anticipate and avert sexual advances deftly and even pleasantly.)
- How to get and use protection, usually condoms, if already sexually active
- How to develop, through practice, confidence that the skills being learned will surely work in real-life situations

How They Teach It

The teacher, who is specially trained to do so, personalizes instruction with specially designed games and exercises. These maintain student interest and reinforce learning.

Role-Playing

The following role-playing exercise is from a much longer scenario developed by Kirby and his associates at ETR:

Scene: Harold and Thelma, dating for a few months, are at a party.

Harold: Let's get out of here, so we can talk. It's too crowded. (Students learn to detect this line as dangerous.)

Thelma: Yes, it is crowded in here, but the porch is empty.

Harold: If I'd known you'd do this, I wouldn't have come here with you.

Thelma: (Stands up straight, faces him squarely. Her tone is clear, not wimpish.) Maybe not, but I know we can have fun. Let's get something to eat in the kitchen.

Games

Games also teach interaction. In the old sex ed courses, a teacher might say: "If you have intercourse once a month, your chances are 1 in 6 of becoming pregnant." Such a dry approach soon loses teenagers' attention. Instead, today, the teacher starts a game:

Teacher: Class, write down any number from 1 to 6. Now I'll draw a number from this box. (Draws and reads.) Number 6. All those who picked number 6, please stand up. You or your partner just got pregnant. Remain standing. OK. Now I've drawn number 3. All those with a 3, please stand. You just got pregnant."

Soon, all the students are standing. The lesson: Frequent, unprotected sex raises your chances of pregnancy.

Homework

Teacher: At home, discuss sex with one or both of your parents. Interview them. Try to learn what their values are. Ask whether and at what age they think you should start having sex. Try talking about contraception. It may be difficult, but our experience is that parents want to be part of the process.

Feeling the Cost

Teenagers often have a distorted view of what it means to be an unwed parent. This exercise helps bring that cost home:

Teacher: Write down all the things you do in 24 hours. Extend the list to 3 months. Review it and check the things you couldn't do if you had a baby. (Discussing the lists soon shows how parenthood can affect their lives.)

Teaching Abstinence

A 1991 Gallup poll reported that 87 percent of Americans said they want sex ed for all schoolchildren. Most states recommend or require it in some form.

Among those who disagree is Phyllis Schlafly. She is the founder of Eagle Forum, a group based in St. Louis that promotes 100 percent abstinence. She estimates membership is 80,000. Mrs. Schlafly contends that, as taught in schools, sex ed has failed because it has not reduced teen pregnancy.

"To reduce teen pregnancy," she says, "we should teach kids it is shameful to have sex outside marriage."

Marianne Whatley, professor of curriculum and instruction at the University of Wisconsin, demurs. "There is no proof that abstinence-only programs work," she says.

With the help of federal funding, four 100 percent abstinence programs—Sex Respect, Teen Aid, Living Smart, and FACTS—hired experts to evaluate their groups' effectiveness. When a team from the Public Policy Office of the American Psychological Association later evaluated this research, they found it didn't meet scientific standards and so was inconclusive.

School behavioral programs do remind students that total abstinence is the only foolproof way to avoid early pregnancy and disease. For sexually active students, teachers stress protection. Younger students are taught that delaying first intercourse is a wise thing to do. And research shows they *do*.

Does Behavior-Related Training Work?

Having shown that teens can learn to delay intercourse, use condoms, and have fewer sex partners, scientists must also prove that this behavior will lead to fewer cases of unwanted births and disease. In 1996 ETR and the University of California at Berkeley were evaluating Education Now and Babies Later (ENABL). This statewide program, begun in 1992 by the California Department of Health Services, included Postponing Sexual Involvement, a sex ed program for 12- to 14-year-olds, and a media and public relations campaign. Researchers are comparing the behaviors of students in that age group, who were exposed to the sex ed or media campaign with that of a control group of students who were not.

Sex education alone won't halt teenage pregnancies. Much help is needed from parental involvement, community activities, and social support groups. Still, progress has been made. If research truly connects less teenage pregnancy with a change in behavior inspired by sex ed, we may soon see a reduction in disease, unwanted pregnancies, and unwanted, uncared-for children.

Fertility

AS THE BABY PUSHES ITS TINY, WET HEAD OUT into the universe, the birth of a child makes us gasp at the wonder of the creation of life. But that wonder is denied to between 3 million and 4 million American couples who cannot achieve pregnancy. They are infertile.

I am amazed that our species has survived the delicate balance of fertility. Before conception takes place, a dozen different organs in the husband and wife must mesh their output.

Despite recent successes with surgery and drugs, one couple in five still fails to have children. Undaunted, scientists are developing newer, bolder techniques that have given babies to thousands of childless couples and offer hope to thousands more. In less than a decade, doctors have achieved breathtaking results with the following techniques:

- Microsurgery that opens blocked or destroyed egg and sperm ducts
- Radioactive tests of sex-hormone levels to treat the lack of eggs and sperm; new hormone preparations that induce the sluggish ovary to ovulate—that is, to produce and release eggs
- The sonogram, a sound-wave picture that enables doctors to see eggs sprouting and to monitor drugs' effects on the ovary

Many of these advances are part of a new era of infertility treatment, which burst on the world on July 25, 1978, with the birth in Oldham, England, of 5-pound, 12-ounce Louise Brown, the world's first test-tube baby. She was conceived in the laboratory, where her mother's egg joined her father's sperm in a glass petri dish. The fertilized egg was then implanted in Mrs. Brown's uterus, where it grew normally for 9 months. Scientists call this method in vitro (meaning "in glass") fertilization, or IVF.

Common Fertility Problems for Women

Ovulation actually begins in the woman's brain, where the hypothalamus releases chemicals that stimulate the pituitary gland. In turn, the pituitary, just under the brain, releases hormones (chemical messengers) that trigger the ovaries to make and release eggs.

No Eggs, No Babies

It's called *anovulation*. And there are many reasons that a woman produces no

237

eggs. Mostly, it's because her hormones are out of balance. This can be caused by malnourishment, certain medications, emotional stress, infections, or chronic illness.

When the pituitary fails to release enough ovary-stimulating hormone, doctors usually prescribe "fertility drugs," such as Clomid and Pergonal, to provoke egg production. The drugs work nine times out of ten, but Pergonal treatment sometimes results in several eggs, causing the birth of triplets, quadruplets, quintuplets, and even sextuplets!

The Fertility Pump

Some women's brains do not make enough pituitary-stimulating hormone. Doctors have attached an experimental fertility pump to women. Through a catheter inserted into a vein, the pump injects a synthetic form of the hormone around the clock. Ovulation has returned to 80 to 90 percent of the women, and several pregnancies have been reported.

Blocked Tubes

Infections of the ovaries, fallopian tubes, and pelvis—called pelvic inflammatory disease—frequently scar or destroy the tubes, blocking the egg's path. Today, microsurgery is overcoming the damage that infections inflict. Dr. Luigi Mastroianni, Jr., of the University of Pennsylvania in Philadelphia, a pioneer in repairing blocked or damaged tubes, says that the success rate can be as high as 80 percent if there is only light scarring.

Endometriosis

Studies show that in half of all women, pieces of the inner lining of the uterus (the endometrium) grow outside the uterus after menstruation each month. In severe cases, the tissue spreads over the ovaries and fallopian tubes. Called *endometriosis,* this condition can cause severe pain during menstruation and intercourse.

But worst of all, a third of the women stricken with endometriosis become infertile—exactly how is unknown. And because the risk of endometriosis increases with age, it may be a major cause of infertility in older women.

The drug Danocrine helps some women. In others, surgery removes the wandering tissue. Pregnancy practically cures the disease by stopping the growth of endometrial tissue, but the problem is to get pregnant in the first place. Likewise, treatment with birth control pills, which induce artificial pregnancy, can clear up the condition.

"Sperm Allergy"

About 10 percent of women are infertile because their immune system attacks their husbands' sperm. Bonnie Marangoni, 28, an attorney from East Meadow, New York, tried to conceive for years. One pregnancy ended in miscarriage. Dr. Richard Bronson of North Shore University Hospital in Manhasset, New York, discovered that Mrs. Marangoni produced antibodies that stopped her husband's swimming sperm. He treated her with a hormone that suppressed the allergic response. In August 1983, Jillian was born. "She's adorable," says the proud mother. Dr. Bronson reports 40 percent success.

Surrogate Mothers

Some infertile wives hire women to bear children conceived with their husbands' sperm. The surrogate mother agrees to release the child to the couple for adoption. The legal, moral, and ethical problems surrounding this procedure have made the use of surrogate mothers rare.

Beyond IVF—Embryo Transfer

Since the birth of Louise Brown in 1978, in vitro fertilization has produced more than 300 babies around the world, and the number grows daily as new clinics open. Louise has an IVF sister, Natalie Jean, born in 1982. But the success rate of in vitro fertilization is less than 20 percent. To increase the possibility of a "take," doctors use fertility drugs, fertilize several eggs, then reimplant all of them. This approach also ups the chances of a multiple birth, as Todd and Nancy Tilton of Sea Cliff, New York, discovered. Mrs. Tilton underwent in vitro fertilization at the Eastern Virginia Medical School in Norfolk and gave birth to IVF twins.

In vitro fertilization can cost up to $15,000 before a pregnancy is achieved, and it may be useful to fewer than 5 per-cent of infertile women. Nevertheless, the success of IVF has inspired doctors to pursue even bolder, more remarkable solutions to infertility.

One such answer is embryo transfer. In 1983, Australian scientists announced the birth of an IVF baby (that is, fertilization took place outside the body in a glass dish) from an egg donated by one woman to an infertile wife.

More remarkable still, Dr. John Buster and his colleagues at Harbor–UCLA Medical Center in Los Angeles, California, delivered to one mother a baby who started life inside the womb of another woman. Doctors inseminated the husband's sperm into the other woman. Five days after the fertilization, a doctor transferred the growing fetus out of the donor's uterus and implanted it into the wife.

"The donors love it," Dr. Buster says. "They feel it is a big thing to give the gift of life to another person."

It's the Man's Problem, Too

A breakdown in the man's reproductive system accounts for as much infertility as does faulty biology in the woman, according to the American College of Obstetricians and Gynecologists. Most cases of male infertility are caused by problems in sperm production and quality.

Weak or Missing Sperm

Only one healthy, active sperm is needed for fertilization to take place. For insurance, however, nature creates at least

100 million sperm in every ejaculation in the normal male. If the man makes too few sperm or only weak, slow-moving sperm, the chances of fertilization drop dramatically.

Causes and Treatments
Hormonal imbalances and blocked tubes can destroy, weaken, or otherwise damage sperm. Microsurgery can repair a man's damaged sperm ducts. Hormone therapy works only when a specific hormone deficiency has been diagnosed. Treatment with hormones that stimulate testosterone—the male hormone responsible for sperm production—increases sperm count. But treatment with actual testosterone does not. Other hormone treatments are still in the experimental stages.

Most frequently, the quality of a man's sperm declines because one testicle has a varicose vein, called a *varicocele*. Like most veins, the ones in the testicle have little valves that prevent backflow of blood. If that valve cannot close or is absent, blood flows backward and the vein swells. This heats up both testicles. Heat interferes with sperm production.

Dr. Richard D. Amelar, of the New York University Medical Center, blames 40 percent of male infertility on varicoceles. With a simple half-hour operation, he and Dr. Lawrence Dubin blocked off the damaged delicate veins in almost 1,000 men whose sperm was otherwise normal. Sperm quality improved in three

of four men. For more than half, the wives became pregnant.

A nonsurgical treatment for overheated testicles was developed by Dr. Adrian Zorgniotti of the New York University School of Medicine. He fashioned a water-cooled jockstrap that the man wears for several months. Of 26 patients, Dr. Zorgniotti reports, 10 became fathers.

Infertile Couples
Jayne and Dr. Lawrence Reed of Houston are parents to two adopted children. They have tried to have a child of their own for 10 years. They went through countless tests and treatments. Dr. Reed's sperm was normal. Mrs. Reed ovulated, but irregularly. Then one doctor discovered that she had too much testosterone. (All women produce this male sex hormone.)

The physician prescribed Prednisone, a hormone that depressed the adrenal output. Mrs. Reed conceived three times, but each pregnancy failed. Something else was wrong that escaped science.

"We want more children, and my time is running out," says Mrs. Reed, who is 37. "We have a huge house that we built so we could have a large family." They're still trying.

In 20 percent of infertility cases, the problem lies with both the husband and the wife. They may be having sex too infrequently. Or, if the husband's sperm count is just below the normal range and the wife ovulates intermittently, the couple could be infertile.

Artificial Insemination

Doctors occasionally collect the husband's lazy sperm and place it at the mouth of the wife's womb or even inside the womb itself to raise the chances of fertilization. Here, too, doctors borrow from IVF technology. Before insemination, the sperm is placed in the same fluid used for in vitro fertilization. This seems to increase chances of a "take."

When the husband has no sperm at all or a sperm count so low that fertilization is impossible, many couples rely on artificial insemination with sperm from an unrelated donor whose identity is un-

known to them. In recent years, thousands of couples have "adopted" sperm from a sperm bank.

The late Dr. Sophie Kleegman, the New York gynecologist who 40 years ago pioneered sexual and fertility studies, said, "Infertility patients are not sick, but they are heartsick, and the help they seek is, to them, as urgent as any in medical practice." At last, doctors have heeded those words.

For further information on where to get help for infertility, send a self-addressed, stamped envelope to RESOLVE, a national self-help organization, 1310 Broadway, Somerville, MA 02144-1731. Or call their help line at (617) 623-0744.

You Don't Have to Be Childless

SCIENCE NOW OFFERS THE GIFT OF PREGNANCY to "infertile" couples wanting to have a baby—almost without exception—whatever the barrier to conception might be. Their becoming expectant parents depends on how far they may want to go to solve their problems and achieve their goals.

Solutions include these:

- Surgery to repair damaged anatomy
- Drugs to heal interfering infections

- Drugs to normalize hormone levels
- Fertilization in a glass dish
- Frozen embryos
- Borrowed sperm
- Borrowed eggs
- A "borrowed" uterus

Not every couple wants to opt for the most exotic of infertility treatments. But most of those who desperately want a baby will consider any effort at any cost. Susanne and David Johnson of

Chesapeake, Virginia, both 37, spent $40,000 over the course of 14 years before their son, Richard David, was born in 1988.

Mr. Johnson, a police sergeant, was tested—inconclusively—for a low sperm count. Doctors also tried to repair Mrs. Johnson's fallopian tubes, damaged by an infected, ruptured appendix when she was 13. The operation failed, and the surgeons had to remove her tubes, leaving no way for an egg to get from her ovary to her uterus.

So the Johnsons went to the Howard and Georgeanna Jones Institute for Reproductive Medicine at Eastern Virginia Medical School in Norfolk, Virginia. It was the first clinic in the United States to succeed with in vitro fertilization (IVF). In vitro fertilization means that sperm and egg are joined in a glass dish. (*Vitro* in Latin means glass.)

The doctors gave Mrs. Johnson drugs that stimulated her ovaries to produce eggs. With simple surgery, they recovered those eggs and mixed them with her husband's sperm in a glass dish. The sperm entered and fertilized the eggs and produced several embryos. These were implanted singly into Mrs. Johnson's uterus. After six attempts in 18 months, an implant succeeded. Nine months later, Richard David was born without a hitch.

"We're ecstatic about our baby," says Mrs. Johnson. "He is a dream come true. He is a picture of his father. He has our personality and our disposition. That's why we wanted our own child."

More than 15,000 IVF babies have been born worldwide since British doctors brought Louise Brown into the world in 1978 as the first "test-tube baby."

Dr. Larry Grunfeld, a fertility expert at Mount Sinai Medical Center in New York City, says he sympathizes with the Johnsons: "The most difficult job I have is telling a couple to stop trying." He adds that many fertility problems went unidentified and unsolved 20 years ago. "Today," he says, "we have something to offer nearly every infertile couple."

Dr. Grunfeld says science now can figure out the cause in 85 percent of infertility cases and that, with further testing, causes for infertility could be found for the rest. Forty percent of the time the problem lies with the man; 40 percent, the woman. The remaining 20 percent are man-woman difficulties— her body rejects his sperm. Her womb may create antibodies to the incoming male sperm, or her mucous may block all the sperm. A man's problems are harder to solve. He may have no sperm or poor-quality sperm. Or he may be-impotent—incapable of sexual intercourse.

One in three infertile women may have endometriosis, an overgrowth of the lining of the uterus. That growth invades the pelvis and damages the ovaries and fallopian tubes. One woman in six may have fallopian tubes damaged by infections. Or hormone difficulties may interfere with egg production.

But science has new ways to bypass these obstacles. For example, with IVF, the sperm bypasses the woman's hostile antibodies to fertilize the egg in vitro.

In 1984, scientists at the University of California at Irvine developed another way of joining egg and sperm called GIFT, which stands for gamete intrafallopian transfer. Instead of mixing sperm and eggs in a glass dish, the scientists insert a thin plastic pipe carrying the sperm and eggs into the fallopian tubes, where they unite just as they would in a normal pregnancy.

After 8 years of trying all sorts of techniques, GIFT worked for Jerry and Susan White, both 38, of Mission Viejo, California. He's a police officer; she's a flight attendant.

"We had every test possible," Mrs. White recalls. "Doctors could not pinpoint the problem. The sperm were not reaching my tubes. There was nothing physically wrong with either of us."

In 1987, Mrs. White received the eggs and sperm directly into her tubes. Two weeks later, she got the word: she was pregnant. Two weeks after that, sound-wave pictures revealed that she was carrying twins. "I was in total disbelief," she says.

It was a difficult pregnancy: anemia, high blood pressure, diabetes, and a 12-hour labor 5 weeks early. On January 20, 1988, Katie and Sarah, fraternal twins, were born. The girls came from two eggs, two embryos. (Identical twins share one egg.)

Mrs. White, who is Roman Catholic, was able to have her babies with church approval, since fertilization occurs naturally

in the fallopian tubes with GIFT. However, the church's stand against IVF and other "artificial" techniques—as well as fear of opposition from other religions and anti-abortionists—has had an influence on federal support and regulation of fertility research, including the use of human embryos. For example, the National Institutes of Health (NIH), the leading supporter of medical research in the United States, provides no money for IVF research.

Pro-choice and anti-abortion forces have turned IVF research into a political battleground. In 1996, the Republican-dominated Congress passed a law that blocked NIH funds for research on embryos and fertilized eggs. However, the law still permits scientists to explore fetal tissue from induced abortions. Such tissue could lead to cures for Parkinson's disease, Alzheimer's, and diabetes. Paradoxically, the NIH may not fund work that could show whether fertility techniques are safe.

The lack of funds and leadership dismayed many scientists at the National Institutes of Health, but they do not speak out for fear of reprisals.

Says Dr. Jon Gordon, who does extensive fertility research at New York's Mount Sinai Medical Center, "It's irrational. It slows the progress of science. It's very frustrating to me that I cannot get NIH funds. Those who want to limit this research stand to lose as much as patients who want and need the research."

Judie Brown, president of the American Life League, opposes using human embryos in research. "They are human beings," she says, "not property. We are opposed to technology that risks the life of an innocent person. These are moral absolutes. You don't kill an innocent person. Science has advanced beyond its moral limits."

The ethics committee of the American Fertility Society counters that the embryo used in IVF is a "preembryo" that "should not be treated as a person, because it has not yet developed . . . and may never realize its potential." Preembryos, however, do take on some advanced features of an embryo after 14 days.

Father Richard McCormick, professor of Christian Ethics at Notre Dame University, says, "I believe a good case might be made for preembryo research up to 14 days if it promised great medical benefits not otherwise attainable." He urges appointing a national ethics board. "This is too important to leave up to individual hospitals and medical centers," he asserts.

When Bill Clinton became president in 1993, he wiped out the ban against using fetal tissue in scientific research or treatments such as IVF. With a presidential order, the government reinstituted research into methods of improving fertility and other uses of fetal tissue.

In September 1989, a Tennessee judge ruled that embryos were human beings existing as embryos. He assigned temporary custody of seven frozen embryos to Mary Sue Davis of Knoxville, who had gone through the in vitro program with her husband, Junior Davis. But before the embryos could be used, the couple divorced. Junior Davis said he didn't want his ex-wife to bear his child after their divorce. However, the judge's ruling can still be appealed, and the U.S. Supreme Court has yet to rule on such a case.

Dr. Sherman Silber, of St. Luke's Hospital in St. Louis, and a colleague developed a method for helping men whose sperm is trapped in the body because the testicles lack vas deferens tubes to provide an exit.

Ed Gruetzemacher, 44, an aviation officer for the Missouri National Guard, had such a problem. When he married Jeanie, now 39, who works for the Missouri Women's Council, they considered adoption. They live in Jefferson City, Missouri.

But their physician, Dr. Silber, decided on surgery to remove sperm from Mr. Gruetzemacher's testicle, then mix it with his wife's egg in a dish and place the fertilized embryo in her tube just as they do in GIFT. They had to use the dish for joining egg and sperm because the surgically removed sperm were weak. Mrs. Gruetzemacher conceived in August 1987 but then miscarried. The couple tried again in February 1988, and Eve Cristine was born that November.

"Having the kid is the greatest thing I ever did," says Mr. Gruetzemacher. "It's up to each individual to say how much effort they want to make."

What about the opposition some have because the technique is "artificial"? Says

Mrs. Gruetzemacher, "No one who has tried to have children and failed would raise that question. You can't understand what it means to us."

Doctors successfully transferred eggs from anonymous donors to women who can't produce eggs. Mount Sinai's Dr. Gordon has punched small holes in the soft shell surrounding the egg. That makes it easier for weak sperm to penetrate.

Dr. Gordon's colleague, Dr. Daniel Navot, invented a test to determine whether a woman can conceive. He gives her clorniphene, a drug that stimulates the ovary to produce eggs. By checking a woman's hormone levels, he can predict the potential of the ovary to produce healthy eggs and the chances of pregnancy.

Some infertile women (1 to 2 percent, estimates Dr. Navot) don't produce eggs because they have too much of the hormone prolactin, which controls the production of breast milk. Too much prolactin stops the production of female sex hormones and, consequently, the production of eggs.

A drug called bromocriptine (trade name: Parlodel) lowers the prolactin level and restores the normal hormonal balance. Reported pregnancy rates among users are 38 to 81 percent.

New treatments for endometriosis, infections, and low sperm counts promise to cut the infertility rate even more. It's all a question of how much a couple really want a baby—of how much they will pay, how far they will go. Science does have the answers.

If You're Trying to Have a Child ...

IN 1977 TWO BRITISH SCIENTISTS CAPTURED several eggs from the ovary of a woman who had been told she would never have children. Her fallopian tubes were blocked, and her eggs could not travel from her ovary to her uterus. The scientists slipped the tiny globs of potential life into a glass dish filled with liquid. They collected the husband's sperm and poured it into the same flat saucer. After a few days of incubation, the physicians inserted the embryo into the woman's uterus.

Nine months later, Louise Joy Brown came into the world. She was the first "test-tube baby." Since then, more than 65,000 children around the world have found life in a glass dish. The United States alone has produced 44,000 such babies.

At the start, the procedure—called in vitro fertilization, or IVF—yielded only one live baby out of every 16 attempts, a 6 percent success rate. Today, however, the overall success rate has climbed to more than 18 percent. And new variations of the method have boosted many couples' chances even further. More than 300 hospitals and clinics around the country offer a wide range of infertility services. At the best treatment centers, the success rate for IVF or one of its technical cousins is almost 40 percent.

There is more good news: The price has dropped. Fifteen years ago, a couple could spend about $100,000 in efforts to have a baby, with no guarantees. Today, the price for IVF or other assisted reproductive technology hovers between $10,000 and $20,000. And it is still coming down, according to Dr. Alan DeCherney, president of the American Society for Reproductive Medicine. The cost may be covered in whole or in part by insurance.

The new technology has helped thousands of couples fulfill their dreams of having children. But there are still difficulties to overcome. Getting pregnant the new way may mean taking powerful chemicals, the long-term effects of which are unknown. And women who undergo IVF tend to have a higher rate of miscarriage. Moreover, even though the price has dropped, going through infertility treatments can put a big dent in the family budget. Successful couples invariably say that the investment was the best they ever made. Failing couples, however, have likened the process to playing a slot machine with a $2,500 minimum bet.

"The most important factor in determining success is the age of the woman," explains Dr. Zev Rosenwaks, director of the Division of Reproductive Medicine and Fertility at New York Hospital. "Women younger than 34 have a 45 percent to 50 percent success rate. This figure drops until, by age 44, the success rate is 2 percent to 3 percent."

Theresa and Ken Pope were lucky. When the Boston couple—both musicians in their mid-30s—tried to have a baby 7 years ago, they discovered that Theresa's fallopian tubes were blocked. Surgical repair was impossible. In 1992, Theresa took drugs that stimulated her ovaries to produce seven eggs. Six were fertilized with Ken's sperm. Four embryos were transferred into Theresa's uterus, and two were frozen for later use if the first try didn't work. Both attempts failed. The Popes were devastated.

"Each failure brought a new animal into our home," Theresa remembers. "We now have eight cats and two German shepherds." Finally, after three attempts, Theresa became pregnant with twins in May 1993.

In the first round, the Popes' flight into high-tech medicine cost them $8,000, because they were not fully insured. Last August, the couple went for another try to have more children, and their HMO is now paying almost the whole bill. The Popes live in Massachusetts, one of six states—along with Arkansas, Hawaii, Illinois, Maryland, and Rhode Island—that require insurance companies to cover fertility treatments. Many other states are considering similar laws.

Though the Popes went straight to IVF, fertility treatments often do not begin with in vitro or its variations. In fact, only 11 percent of infertile couples ever reach the IVF stage. Before plunging into costly high-tech methods, couples first undergo diagnostic tests to learn the cause of infertility. Then they may be treated with relatively simple (and less expensive) techniques.

Women who do not shed enough eggs, for example, can be treated with clomiphene (one of a number of ovary-stimulating drugs) or hormones. They may become pregnant in 6 to 9 months, at a cost of about $4,000. If blocked fallopian tubes are the problem, surgery often can be used, at a cost of between $5,000 and $10,000. In another scenario, women may be producing harmful antibodies—chemicals that can destroy or injure sperm entering the vagina. The condition may be treated with potent steroids like cortisone.

About 40 percent of the burden of infertility lies with the man. Women account for another 40 percent; the remainder may be a result of both partners or may have unknown causes. One common cause of male infertility is a swollen vein in the testicles, called a varicocele. It can be corrected with surgery.

If these treatments do not work, doctors may try a high-tech method. In 1993, about 41,000 such procedures were performed in the United States, according to the American Society for Reproductive Medicine. Although traditional IVF was by far the most common, accounting for 81 percent of all procedures, other methods increasingly are being used. Here are some of the latest variations and their success rates:

• GIFT and ZIFT. The letters stand for gamete or zygote intrafallopian transfer. With GIFT, doctors surgically insert an egg and sperm (or gametes) inside the fallopian tube. Once there, the sperm is supposed to fertilize the egg, forming an embryo, which then travels to the uterus. ZIFT is similar: Instead of placing the sperm and egg immediately into the fallopian tubes, the doctor places them into an incubator for 24 hours. Then the fertilized eggs are put into the fallopian tubes. The success rate for both techniques is around 24 percent, although that figure, along with the cost, can vary considerably from clinic to clinic.

• ICSI—intracytoplasmic sperm injection. One of the most promising new treatments for male infertility is ICSI. Doctors take a single sperm and inject it into a single egg; the resulting zygote is then transferred into the uterus. About

1,000 ICSI procedures are performed each year, and the success rate is around 24 percent. ICSI costs $10,000 to $15,000.

Jeffrey and Amy Hill of Minneapolis used GIFT to help them give birth to two daughters: Kate Lynn, now 7 years old, and Julia, almost 4. The couple spent $22,000 on their fertility program.

"We depleted our savings," Amy, 41, recalls. "My husband was out of a job. [Jeffrey, 44, is now president of a water treatment company.] We had to make a major decision on whether to gamble. But it was in our plan, in our hearts, and it would have been a real sting if it had not worked.

"But we have two beautiful, healthy daughters. We never really believed we'd have a baby until we had Kate Lynn in our arms. We were in total awe of her."

For more information, write to the American Society for Reproductive Medicine, 1209 Montgomery Highway, Birmingham, AL 35216-2809.

When Is a Cesarean Really Necessary?

NEARLY ONE IN FOUR AMERICAN BABIES IS exposed to its first light in an operating room, with masked doctors and nurses peering into its mother's womb as a surgeon cuts open the uterus to remove the baby.

Although often lifesaving for both mother and child, surgical delivery—also called a cesarean section or C-section—has become a multi-billion-dollar business for both doctors and hospitals. The fee is higher for surgery than for a vaginal birth. Hospital bills are higher too: the mother stays longer and requires more services and drugs.

Public Citizen's Health Research Group, consumer advocates in Washington, D.C., analyzed the cesarean situation. Since 1970, they report, C-sections have surged from 6 percent to almost 25 percent of all births. The group found 56 hospitals nationwide with more than 40 percent C-sections; some hospitals exceeded 50 percent. The Abrom Kaplan Memorial Hospital in Kaplan, Louisiana, topped the list, with a cesarean rate of 57 percent. The Health Insurance Association of America says the average cost for a cesarean in this nation in 1991 was $7,826, compared to $4,720 for a vaginal delivery. More than $7 billion was spent in the United States on nearly a million cesareans. Public Citizen's Health Research Group estimates that half of these surgeries were unnecessary.

There is a rising clamor within and outside the medical community for doctors and hospitals to reject surgery as the first answer to birth problems.

In an interview shortly before he died, Dr. Mortimer Rosen, chief of obstetrics at Columbia-Presbyterian Medical Center in New York City, called the cesarean explosion a dangerous national scandal. He was a leader in the effort to reduce birth surgeries. "Cesareans are costly, dangerous, and painful," Dr. Rosen told me. "This is not a neat, simple procedure. It is big-time, major surgery. The floor of the operating room is covered with blood and fluids. A woman loses two units of blood, undergoes anesthesia. She is scarred internally and externally."

A C-section *can* be a lifesaver, however. Liz Baldwin, 41, of Miami, says she is sure surgery saved the life of her first-born son, David. Labor contractions were lowering David's blood supply in the womb by pushing against his defective birth cord. A cesarean was performed, and David was saved. Still, Mrs. Baldwin recalls the aftereffects: "For 2 to 3 weeks, I had the most horrible pain." She was determined that her next baby would have a vaginal birth. But her first doctor said that a vaginal birth after a cesarean would endanger the baby's life and hers also.

Many obstetricians maintain that a surgically scarred uterus can rupture under the pressure of labor contractions. However, Dr. Bruce Flamm, of Kaiser Permanente Medical Center in Riverside, California, says the risk of rupture is less than 1 percent. Dr. Flamm led the research for a 5-year study on the risk of uterine rupture after C-section. The study, involving 5,733 women, ended in 1988.

Mrs. Baldwin found another doctor and, 4 years later, had Billy by vaginal birth. "It was the most wonderful experience," she says. "I wept tears of joy for 3 months, just thinking of it."

Lots of women must feel that way: A survey of doctors by the American College of Obstetricians and Gynecologists shows that in 1970 only 2.2 percent of women who'd had cesareans later delivered vaginally. By 1991, that figure had leaped to more than 25 percent. Dr. Richard Porreco, director of the perinatal program at Presbyterian–St. Lukes Medical Center in Denver, says, "To get cesareans below 10 percent, you need to give almost every woman who has had a C-section the *chance* to go into labor."

No single cause explains the burgeoning of surgical births. As noted earlier, profit is one motive. So is fear.

Fearful doctors mean more cesareans: They want neither to be blamed nor to have to blame themselves for damaging an infant by letting labor continue if either baby or mother is in danger. Sometimes the problems are genetic, not medical. John J. Bower, a New York lawyer who has been trying malpractice cases for four decades, says, "People think the doctor is delivering a product, and they want a perfect product. But in medicine, the doctor isn't always in control. Even with the best techniques, things can go wrong."

The fear of malpractice suits seems justified. A 1992 survey conducted by the American College of Obstetricians and Gynecologists showed that 80 percent of obstetricians had been sued at least once. One-fourth of those doctors said that they reduced the number of high-risk patients they cared for. In some states their malpractice insurance cost more than $100,000 a year. Small wonder that in 1992 more than 12 percent quit the profession.

Some women get C-sections because they need them, some because they want—and can afford—them. Dr. Jeffrey B. Gould, chief of a program for maternal and child care at the University of California at Berkeley, says, "Affluent women are better at telling doctors what they want." It's the private hospital that might end up with as many as one in two born under the knife. In public hospitals, cesareans are more likely to meet the ideal rate of 12 percent, because the uninsured poor can't demand such costly elective services.

Why would women demand cesareans? Some want to avoid labor or ensure a convenient time for the birth. (Doctors, anxious to keep their patronage, don't refuse.) Still others are attracted to C-sections by the anesthesiologists' epidural "spinal block." With it, the mother is awake during childbirth, yet she feels no pain.

Prolonged labor is a good reason for a cesarean. Some obstetricians charge that epidural painkilling slows the birth process—that the mother, feeling no pain, fails to push hard enough to squeeze her baby out. Many anesthesiologists argue that epidurals speed some deliveries by reducing pain's stress. But Dr. Ezzat Abouleish, professor of anesthesiology and obstetrics and gynecology at the University of Texas Medical School in Houston, says data from England show epidurals don't affect labor's duration. Janet O'Driscoll, 36, of Cleveland, says she feels she had an unnecessary C-section. "I was given an epidural. I could not feel the contractions. I could not push. The baby was coming down, but the doctor decided that the baby was too big. So cesarean surgery was performed. The baby weighed 8 pounds, 5 ounces."

Mrs. O'Driscoll had two more children easily, by vaginal birth—one weighing 7 pounds, 8 ounces, the other 10 pounds, 1/2 ounce. "I think my first baby could have come out with the proper encouragement," she says.

Despite the campaign to lower the number of unnecessary C-sections, many conditions do make them necessary, says Dr. Flamm. For example:

- Slowed labor—the baby isn't seen to be progressing down the birth canal.
- Small pelvic bones—the mother's frame is too small for baby's passage. (But normal births have succeeded in hundreds of cases.)
- Breech birth—when the baby is not coming through headfirst. If the doctor cannot turn the infant from a buttocks- or legs-first position, a C-section may avoid damage to mother and child.

To avoid unnecessary and dangerous birth surgery, first ask the doctor about his or her rate of cesarean deliveries. If the rate exceeds 15 percent, you might do well to look for another physician. Otherwise, you risk having surgery performed at the first sign of even the slightest trouble.

Research shows that if you have a vaginal birth after cesarean surgery, 99 percent of the time your baby should be at least as healthy as if delivered by surgery. And you will be playing the key role in your child's destiny.

However, if the doctor advises a C-section during your labor because you or the baby are not faring well, your best bet is to follow that advice.

Are Births As Safe As They Could Be?

A REVOLUTION IN HEALTH CARE HAS CAUGHT Americans off guard. New research tells us that much of what our doctors and hospitals do for pregnancy and birth is wrong, expensive, and dangerous. That same research has found good, inexpensive, and safe methods for bringing babies into the world.

Although the United States may offer some of the finest medical technology on earth, millions of our citizens suffer inadequate health care. And the cost of medical care has zoomed to $810 billion a year—a sum to stagger any treasury.

Add to this the fact that of the 4.17 million babies born in the United States each year, 39,000 die before their first birthdays of ills that are largely preventable. As for infant safety worldwide, statistics show that the United States has 9.7 deaths for every 1,000 births—ranking a lowly 22nd. Japan is first, with only 4.4 deaths per 1,000; Sweden is second, with 5.7.

But the new science of birth could improve that. A research team led by Dr. Murray Enkin has produced perhaps the world's most careful and systematic study on childbirth. For 10 years, this team searched the world for solid scientific data on what's wrong and what's right in the handling of pregnancy by hospitals, doctors, midwives, nurses, and pregnant women themselves. Dr. Enkin is professor emeritus of obstetrics at Canada's McMaster University in Hamilton, Ontario, and a principal researcher for the pregnancy project at Oxford University in England.

Much confusion surrounds pregnancy, Dr. Enkin says. "There are old wives' tales, old doctors' tales, medical textbook statements, doctors' beliefs, scientific data, and communal myths."

Although many caregivers do a great deal of good for both mother and baby, Dr. Enkin's team found that several do not. For example, he says, it is very important to provide a pregnant woman with social and psychological support. It reduces her anxieties about an easy and successful delivery, about the baby's health and her own, and about the running of the family after the baby is born. However, Dr. Enkin adds, too many physicians fail to provide such support.

The Oxford team also discovered that hospitals and the staff members who oversee births—primarily doctors and nurses—routinely employ some methods of care that ultimately not only offer little benefit to mother or infant but actually can be dangerous to them. For example, some hospitals put healthy newborn babies in nurseries to prevent their mothers from passing on infections to them. However, evidence shows that generally it is much safer for the infants to room with their mothers, in whose bodies, after all, they were carried and nurtured, and very likely instilled with immunities. In the nursery, on the other hand, germs spread to the healthy infants from the sick ones.

Research shows that keeping mother and child apart for 4 hours or more can have dire effects, such as the failure of breast-feeding and the restriction of maternal affectionate behavior. How such separations affect maternal behavior has been the focus of much of this research. Urging that mother and newborn share a room, rather than be separated, the Oxford team cites a study suggesting that such routine hospital separation policy has led to an increased risk of child abuse and neglect among socially deprived, first-time mothers.

The research team—about 40 doctors, mathematicians, and public health experts—rated the effectiveness or danger of 285 forms of care, including pregnant women's diets, the birthing position, episiotomy (cutting the skin and underlying tissue at the bottom of the vagina to prevent ragged tearing during delivery), and keeping a newborn in the hospital nursery or in a crib near the mother's bed. Here are some of the results:

- 100 of the 285 forms of care studied were rated successful and safe.
- 37 were rated possibly effective, needing more exploration.
- 88 had unknown effects, requiring more research.
- 60 were rated "should be abandoned—they do little good and produce danger."

The study's data and results are available in three forms: for computer use as *The Oxford Database of Perinatal Trials;* as a two-volume set of scientific papers; and as a paperback book, *A Guide to Effective Care in Pregnancy and Childbirth*. All three discuss the findings for doctors, nurses, midwives, and informed laypeople. And all come from the Oxford University Press, authored by Drs. Iain Chalmers, Marc J. N. C. Keirse, and Murray Enkin.

The study criticizes the birthing position common in most urban hospitals—women lie flat on their backs or put their feet in stirrups, with the pelvis slightly tilted. Research suggests lying on the back can adversely affect labor by interfering with the blood supply of mother and baby.

When the mother is *allowed* to select positions during labor, she is likely to choose standing or walking for the first stages. She will feel less pain and need less pain medication if the birth canal is open wide. If she needs to lie down, she will elect to lie on her side during delivery, or she may squat and deliver the baby with her own hands. Although many cultures use the squatting posture, little scientific evidence supports its use in preference to standing or lying on one side.

Try this quiz: Test your knowledge—your doctor's too. To answer, circle T or F for true or false:

1. **T or F?** A medical doctor must supervise the entire pregnancy and delivery in case something goes wrong.
2. **T or F?** It is really much safer to have your baby in a hospital, using the latest equipment and know-how.
3. **T or F?** Hospital nurseries protect newborns from germs.
4. **T or F?** Episiotomy eases birth, and suturing (sewing) the cut afterward prevents pain and infection.
5. **T or F?** Once you have a cesarean, or C-section surgery, all later births must be by C-section, too.

As you may have guessed, all the answers are false. But many obstetricians and other doctors still insist they are true. And that is sad, because all of these long-established procedures can cause harm. The researchers found that episiotomies, for instance, often do not help and actually injure the vagina.

Hospitals are dangerous for both mother and baby, says Dr. Keirse. "Having a doctor involved in *all* pregnancies can be a bad thing. You get more technology, more hospital infections, more unhappy mothers—and more cost.

"It comes down to whether you consider pregnancy and birth pathological [disease] or physiological [normal] events," he says. "As soon as a doctor shows his face, everything turns toward disease. It's hard to accept that having obstetricians at all deliveries is a bad thing. Yet, if you have well-trained midwives, very few deliveries need a specialist present. In the Netherlands, 30 percent of all women deliver safely at home."

This is borne out in the following experience one American woman shared with us. She has delivered two children—one by traditional means with a doctor in charge at a hospital in New York, and the other by a midwife at a women's center in Florida.

She is Deborah Namath, 33, of Tequesta, Florida—the wife of the legendary New York Jets quarterback Joe Namath, 52.

"I had focused on one fear," Mrs. Namath relates. "I was terrified of having the episiotomy. I asked the doctor, 'Please don't do it.' He assured me that he wouldn't do it unless necessary." But, she says, forceps and an episiotomy became necessary, in his view.

"I was on my back," recalls Mrs. Namath. "It was not even suggested that I could be in any other position. I was lying down with my feet in stirrups. That day, Jessica, who is now 10, was born."

"With my second child, Olivia, now 5, I absolutely knew that I did not want to give birth in a hospital. Joe was concerned: he didn't think we'd be OK outside a hospital. We went to a women's center, and Joe became an active partici-pant. When labor began, I stayed upright—on my feet. I was comfortable only on my feet. At the last moment, I lay down on my left side, to push the baby out. In three pushes, she was out.

"We—Joe and I—pulled her out as a team. At the hospital in Manhattan, Jessica and I were kept apart. They wouldn't bring me my baby. But with Olivia, in Florida, we all slept in one big bed—me, Joe, Jessica, and my newborn. This was my heaven."

The Oxford team found that the use of metal forceps to pull the baby from the birth canal damages both the baby and the mother. The team recommends the use of a suction cup by well-trained individuals. The cup fits on the baby's head, and a vacuum pump firmly fixes it there. The doctor or birthing assistant gently pulls to draw the infant out. It sounds strange, but it has been proved quite effective.

Carol Markoski, 30, of Moreno Valley, California, delivered an 8-pound girl, Kelsie, with the aid of a suction cup. "The baby was stuck," she says. "I'd had an episiotomy. I just wanted her out."

Mrs. Markoski's husband was there and recalls, "After doing the episiotomy, the doctor attached the cup, and the baby came out in minutes."

The Oxford team's research also revealed that the surgery and suturing involved in an episiotomy lead to more bleeding, infection, and tearing of tissue than when no episiotomy is done.

As for cesarean deliveries, there is mounting evidence that more than half of all C-sections performed in this country may be unnecessary.

In the United States, C-sections exceed 30 percent of all births. In England, they total 9 percent. As do many American researchers, the Oxford team says that there is no reason to rule out natural vaginal birth for a mother just because she has had a cesarean.

How did the Oxford team members arrive at the findings? They focused on studies on childbearing done from 1950 onward that were published in 60 key scientific journals, then wrote to the authors of these studies and to 18,000 obstetricians to obtain unpublished data.

Finally, they subjected the studies to meticulous mathematical evaluations. In particular, they were looking for research that used *random and controlled* techniques.

For example: Suppose a researcher wants to evaluate the safety and effectiveness of shaving pubic hair before birth. (Such an experiment was conducted in 1922.) As women come through the hospital, they are assigned by a coin toss: shaved or not shaved. That makes their selection *random,* eliminating bias in selection. The effects are evaluated later by individuals unaware of who was and was not shaved: they were "blinded" with respect to who received what. This prevents conscious or unconscious bias. The unshaved patients become the comparison or *control* patients. A statistician later sums up the results. If there is no difference between shaved and unshaved patients—as the 1922 test concluded—then shaving should be abandoned. (Of course, in any trial, if the number of subjects is too small, it cannot be concluded that there was no difference between them.)

Frederick Mosteller of Harvard University, one of the nation's leading statisticians, strongly endorses the Oxford methods. "I am very impressed with the magnitude and strength of the effort and experts brought into play," he says. "One of the things I like about their work is that they cared deeply whether the patient was pleased. This more tender and humanitarian interest is quite surprising in a book concerned with quantitative analysis. They emphasized letting the patient participate in decisions."

Despite the findings of the Oxford team and others, many obstetricians and pediatricians—especially those with practices away from large research centers—have been slow to change their methods.

"I am shocked that 10 percent of Canadian hospitals still shave women," says Dr. Enkin, "or did so until very recently. Though the story on shaving has long been known, doctors didn't change their habits until women began to complain and ask why it was being done."

"If a doctor believes that our data do not tell the truth," Dr. Keirse asserts, "then that critic must mount his own randomized, blinded, controlled trials to prove he is right and we are wrong."

Daniel M. Fox heads the Milbank Memorial Fund, based in Manhattan, which is sponsoring conferences and an information network to encourage putting the study's results to work.

"As the medical world learns more of what this Oxford team has done," Mr. Fox says, "there could be a revolution in obstetrical practice. And that could save many babies and mothers, and billions of dollars."

Here are some other new views their research has provided:

• Diet and pregnancy-induced hypertension (pre-eclampsia). There is no evidence that dietary intervention prevents this condition.

• Routine use of iron supplements. It is unnecessary and probably harmful.

• Giving steroid hormones to mothers in labor to relieve breathing problems in their low-weight babies. Proponents say this could save billions by replacing more costly care for the infants later.

As the Oxford team's work gains recognition, it seems logical that we will be seeing more infants born at home or in birthing centers, attended to by midwives or physicians' assistants. Hospitals will provide emergency backup for births, but their primary role will be to provide care for high-risk patients.

Hormones

Should You Take Estrogen?

IN THE 1960s, A SMALL GROUP OF PHYSICIANS asserted that a drug called estrogen, taken in pill form to supplement the natural female hormone estrogen, could keep women young—retaining smooth, un-wrinkled skin, strong bones, and youthful sexual capacity. Moreover, they said, the estrogen supplement eliminated or limited such menopausal symptoms as hot flashes, increased facial and body hair, mood swings, insomnia, and night sweats.

Then came the bad news: Studies suggested that estrogen caused cancer and also would stimulate the growth of estrogen-dependent cancers of the breast, ovaries, and uterine lining in meno-pausal women. After that, doctors quickly dropped estrogen for treatment of menopause. But the doctors also assured women under age 35 that estrogen sup-plementation was safe for them and that they ran a low risk of breast cancer. So young women kept using birth control pills with estrogen. Later studies revealed that the birth control pills even protected young women against some malignancies.

Now supplemental estrogen again is being hailed for keeping women not only young but also alive and healthier longer. Studies show that menopausal women taking estrogen gain two or three extra years of life. Estrogen also has been shown to lower cholesterol buildup and to delay heart disease, which kills 923,000 Americans yearly and affects about half of those over age 55.

Dr. William Castelli, who heads the Framingham, Massachusetts, study of heart attack risks, points out that 90 per-cent of heart attack victims do not die but struggle on, disabled, for years. "If I can delay or eliminate that heart attack or stroke," Dr. Castelli says, "I can save many older people years of pain and dis-ability. Prescribing a supplement of the female hormone estrogen is proving to be one way to do that for many women."

Numerous studies now show that, after menopause, older women face at least 15 times the risk of dying of heart disease than of estrogen-dependent can-cers. These studies also show that estro-gen supplementation reduces the risk of heart disease in women of normal health with no family history of heart disease.

Estrogen supplementation also has been shown to help protect against osteo-porosis, the thinning of bones—a condi-tion that affects about half of all menopausal women. Loss of bone matter speeds up rapidly in the first few years of menopause.

A woman's ovaries normally produce the hormones estrogen and progesterone from the onset of menstruation in adolescence through menopause, when menstruation stops, generally between the ages of 45 and 55. In estrogen replacement therapy (ERT), only estrogen is replaced. In hormone replacement therapy (HRT), both estrogen and progesterone are replaced. Studies show that combining the hormones seems to provide better results.

Doctors caution that some women will be at risk from either therapy, but Dr. C. Wayne Bardin, former medical director of the Population Council, a non-profit research organization, is an expert on estrogen and emphatic in his praise: "It looks like the overall benefits of estrogen treatment far exceed the risk," he says. "Not only does it benefit the heart, it can slow down the escape of calcium from bones, preventing fractures of the hip and spine. Nursing homes are filled with osteoporotic women, confined to bed and unable to help themselves."

Denver resident Barbara Silverman, 61, began taking estrogen at age 54. "I'm scared to death of osteoporosis," she explains. "My mother, who died last year at the age of 90, suffered from osteoporosis. In her early 60s, her back started to curve. She had to use a walker for 15 years. My mother had broken her hip three times and had two hip replacements. She had no real life for 30 years—the last third of her life."

Dr. Brian E. Henderson is president of the Salk Institute in La Jolla, California. In 1981, with his colleagues, he studied 8,881 menopausal women from Leisure World, a retirement community. Each woman filled out a health questionnaire. Following up on the participants in 1989, he made an astonishing finding. The death rate for those who took estrogen was 20 percent lower than for those who never took it. Those taking estrogen for more than 15 years had a mortality rate that was 40 percent lower than others in the same age group. Dr. Henderson also found that women who took estrogen had fewer deaths from heart disease.

A number of studies conclude that estrogen treatment of older women raises their risk of breast cancer and uterine (endometrial) cancer, but estimates vary. Dr. Karen K. Steinberg headed a team at the Centers for Disease Control in Atlanta that researched 16 investigations of estrogen and breast cancer in older women. These investigations dated to the early 1970s.

"After 15 years of estrogen use," Dr. Steinberg says, "we found about 1,500 extra breast cancer deaths a year among 3 million women, ages 45 to 64, who had been exposed to estrogens for 15 years. From a research vantage point, the protective effect on heart disease may outweigh the breast cancer risk. But not, certainly, from the viewpoint of the women who get breast cancer. Most women are frustrated that we can't give them a bottom line on breast cancer, because we don't have the data."

Should You Take Either of the Hormone Therapies?

There are no clear answers in the research. Some studies showed a correlation between the length of ERT and breast cancers. Other studies showed contradictory results—no risk for up to 15 years of ERT; increased risk of 30 percent or more after 15 years. Hormone replacement therapy has been shown to protect certain women from heart disease and stroke. Some scientists say that women with high blood pressure or a family history of stroke should avoid ERT and/or HRT. Most experts say each woman must make her own decision, based on family history and her response to the replacement therapy prescribed.

Are You at Risk for Osteoporosis?

Probably—if your mother had it, if you began menopause early (at age 42 or so), or if you are small-boned and sedentary. Hormone supplements should help you.

Dr. Daniel Mishell, head of obstetrics and gynecology at the University of Southern California, says that nearly all postmenopausal women need supplemental estrogen for protection against osteoporosis. He cites 300,000 hip fractures yearly in these women at a health care cost of $6 billion, adding that 10 percent of the patients die within 6 months.

What about cancer and heart attacks? When it was found that patients receiving ERT developed cancer of the endometrium, the lining of the uterus, doctors added the hormone progesterone to reduce that risk. Progestin, the prescribed form of progesterone, seemed to reduce that cancer risk. Some scientists speculated that, when combined with estrogen, progestin also could reduce the threat of cancers of the breast and ovaries, which are estrogen-dependent. There is no proof that progestin actually can prevent cancer.

Estrogen is said to help the heart by raising the body's levels of "good" HDL cholesterol and preventing the "bad" LDL cholesterol from clogging arteries. But evidence indicates that, in some doses, progestin can increase cholesterol—a point to consider if cholesterol is a problem for you or threatens to become one.

You and your doctor must weigh the pluses and minuses for you. To help clarify the issue, the National Institutes of Health began a study in 1987. It involves 875 women receiving either estrogen therapy, or both estrogen and progestin, or a placebo. The results are not yet available.

Fighting Hot Flashes

With the onset of menopause, many women suffer from hot flashes and night sweats. Arlene March, 56, a Los Angeles psychotherapist, says she started getting hot flashes 5 years ago. "I'd be working," she recalls, "and suddenly feel intense heat all over my body. I'd break out in a sweat. I'd have to stop work. Then Dr. Mishell prescribed estrogen pills, and I've not had a day of discomfort."

Some women experience a drying and thinning of vaginal tissues in the absence of estrogen, making sex painful. They also might suffer urinary tract infections and incontinence. Estrogen therapy often helps.

Among the physicians consulted, the most cautious was Dr. Morris Notelovitz, founder of the nation's first Menopause Center, at the University of Florida, and head of the Women's Medical and Diagnostic Center in Gainesville, Florida. He says each symptom needs a different treatment and advises that genital tract problems be given estrogen treatment for a couple of years at most. He also urges special measurements of the bones before prescribing estrogen therapy for osteoporosis.

The Patch

If a woman is at risk of heart disease because of family history or a risky cholesterol pattern, Dr. Notelovitz says, he probably would put her on estrogen for the rest of her life. The leading form of estrogen is Premarin, extracted from the urine of pregnant mares. More recently, doctors have prescribed a plastic bandage-type patch, usually affixed to the buttocks or abdomen. It delivers a synthetic estrogen through the skin. The patch is changed twice weekly, and so is its location, if a skin rash occurs.

When estrogen is taken in pill form, its level in the blood rises after the pill is taken, then falls as the day passes. But with the patch, a steady estrogen level is maintained, usually causing fewer side effects.

Valene Crumpley, 55, a registered nurse in Salt Lake City, had her ovaries surgically removed at 37. Ensuing hot flashes were not relieved by estrogen pills. She has used the patch since its introduction 6 years ago. As a result, she says, she has "no hot flashes at all."

In 1966, when Dr. Robert A. Wilson advocated estrogen therapy in his book *Feminine Forever,* most doctors pooh-poohed his ideas, but some researchers took them up. Now it's the treatment of choice for most menopausal women.

How Your Body's Secret System Works

AS YOU WALK DOWN THE STREET, A LARGE, ferocious dog suddenly jumps from behind a bush and directly in your path. Your heart begins thumping wildly.

Your blood pressure peaks. Your body mobilizes its energy resources. You are ready to stand firm and do battle or to flee—ready for fight or flight.

Your body contains a marvelous system of glands and nerves that quickly organizes your heart, lungs, liver, kidneys, blood vessels, and bowels, causing them to work at top efficiency in an emergency. And when the threat ends, that same glandular system calms everything down.

Of course, your brain acts first. Through your senses, generally your eyes, the brain recognizes the dog as a threat, sizes up the danger, and then releases chemicals to trigger the complex web of glands posted throughout your body. The glands pour out more chemicals—messengers that start the other organs working at top speed.

These chemical messengers are called hormones (from the Greek *hormon*, meaning to stimulate). Until 15 years ago, scientists had found only about 20 hormones; now they believe that more than 200 hormones course through our veins and arteries.

"Recently, we have had an explosion in our knowledge of hormones," says Dr. Charles Hollander, director of endocrinology (the study of glands) at New York University Medical Center. "Through endocrinology, we have new understanding of cancer, diabetes, heart disease, depression, and a host of other diseases."

The fight-or-flight hormone network takes care of just one of your needs—the survival response to danger. Your glands also release hormones to

- regulate your sexual development (ovaries and testes),

- influence your blood pressure and heart rate (adrenals),
- adjust your growth (pituitary),
- control energy use (thyroid), and
- govern how your cells burn sugar (pancreas).

In 1983, Ruby Hunt-Russell of Torrance, California, was born without a thyroid gland. Had she come into the world 4 years earlier, the lack of thyroid hormones would have irrevocably damaged her brain. But she was lucky. In 1980, California implemented a law requiring that every newborn get a thyroid test. Today, most states have such a law.

When Ruby was 2 days old, doctors took a sample of her blood. No thyroid hormone showed in the sample. X rays of the base of her throat, the site of the thyroid, revealed no thyroid gland. In this country, one baby in 4,000 is born with a defective thyroid or is lacking one. Doctors prescribed that thyroxin be given to Ruby in her milk. She will take the hormone in pill form for the rest of her life.

"She is totally normal, physically and in intelligence," says Lyn Hunt-Russell, Ruby's mother, a schoolteacher.

Ruby today is a striking blond child, with giant brown eyes and a California tan. Without thyroid hormone, she would have become a mentally retarded dwarf.

Scientists also have learned that glands strongly influence both your physical life and your moods and thoughts. Too much or too little hormone secretion by glands can cause anxiety (nonstop fear or depression) and uncontrollable sadness and moroseness, or impair the ability to think clearly.

More news: Other organs, in addition to your glands, make important hormones. Your kidneys make erythropoietin, a substance that spurs the growth of red blood cells. Scientists have made this hormone artificially to help produce blood in people without kidneys.

Your heart pours out atrial natriuretic factor, a hormone that controls blood pressure. Some doctors believe this hormone may be the most powerful medicine yet discovered for high blood pressure. Your stomach secretes cholecystokinin, which tells your brain that you have had enough to eat. If scientists can find ways of making this substance in quantity, they may have the drug that will end the need for dieting forever.

The new knowledge about hormones has given doctors powerful new treatments for ailments that had resisted cure. Among them are synthetic growth hormone to make dwarfs grow to near normal height, tests to show whether depression has a glandular cause, hormone techniques to treat infertility, and hormone treatments for menopause symptoms.

They also have found inhibin, a hormone that could be a male contraceptive. Inhibin is made by the testes and ovaries. But its commercial production for general use could be years off.

At the Salk Institute in La Jolla, California, Dr. Roger Guillemin, a Nobel Prize winner, and his colleagues have isolated what Dr. Guillemin calls "perhaps the most important molecule ever characterized." Called fibroblast growth factor (FGF), it speeds up the healing of wounds, stimulates the growth of new blood vessels after menstruation, and helps restore damaged nerves. It may be involved in stimulating blood vessel growth to feed new blood to the heart after a heart attack or to the brain after a stroke.

Scientists are trying to create FGF by genetic engineering as a possible treatment for heart attack or stroke patients.

Scientists already have created two kinds of hormone that make children grow—one that normally comes from the pituitary gland at the base of the brain and the other from the brain itself. The pituitary chemical, called growth hormone (GH), can stimulate growth in children whose pituitary gland cannot naturally make it. The brain chemical called growth hormone releasing factor (GHRF) stimulates the normal pituitary gland to release growth hormone. It was first isolated by Dr. Guillemin and his colleagues.

At age 7, Scotty Floyd of Buena Vista, Virginia, stood eye-to-eye with 4-year-olds. "I'm just barely 5 feet tall and my husband, Larry, is average height," says Scotty's mother, Donna. "So we thought Scotty would be short."

Scotty's pediatrician sent his young patient for tests by Dr. Michael Thorner, an endocrinologist at the University of Virginia Medical School in Charlottesville. Dr. Thorner found a cyst in Scotty's brain that stopped GHRF from getting to his pituitary.

Scotty began wearing around his waist a special medicine pump that contained the hormone. Every 3 hours, the pump automatically fed a dose of GHRF through a needle in Scotty's skin. In the first 3 months of treatment, Scotty grew 3 inches. Now 12, he alternates by wearing the pump for 6 months, then removing it for 6 months. When Scotty wears the pump, he grows 2 or 3 inches during the 6-month period. When he removes the pump, he grows less than an inch during the same amount of time. He will continue this treatment until he's 17.

"There have been no side effects," says Mrs. Floyd. "He doesn't even notice the pump. Scotty plays sports, except contact sports. And he grins a lot, now that he's growing."

The Brain—Your Most Powerful Gland

In the last 20 years, scientists have discovered that the brain puts out scores of hormones to control other glands and organs. Not all of these speedy messengers are known or named.

The brain acts as a switchboard between your mental and physical lives. By releasing hormones to travel to distant organs, your brain translates your emotional upsets into physical responses—a rapid heartbeat, a stomachache, inflamed intestines.

The brain controls, first of all, the master gland—the pituitary. Just above the pituitary lies a tangle of nerves known as the hypothalamus. The hypothalamus spews out several chemicals that release the major hormones from the pituitary. Here's a brief summary of the process:

The growth hormone releasing factor triggers growth hormone from the pituitary. This is the substance that is enabling Scotty Floyd to grow to normal height.

The growth hormone inhibiting factor controls the release of growth hormone from the pituitary. Called somatostatin, it helps regulate our growth and probably protects us from becoming giants.

Several new drugs—somatostatin-like compounds—are effectively treating disorders linked to this hormone.

The thyrotropin releasing factor lets thyrotropin go to the thyroid. It's like a double play in baseball: the brain triggers the pituitary, which, in turn, triggers the thyroid gland to produce its thyroid hormone.

The gonadotropin releasing hormone (GnRH) does the same for the sex organs: brain to pituitary to sex glands. Doctors give this hormone to women who cannot ovulate. In some infertile men, the hormone increases sperm production.

Chemists have developed artificial cousins of GnRH that are even more powerful. These substances are being tested against prostate gland cancer. Male hormones stimulate the growth of this cancer. By giving the hormone steadily and in large doses, doctors can shut off the testes' production of male sex hormone and slow the cancer. In women, these sex hormones could be used to treat premenstrual tension and a disease called endometriosis, in which tissue from the lining of the womb invades other parts of the pelvis.

Corticotropin releasing factor (CRF) is a major stress control hormone. First isolated from human tissue in 1981 by Dr. Wylie Vale of the Salk Institute, CRF may be the key to understanding chronic stress and whether it is of psychological or physical origin.

CRF triggers the pituitary to secrete cortisol (an adrenal hormone) and also stimulates the brain to activate the fight-or-flight response.

"In the short run, your body response mechanism is good for you," says Dr. Vale. "You are ready to act. But if you are chronically under stress, you suppress your immune system, your appetite, and your reproductive system. Chronic stress also suppresses growth in children."

To counteract this suppression, Dr. Vale and his associates developed the first agent that blocks the action of the hormone, called a CRF blocker, in the hope that resultant drugs will be able to relieve patients who overrespond to stress situations.

The Pituitary—Master Gland

Snuggled under your brain is the pituitary, a tiny lump of tissue that squirts out a variety of hormones that control nearly every major biological system.

I already have told you about GH, the hormone that stimulates growth. Doctors succeeded in isolating that hormone from human cadavers and injected it into children whose pituitary glands could not produce the chemical. But tragedy occasionally accompanied this treatment: Some researchers believe that a virus that causes severe brain damage sometimes "piggy-backed" with the human hormone and invaded the patient, destroying the child's ability to think. A safe form of the hormone is now made in the laboratory by genetic engineering.

The pituitary also puts out gonadotropic hormones, chemicals that head for the ovaries or testes—our gonads, or sex glands. (*Gonad* means seed; *tropic* means turning.) In women, these hormones control the ovaries' production of eggs, menstruation, and the release of female sex hormones, such as estrogen and progestin. In men, the hormones stimulate the formation of sperm and the manufacture of male hormones, such as testosterone.

Doctors now use these gonadotropic hormones to stimulate egg production in infertile women. They also inject them to induce eggs from the ovaries for in vitro fertilization. The employment of these hormones has also produced many more multiple births: triplets, quadruplets, quintuplets, and even sextuplets.

Thyrotropin stimulates the thyroid gland to release its hormone, thereby controlling the body's energy levels. Too much or too little thyrotropin also may contribute to mental depression.

In addition, the pituitary produces adrenocorticotropic hormone (ACTH), which switches your adrenal glands on and off. In response to ACTH, the adrenals (one astride each kidney) create several hormones that increase blood sugar, turn off inflammation, lower immunity, and trigger the production of male sex hormones.

Perhaps most intriguing of all, the pituitary makes beta-endorphin, a natural, opium-like substance that reduces pain, gives a feeling of pleasure, and may help counter depression.

Clearly, trouble in the pituitary gland spells trouble throughout your body. However, doctors now have powerful treatments to reverse or head off the troubles.

Your Hormones at a Glance

The following table is just a small sample of the number of hormones racing through your body. Their functions interlock. A decline in one hormone triggers a decline in another and another until the system is back in balance. It seems that new hormones are discovered nearly every week.

Hormone	Gland/Organ	Function
Thyroxin	Thyroid	Stimulates energy use
Erythropoietin (EPO)	Kidney	Stimulates blood formation
Atrial natriuretic	Heart	Controls blood pressure
Cholecystokinin	Stomach	Controls appetite
Inhibin	Testes; ovaries	Controls sperm and egg output
Fibroblast growth factor (FGF)	Various	Speeds wound healing
Growth hormone (GH)	Pituitary	Controls growth
Growth hormone releasing factor	Brain	Stimulates pituitary to release GH
Cortisone	Adrenal	Acts as an antiinflammatory
ACTH	Pituitary	Releases cortisone from adrenal gland

A Cure for Diabetes?

FOR THE FIRST TIME, SCIENTISTS ARE TALKING seriously about a cure for diabetes, the "sugar disease" that afflicts 13 million Americans and each year kills 300,000. Five million of those who have diabetes don't know it. You could easily be one of them.

Diabetes starts insidiously with excessive thirst, frequent urination, and fatigue. As the years roll by, the disease damages blood vessels, nerves, the heart, kidneys, and eyes. Diabetics are twice as likely as unaffected people to suffer from coronary heart disease and strokes. They may die of kidney failure, are often

blinded, and have an amputation rate 40 times higher than that of nondiabetics. With its complications, diabetes kills more Americans than all other diseases except heart disease and cancer.

Noreen Harmer's victory over diabetes is one example of how the bold new researchers are making inroads toward a cure. Ms. Harmer is one of about 500 recipients of a transplanted human pancreas. The organ puts out the vital hormone, insulin. It enables Ms. Harmer to turn the foods she eats into energy. After 25 years of daily injections of insulin—sometimes as many as four a

The History of Diabetes

1922

After 3,000 years with no effective treatment, diabetes is no longer a quick death sentence. Canadian researchers extract insulin from a dog, inject it into a 14-year-old diabetic boy, and extend his life.

1935

Researchers advance the theory that diabetes is not a single disease and divide it into two categories: insulin sensitive (what we call Type I) and insulin insensitive (Type II).

1956

The first antidiabetes pill, an "oral hypoglycemic agent" called Orinase, is introduced in the United States, making it possible for some diabetics to control their blood sugar without insulin injections.

1966

The first successful pancreas transplant is performed by Dr. Richard Lillehei at the University of Minnesota. The body rejects the organ, but doctors have new hope—and much work still to do.

1970

Dr. Paul Lacy of Washington University in St. Louis proves that transplanted insulin-producing cells can survive and control blood sugar in rats. Is this an alternative to pancreas transplants?

1975

Dr. Gian F. Bottazzo, of Middlesex Hospital in London, develops the Islet Cell Antibody Test. This test determines the presence of antibodies in the blood that attack and destroy the insulin-producing cells in Type I diabetics several years before the onset of the disease. This indicates that diabetes may be caused by the body's own immune system.

1977

The Hemoglobin A_1c Test, the "report card" of blood tests, gives diabetics a more complete picture of their condition by indicating blood sugar control over the previous 90 days.

1978

Improvements in the form and features of the insulin pump make the use of these "mechanical syringes" more common and desirable. Today, about 8,000 diabetics nationwide wear pumps round-the-clock. . . . The first successful long-term pancreas transplant is performed by Dr. David Sutherland at the University of Minnesota. The woman patient seems healthy and free from diabetes.

1980

Human insulin is produced in the lab through genetic engineering. For the first time, diabetics can be treated with insulin identical to that made in the body, instead of from cows and pigs.

1981

Dr. David Jenkins and his colleagues at the University of Toronto discover that different forms of starches raise blood sugar at different rates. Time-honored diabetic diets must be reevaluated.

1984

Dr. Daniel Mintz and colleagues at the University of Miami transplant islet cells into diabetic dogs and "cure" them. Hopes are rekindled that such transplants will soon be possible in humans. . . . Doctors at the University of Western Ontario "cure" newly diagnosed diabetics with cyclosporin. This advances the theory that diabetes may one day be wiped out by treating the patient's immune system.

1991

Results of a nationwide study reveal that diabetics who take tight control of their blood sugar levels suffer fewer complications of the disease, such as heart attacks, vision difficulties, and kidney problems.

day—she had no sign of diabetes after her transplant.

"I didn't know what the outcome of the transplant surgery would be," says the 35-year-old part-time waitress from Howell, Michigan. "But I did know what the long-term outcome of diabetes would be. I'm one of the lucky ones."

Pancreas transplants are still largely experimental. Other advances on the road to a cure for diabetes are as follows:

• New hope of transplanting insulin-producing cells into diabetics where they will grow, produce insulin, and wipe out the disease

• New insights into the viruses that may cause diabetes by triggering the body's immune system to destroy the insulin-producing cells in the pancreas

• A new use for cyclosporin, the drug that revolutionized organ transplant surgery. Cyclosporin clamps down on the immune system. In diabetes, it is believed that the body's own strong immune system may destroy the insulin-making cells. It may lead to remission in new cases of one type of diabetes.

• New technology that enables the patient to monitor her condition closely at home by performing blood tests that were once confined to the laboratory

• New diets full of starches (the foods once forbidden to diabetics) and fiber, which help regulate blood sugar levels

What is diabetes, anyway? Simply, diabetes is a chronic, metabolic disorder in which the body is unable to turn digested food into energy. The hormone insulin is the key. Normally, the body metabolizes, or breaks down, the carbohydrates we eat into the most basic glucose. Without insulin, the glucose cannot be used by the cells as a source of energy. This unused glucose piles up in the blood to very high levels. The glucose attaches itself to blood and other proteins. The sugar coating makes the big proteins stick together in clumps. Because these proteins are, in a sense, sugar poisoned, they cannot carry out vital cell chemistry, which leads to complications.

There are two types of diabetes. Type I, of which there are estimated to be more than 500,000 victims in the United States, was formerly called juvenile diabetes because it usually strikes children and young adults. Their pancreases stop making insulin, so patients need daily injections to survive.

Type II, once called adult-onset diabetes, usually affects people 40 or older who are overweight. Because the pancreas functions abnormally, it makes an insufficient amount of insulin or the body is unable to use properly the insulin that the pancreas makes. Type II diabetics usually are treated with oral drugs and diet.

The Special Problem of "Hidden Diabetes"

Of the estimated 12 million Americans with Type II diabetes, at least half do not know that they are victims. If left untreated, life-threatening complications can result.

If you are over 40, overweight, or have relatives with diabetes, you should be checked by your doctor periodically. However, you should see your doctor immediately if you are thirsty and urinate excessively; tire easily; have blurred vision or cuts that are slow to heal; feel tingling, numbness, or cramps in your legs, feet, or fingers; or have frequent skin infections or itchy skin. These are all classic symptoms of diabetes.

Injecting Insulin-Making Cells

In September 1984, in one of the most promising advances, researchers at the University of Miami transplanted the insulin-making cells of the pancreas (called islets) into dogs with diabetes. Their disease was completely and permanently reversed. Human patients now are being prepared for these revolutionary experiments. If the scientists are successful, they will, in effect, have done a pancreas transplant without surgery—only an injection of cells into the patient. Experiments are being carried out at a dozen institutions. As of this writing, scientists are still struggling to make transplants work for a long time in humans.

Another promising method involves wrapping the insulin-making cells in plastic. The plastic has microscopic holes that allows small molecules to enter the space where the cells are. The small energy-containing molecules can seep in to feed the cells. But the tiny holes will not allow larger, cell-killing molecules to attack the insulin-producing cells.

The Viral Connection

Scientists now have evidence that Type I diabetes may be caused by viruses that invade the islets in the pancreas. Then, in some mysterious way, the body's immune system attacks and destroys the islets.

Dr. H. Peter Chase, of the Barbara Davis Center for Childhood Diabetes in Denver, is studying families who show signs of these antiislet antibodies. And researchers at the Mount Sinai School of Medicine in New York have found that these antibodies appear several years before the patient develops diabetes. These early warning signs may one day help scientists prevent diabetes by using drugs that suppress the immune system.

A Drug Offers New Hope

One such drug already has "cured" diabetes, in a sense. Dr. Calvin R. Stiller and his colleagues at the University of Western Ontario in Canada treated 30 newly diagnosed Type I diabetics with cyclosporin. This is the drug that prevents organ rejection in heart and kidney transplants. In 16 of the patients, cyclosporin suppressed the body's destruction of the islet cells. The patients continued to secrete insulin and no longer needed injections.

The researchers believe that if cyclosporin is prescribed soon after diabetes manifests itself—and before all the islets are destroyed—it can arrest the development of diabetes.

Better Control, Tight Control

Thanks to battery-operated blood-reading meters and color-coded testing strips, the diabetic patient today can get an accurate reading of his blood sugar at home within minutes by pricking a drop of blood from a finger. He then can adjust his medication, food intake, and exercise to bring his blood sugar levels back under control.

This new technology comes at a time when doctors are advancing their stand on "tight control." This means that the diabetic must keep his blood sugar levels as close to normal (between 80 and 120 milligrams) as possible at all times. Doctors believe that tight control can reduce or eliminate the long-term nasty effects of diabetes.

Insulin Pumps

Scientists also are seeking more efficient insulin-delivery methods.

The insulin pump, a small battery-powered machine that delivers insulin through a tube inserted under the skin, is an improvement over injections because the pump drips a steady flow of the hormone into the body all day long.

Adam Boroughs of Wallingford, Pennsylvania, was once taking up to six insulin injections a day, but his blood sugar was still out of control. Then his doctors prescribed the pump. "I feel a lot better," says Mr. Boroughs. "I hang my pump on my belt, or else I wear a special T-shirt with a hole in the pocket so the tube is less noticeable. Sometimes, when I play sports, the pump gets in the way. But my friends don't care at all."

Patients who wear pumps, however, must do several blood tests every day to ensure that the right amount of insulin is being delivered. A study at the Mason Clinic in Seattle revealed that pump patients suffer more infections at the needle insertion site and more toxic reactions from too little insulin.

Scientists in Japan are working on a pump that works just like the pancreas. It measures the blood sugar and then releases precisely the right dose of insulin. This system has turned out to be more difficult than the developers first thought. There is still no foolproof way of measuring the sugar in the blood by a device.

At the University of Utah, researchers are infusing insulin safely, painlessly, and directly into the abdomen. They implant a small silicone rubber container just under the abdominal wall. The patient injects the insulin directly through the skin into the container, from which it flows into the abdominal cavity and is quickly absorbed.

New Findings about Food, Weight, and Exercise

Formerly, the diets prescribed for diabetics allowed very few carbohydrates but lots of proteins and fats. Then doctors discovered that such diets probably contributed in part to diabetics' increased risks of heart disease and stroke.

Doctors now know that diets comprised of fiber and complex carbohydrates (fresh fruits instead of fruit juices, whole grains, legumes, pasta) can actually smooth out the body's absorption of digested sugars into the bloodstream.

Dr. James Anderson of the University of Kentucky prescribes a diet in which about 50 percent of daily calories come from complex carbohydrates—starches. The diet is primarily fresh vegetables and fruits, plus dried beans, lentils, and peas.

Dr. Anderson says he can get the majority of Type I diabetics off insulin and can reduce the need for insulin by a third for Type II diabetics. "We have good evidence that the diets increase the sensitivity of the body to insulin," he reports.

Essentially, the insulin molecule works by attaching itself to the molecules of the cell membrane, like a key fitting into a lock. The cell membrane is like a wall. The molecules attached to the "wall" are called receptors. They change in size and number. Studies at Yale University by Drs. Philip Felig and Ralph A. DeFronzo have found that the number of insulin receptors increases—and blood sugar levels drop—in diabetics who exercise regularly.

Doctors have always known that obesity increases the risk of developing Type II diabetes. Now they also know that overweight diabetics have fewer insulin receptors and that weight loss somehow reduces blood sugar levels by increasing the number of receptors.

Research into ways of stopping the death of the insulin-producing cells is going forward at a breathtaking pace. New treatments are constantly tested. The scientists are confident that they will find ways of controlling this killing disease.

A Real Chance for Diabetics to Live Longer, Better

A NEW APPROACH TO DIABETES WILL SOON allow the nation's 13 million patients to look forward realistically to longer lives and fewer years of illness. Leading diabetes researchers believe they are close to fashioning a grand weapon against diabetes. At last they developed solid evidence that they can reduce dramatically the often fatal or profoundly damaging effects of diabetes. They include kidney disease, blindness, sexual impotence, crippling leg pains, gangrene, and even limb amputations.

This optimism comes from a landmark study that showed that diabetics could forestall these complications. To reach this goal, patients must keep the level of sugar in their blood as close to normal as possible.

What Is Diabetes?

In Type I, or insulin-dependent, the insulin-producing beta cells in the pancreas are destroyed. Without daily doses of insulin—by injection or through a pump—blood sugar levels rise dangerously, leading to coma and death. Type I diabetes afflicts about 500,000 Americans. It was formerly called juvenile diabetes because it usually strikes children and young adults. Classic symptoms include frequent urination, excessive thirst and hunger, and weight loss.

In Type II, or noninsulin-dependent, the body makes insulin but too little or too much. Mysteriously, some patients become resistant to the hormone. Type II diabetics are usually overweight and treated with diet control plus oral medicine that stimulates the pancreas to make the hormone. These patients may also take insulin along with the pills.

About 12 million Americans have Type II diabetes. It's also sometimes called adult-onset diabetes because it's commonly found in adults. Half of these people don't know they have it, because they do not immediately have the classic symptoms. The usual symptoms do develop gradually. These patients also evolve hard-to-heal infections of the skin and urinary tract, and itching of the skin and genitals.

Understanding and Controlling Diabetes

Diabetes is the sugar disease. Diabetics have too much sugar circulating because their pancreases do not make enough insulin, a vital hormone. Insulin prepares your body's cells to absorb sugar (glucose) for energy. In the absence of insulin, the sugar piles up in the blood system.

The sugar does its damage to the body's many enzymes. These chemicals carry out the intricate chemistry of the body. Some researchers believe that an overabundance of sugar in the blood allows the excess glucose to stick to enzyme molecules. An enzyme molecule coated with sugar will stick to other sugar-coated molecules. When that happens, the clumped enzymes fail to do their jobs.

Such a chemical catastrophe can shutdown many organs of the body, especially the kidneys, eyes, and nerves. In turn, battered nerves can lead to sexual impotence, severe leg pains, and blindness.

For at least three decades, diabetes experts argued about the need for keeping the blood sugar levels low and close to normal—the same level as nondiabetics achieve without injecting insulin. Pioneering diabetes specialists tried it out on a few patients to see whether low sugar levels could be won with injections of synthetic insulin, diet control, and exercise.

Diabetes patients found the new approach arduous. The system called for sufferers to measure their sugar blood levels four or more times a day. Fortunately, in the 1980s, electronics manufacturers were able to create a blood sugar machine no bigger than a pack of cigarettes. It worked beautifully.

The patient had to stick a sharp needle into one of his fingers. A drop of blood formed on the digit. The patient transferred the red liquid to a small paper stick. He then put the blood-soaked rod into the machine. In about a minute, the sugar reading came up on a small screen.

Depending on the number on the screen, a diabetic could inject more insulin, do some exercise, or have something to eat. It seemed like a thankless and difficult task. But enough diabetics did it to encourage the doctors to do a 10-year study on what is now called "tight control."

"I can think of no other disease where patients can play a more active, direct role in their own care and its outcome," says Dr. Phillip Gorden, director of the National Institute of Diabetes and Digestive and Kidney Diseases. The institute financed the research. Self-management was the key, and the massive experiment was on its way. It was called the Diabetes Control and Complications Trial (DCCT). It involved 1,421 patients and cost $160 million. Half the patients, chosen at random, followed the standard treatment. They used the sugar machine to check their blood sugars once a day and took one or two insulin injections daily.

The other half, the experimental group, strived for tight control—blood sugars in the normal range. They measured their blood four or more times daily, taking at least three injections of insulin a day. For some patients who found four injections a day too difficult, doctors prescribed insulin pumps, which deliver a fixed amount of insulin below the skin.

The idea was not to take more insulin but to deliver it in a way that more closely mimics the body's release of the hormone and to adjust the insulin doses—and sometimes diet and exercise—when sugars are too high or too low. This required working closely with diabetes educators and dietitians.

The result: The tightly controlled group had a 76 percent lower incidence of diabetic eye disease than the other group, 60 percent less nerve damage, and up to 56 percent fewer kidney problems.

Until now, doctors were not certain what caused the complications. Some held to the theory that the crippling effects of diabetes came from defects in body tissues that were part of the basic disease process. Others said it was from the abnormally high blood sugar levels. Dr. Oscar B. Crofford of Vanderbilt University, chairperson of the study, says, "The DCCT proved for the first time that complications of diabetes can be prevented by such intensive diabetes therapy."

The culprit was the abnormally high sugar level.

The DCCT study involved only Type I diabetics. It's the Type II diabetics whose sometimes "casual" approach to diabetes puts them in jeopardy. Dr. James Gavin III of the Howard Hughes Medical Institute in Chevy Chase, Maryland, says, "There is no such thing as 'a little touch of sugar.' Diabetes is serious—whether you take insulin or not. And the DCCT shows us clearly that, to prevent complications, it's important for all people with diabetes to bring their blood sugars close to normal."

Diabetes specialists hope that tight control will also prevent heart attacks and stroke, both of which are very common with diabetes.

Tracy Sankstone, a receptionist at the Mayo Clinic in Rochester, Minnesota, developed diabetes at age 2. She was the first patient in the experimental group of the DCCT, which began in 1983. She reports, "Doing four blood tests and four or more shots a day was tough in the beginning, but I'm used to it now. I feel great, I don't have any complications—and I don't want to get them."

Who Will Foot the Bill?

Better blood sugar control means more than longer, healthier lives for diabetics. It also eventually will reduce the cost of diabetes-related health care in the United States. Some experts estimate that the treatment bill for diabetics now reaches $92 billion a year. Intensive therapy—tight control—does not come cheap, however. The National Institutes of Health places the annual cost of tight control for Type I diabetes (professional-care visits and supplies) at $3,700 a person, compared to $1,700 for conventional therapy. Will private insurance, Medicare, and Medicaid foot the bill for blood-testing supplies, dietitians, and nurse educators for every diabetic?

"If the current health-reform movement is serious about using prevention to save money, here is a case where the proof that prevention is possible has been served up in a profound way," Dr. Gavin says. "What we need now is the availability of the tools for patients to make this kind of prevention possible—and that's in the hands of the insurers at this point. That means covering the cost of blood-testing strips, blood meters, and other monitoring devices and appropriate medication for people who require aggressive treatment of their diabetes. For Type II diabetics, who don't require insulin, aggressive treatment might mean diabetes education, visits to nutritionists, and exercise programs."

Working for Prevention . . . and a Cure

"The fact is that almost anybody with diabetes has a difficult time with it," says Dr. Richard A. Jackson. He heads the Hood Center for Prevention of Childhood Diabetes, at the Joslin Diabetes Center in Boston. "They have to watch what they eat, when to eat it, what physical activities they may do—and none of this ever goes away." But Dr. Jackson and other researchers are making huge advances toward prevention and, ultimately, a cure.

"Even 5 years ago," he says, "no one thought you could prevent diabetes. Today, we can prevent Type I diabetes in animals prone to develop the illness. Our pilot study made me more optimistic."

In the 1970s, researchers in London found antibodies that target the pancreas. In particular, the antibodies destroy the insulin-producing cells. These antibodies appear in the blood up to 10 years before the onset of diabetes. Blood tests to identify these "markers" can predict who will develop diabetes.

Dr. Jackson's pilot study examined 12 close relatives of patients with Type I diabetes; blood tests of all 12 revealed the antibodies. He treated five with small doses of insulin to give the remaining beta cells a rest and prevent their collapse; only one of the five developed diabetes. The other seven relatives turned down the therapy; all eventually became diabetic.

"We still don't have the money to do the things we want to do," says Dr. Jackson. "We need additional support from research organizations and the public in general." Dr. Jackson is part of a nationwide trial seeking to prevent diabetes in those at high risk. The researchers hope to screen up to 40,000 relatives of people with Type I diabetes. If you are related to someone with Type I, you may be eligible to join the study.

Dr. Stephen Leeper, president of the Juvenile Diabetes Foundation, has a son, Mark, diagnosed with diabetes at 7.

"We are convinced that, through research, diabetes cannot only be prevented but also cured—and all of us are determined to make that cure happen in our children's lifetime," he says.

The Juvenile Diabetes Foundation is a voluntary health agency founded in 1970 by parents of children with diabetes. It is dedicated to financing research to find a cure. (Type I diabetes is the most common chronic childhood disease in the United States.)

What You Can Do

Diabetes is the fourth-leading cause of death by disease in the United States. Each year, 650,000 Americans are diagnosed with it. Ask your doctor whether you should be checked for diabetes. And if you have it:

- See a doctor skilled in diabetes.
- Discuss the Diabetes Control and Complications Trial with your doctor. To learn more about it, write to the American Diabetes Association, 1660 Duke St., Alexandria, VA 22314, or call 1-800-DIA-BETES or e-mail http://www.diabetes.org.
- Have your doctor or laboratory draw a glycolated hemoglobin blood test. The test reveals how well your blood sugars have been controlled for the previous 2 to 4 months.
- Check your blood sugar regularly. If you don't have a test kit (blood meter and/or blood strips), get one and use it.
- Tight control is not for everyone (particularly the very young or old), because of the danger of too-low blood sugar, or hypoglycemia. This can cause sweats, confusion, loss of consciousness, shock, and (rarely) death. However, if you are like most people with diabetes, you probably should improve your blood sugar control.
- See an eye specialist experienced in diabetes at least once a year.
- Support research.

Are You at Risk for Type I Diabetes?

A clinical trial to delay and prevent insulin-dependent diabetes is under way at several medical centers across the country. You may volunteer for the trial—which is financed by the National Institutes of Health—if you are the parent, child, brother, or sister of someone with Type I diabetes. The screening and subsequent tests are free. It is not for relatives of people with Type II, or adult-onset, diabetes. To volunteer or for more information, call 1-800-2-HALT-DM, at the Joslin Clinic in Boston.

Immune System

FOR ALMOST A CENTURY, AND WITH DEEP SATIS- isfaction, the nation's health workers watched the tuberculosis (TB) death rate plunge. They thought they had this air-borne killer under control. The germs that caused TB were invading fewer peo-ple. Health workers even spoke of eradi-cating tuberculosis, just as they had eradicated smallpox. Everywhere in the United States, TB was dying out.

Then, about 1989, it became impos-sible to deny that death rates from TB were climbing in the United States for the first time in 80 years. Even more frighten-ing was the discovery that some TB mi-crobes had grown so strong that they now were able to withstand the drugs that formerly had wiped them out.

"TB was noticed again in November 1991, when a prison guard in Syracuse, New York, died of it," says Dr. Lee B. Reichman, an expert in the treatment of TB. "There were stories about his death in newspapers across the country." It was found that the guard had died of drug-resistant tuberculosis—meaning that, al-though the guard had been treated, the drugs couldn't save him.

"There is no question that this resur-gence of TB is a national catastrophe,"

adds Dr. Reichman. "But the tragic part is that almost all TB is eminently treat-able and preventable." Reichman heads the National Tuberculosis Center in Newark, New Jersey. He also is a profes-sor at the New Jersey Medical School.

In 1953, there were 84,304 reported cases of TB in the United States. By 1985, the number had fallen to 22,201. Reported cases began climbing again in 1986 and reached 26,673 by 1992. Though the number of TB cases is on the rise, the average healthy individual usu-ally is not at risk. In fact, 90 percent of those exposed to the disease by inhaling the infectious microbe do not come down with TB. The germ is enveloped in scar tissue, which prevents its spread. The dis-ease then lies dormant and may go un-detected for an entire lifetime. It is in combination with malnutrition or infec-tion with some other disease that the mi-crobes become aggressive and possibly fatal.

When I was in high-school in the early 1940s, 85 percent of my fellow stu-dents, including me, tested positive for TB. That means that those young people had been exposed to TB. For unclear rea-sons those hidden germs remain dormant for the next half century. The germs were effectively trapped. They could not infect anybody else.

As a result, fewer and fewer young people were exposed to the disease. (And, at the same time, the TB death rate plunged.) Today, about 15 percent of the population, mostly in the poor inner city, test positive.

The TB bacterium generally attacks the lungs, but it can spread to other body parts, including the brain, kidneys, or bones. Symptoms include persistent coughing, weight loss, fever, and spitting up blood. If you or someone in your household has such symptoms, see your doctor immediately. A quick test usually can tell whether you have TB. The doctor gives you an injection. If the skin hardens around the area of the injection within a few days, the doctor further examines you for TB. If you have it, you can be treated and made noncontagious within 2 weeks. Often, you can be cured within 6 months.

"It is not easy to catch TB," says Dr. Reichman. "You need, on average, to be in contact with the disease 8 hours a day for six straight months—and even then you have only a 50 percent chance of getting it."

So why is tuberculosis on the rise again? For one thing, Dr. Reichman says, people who have TB don't keep taking their medication as prescribed. He adds that city and state hospitals, lacking money, began to let TB patients leave before they were fully cured, with no way to locate them and no follow-up schedules to make sure the patients were taking their medicines.

As it did 100 years ago, TB afflicts mostly the poor—especially the chronically ill and children. Also highly susceptible are those with AIDS, a disease not fully recognized until the 1980s.

Charles Hooks, 43, lives in Newark, New Jersey. He is HIV-positive and also has TB. Hooks says he is neither gay nor an intravenous drug user—two major routes for HIV infection. When diagnosed with TB, he took his four medications for a few weeks, then stopped. He stopped seeing his doctors too.

To provide follow-up care, the clinic in Newark at which Hooks had been treated assigned Ramona Valentin, a directly observed therapy (DOT) worker, to find Hooks and watch him actually take his medications from then on. He moved a lot. She finally found Hooks at his mother's home.

"At first," Hooks explains, "I didn't want to take my medicines. They made me sleepy. I was going to die of AIDS anyway, I felt, so why take drugs? Now I'm taking them. I feel better." His medications suppress the tuberculosis infection and prevent its spread.

Once Hooks had returned to their care, his doctors took a TB sample from his lungs to learn whether the bacteria had become resistant to the medicines while he'd stopped taking them. Luckily, they had not. So the doctors prescribed the same four drugs he'd taken before—

isoniazid, rifampin, pyrazinamide, and ethambutol—which are recommended by the Centers for Disease Control in Atlanta for the treatment of TB. (Some doctors use streptomycin instead of ethambutol.) Hooks was told to take all four drugs for at least 6 months. It takes about 2 weeks for the drugs to kill enough bacteria so they can't infect other people. It takes 6 months for a cure. Once cured, patients almost never get tuberculosis again.

"DOT workers like Ramona Valentin are modern-day heroes of public health," says Dr. Thomas Frieden, director of the Bureau of Tuberculosis Control for the New York City Department of Health. "They look anywhere to find their clients—in crack dens, under bridges, on park benches. Today, New York has 1,200 patients on DOT.

"In 1992, there were 3,811 cases of active TB reported in the city. In 1993, there were 3,235. That drop of almost 15 percent is the first significant decline in New York City since 1978."

Dr. Frieden credits DOT workers with some of that decrease. He says they give food vouchers, a place to sleep, even cash, to the patients who show up for medication. Yes, this costs taxpayers several hundred thousand dollars a year, but Dr. Frieden contends that it's worth it. "A single case of TB can spread rapidly to hundreds of people and cost millions in health care," he says. "The average bill for each hospitalized TB patient is $25,000."

Dr. Reichman notes that follow-up care is essential. If the TB bacteria become resistant to two of the four drugs prescribed, those particular drugs can't stop the disease; it continues to sicken the patient, and others can catch it. After the four-drug treatment becomes ineffective, more drastic measures must be pursued. They include drugs that are more toxic and expensive and may take as long as 2 years to work, with surgery as a last resort.

In New York City, tests show, many patients have drug-resistant TB. If they refuse treatment, health department workers can detain them under a law that requires hospitalization until the patient is cured. Mark Barnes, an attorney now in private practice, wrote the law when he worked for the city. "Detention is not the first but the last resort," says Barnes.

Private sources are enlisting in the battle against TB. Thanks to a grant of $1.15 million from the Robert Wood Johnson Foundation in alliance with Bellevue Hospital Center, New York City has a program in which outreach workers aggressively track and treat TB patients in poor areas. The foundation underwrites similar projects in Atlanta, Baltimore, San Diego, and southern Florida, all with TB problems in hard-to-reach communities.

Our rising TB statistics give us a grave warning, to be heeded at home and abroad. Globally, tuberculosis kills 2.9 million persons each year. The World

Health Organization sees a bleak future if the drug-resistant strains of the disease get a foothold in countries that lack clinics or hospitals. We can control TB. In 1992, only 10.5 persons per 100,000 in the United States had this disease, according to the Centers for Disease Control. With care, that figure can be made even smaller. With carelessness, it can mushroom, as it did in the 1800s, afflicting not only the poor but the middle and upper economic classes as well.

When Your Immune System Fails

WHEN A PHYSICIAN OR A NURSE INJECTS A FEW drops of measles vaccine into a child, the particles in that liquid set off an incredible chain of events within the child's body. At the end of that sequence, the child is immune to any live, disease-causing measles virus.

The vaccine triggers the child's immune system. And what a marvel that system is. Millions of microscopic blood cells, each smaller than a dust particle, swing into action. They create chemicals designed specifically to knock out the measles virus. They marshal the aid of scavenger cells to chew up the attackers.

Scientists have learned how immunity works and how it fights invading bacteria, viruses, parasites, and pieces of these called antigens. Or how it sometimes turns against the body itself, causing diseases like arthritis, rheumatic fever, perhaps even diabetes. Or how it safeguards you from cancer.

Measles, influenza, and polio no longer kill much of the world, thanks to vaccines. New medications and treatments are coming from research in medicine, chemistry, and genetic engineering.

Scientists today feel overwhelmingly that they have passed the threshold of major discoveries. The way is open to find the causes of cancer and a dozen other diseases, how to treat them, and possibly how to prevent them.

"We are dealing with an unparalleled explosion of information on cancer biology," says Dr. Steven Rosenberg, chief of the surgery branch of the National Cancer Institute.

Sara Brooks, 4, of Sacramento, California, owes her life to this new knowledge. She inherited a defective immune system and had no protection against invading germs from the day she was born. Doctors kept Sara alive for 5 months in a little three-sided box with air filters. Her parents, Steve and Sheryl Brooks, could not touch or cuddle her. A single stray germ could have killed her.

"Sara was pretty sick for a while," says her mother, "but now the doctors consider her cured. We call her a miracle baby."

Dr. Morton J. Cowan of the University of California at San Francisco gave Sara a defect-free immune system by transplanting bone marrow from her father into her body. His healthy bone marrow contained all the cells Sara needed.

Bone marrow transplantation also has been successful in fighting leukemia. It replaces the diseased immune system by producing healthy red cells and platelets and the immune system's white cells. This transplanting occurs after the leukemia is blasted with X rays and chemicals that destroy both the cancer and the patient's bone marrow.

In this same way, bone marrow transplants have helped several workers who received deadly doses of radiation at the nuclear accident at Chernobyl in the Soviet Union. The radiation had destroyed their immune systems.

Although babies born with defective immune systems are rare, the world is experiencing the horror of defective immunity in thousands of people who have AIDS (acquired immune deficiency syndrome). They acquired this condition from infection with a virus that knocks out a key white blood cell in the body's delicate immune system. Without effec-tive immunity, AIDS patients fall prey to bacteria and fungi that live harmlessly on the skin or inside healthy persons. Resultant infections ravage the body. AIDS can kill almost all who contract it, making it the most deadly illness of modern times. In 1996, scientists discovered medicines that slow down the growth of the AIDS virus in an infected person. At the same time, other drugs plus antibiotics control the lethal infections that commonly afflict people with AIDS. This new era in AIDS control has reduced the growth of the AIDS virus to extremely low levels so as to be unmeasurable. People with AIDS, who at first expected to live 2 or 3 years, can now look forward to staying alive for at least 10 years.

The new knowledge about immunity has allowed scientists to move fast against AIDS. The first cases in the United States were reported in 1981 as a strange pneumonia. But, in a year or two, scientists had pinpointed the defect in immunity. In 1984, they isolated the killer virus. Although researchers hailed the identification of HIV as signaling the development of a vaccine, over 10 years have elapsed without a usable one. That's because the AIDS virus is constantly changing (somewhat like the influenza virus, but much more rapidly).

Herpes viruses live forever in nerve cells. Some scientists believe they are triggered by cold, heat, fever, chemicals, or menstruation. The virus grows out of the affected nerve cells and attacks other tissues. Shingles is really the reactivation of an old chicken pox virus, responding, some theorize, to the same triggers.

Four major discoveries have brightened the promise of immunology:

• The unraveling of the complex way in which the different types of white blood cells cooperate to attack foreign substances that get into the body
• The discovery of chemicals released by the cells that give signals for white cell action. Interferon and interleukin, for instance, are both promising cancer treatments.
• The development of genetic engineering. Scientists now know how to alter the biology of common sewage bacteria so that the germs can create unlimited amounts of human chemicals like insulin, interferon, and interleukin.
• The creation of a strange and wonderful cell called a hybridoma. These hybrid cells can produce boundless amounts of antibodies—chemicals that attack invading viruses, bacteria, or fungi. Hybridoma antibodies also hold promise against cancer.

Let's see what these historic advances mean for you.

The White Cell Network

Your blood contains red cells, which carry oxygen, and a clear yellow fluid called plasma that transports chemicals and "food" for the rest of the body, plus several kinds of white cells. The white cells control the immune system.

One species of white cell, called a B cell, manufactures the antibodies. Another, a macrophage (meaning "big-eater"), actually devours germs and cancer cells. Natural killer cells are believed to hunt down and kill cancer cells or normal cells infected with a virus. Another white cell, called a T cell, also issues chemical signals.

Memory cells, which last for life, remember the various germs that have attacked. These cells trigger the immune system quickly if the same germ attacks again. A vaccine is made of a weakened or dead germ, or a part of a germ that "fools" the memory cell into "believing" the live virus has attacked. The memory cell is primed into action by the vaccine without the body experiencing the actual disease.

It would take a much longer chapter to describe in detail how all these cells act to protect you against infection. The action has been compared to an army in battle. Reacting to the invasion of a germ, including viruses and the much bigger bacteria, the immune system deploys millions of different kinds of cells, each a specialist. In a modern military assault, a regiment will mount the battle with foot soldiers, tanks, missile launchers, and airplanes. The immune system activates those marauding, specialist white cells.

Doctors are putting the vaccine reaction to work against cancer, particularly melanoma, a skin cancer that is hopeless once it has metastasized (spread). Dr. Jean-Claude Bystryn, director of the melanoma program at the New York University Medical Center in Manhattan, has created a vaccine against melanoma. It is made from extracts of cancer cells. He hopes that the cancer distillate will "fool" the immune system. Responding to the growth of hidden cancer, the immune system will seek and destroy those tiny cancers.

In 1970, surgeons cut a malignant melanoma from the back of Dolores King, 57, a housewife from Fort Lauderdale, Florida. The cancer returned in 1983, and Dr. Bystryn gave Mrs. King injections of vaccine. Her skin turned red—a good sign. Though Mrs. King says she feels fine now, she adds, "My prognosis is very bad. But I have faith."

"We still don't know if we have cured the melanoma," says Dr. Bystryn. "Now we need to see if the vaccine is safe."

Study of white cells also has led to the idea that many couples are infertile because the wife's immune system destroys the husband's sperm. Worse, the pregnant woman's body may reject the baby in her womb. Sometimes the white cells attack normal body cells. Growing evidence suggests that this happens in the pancreas, which makes insulin. If our insulin-making cells die, we develop severe diabetes. Doctors now give patients cyclosporine, a drug that slows down the immune system. It seems to work in some diabetics—they start producing insulin again.

Dr. H. Peter Chase, of the Barbara Davis Center for Childhood Diabetes in Denver, says that for cyclosporine to stop diabetes, a patient would have to take it a long time, perhaps for life. The drug is expensive ($6,000 a year) and—among other negative side effects—could harm the patient's kidneys.

Other diseases caused by white cells that attack healthy cells include rheumatic fever, rheumatoid arthritis, a strange disease called lupus, and, perhaps, multiple sclerosis.

However, with cyclosporine, doctors have had great success in slowing down the immune system's reaction against transplants of organs from other individuals. Now kidney transplants from unrelated individuals have success rates as high as 95 percent, heart transplants as high as 85 percent, and liver transplants as high as 70 percent.

Immune Chemicals

Interferon, one of the substances secreted by various virus-infected cells, has been approved by the Food and Drug Administration for the treatment of a rare cancer called hairy-cell leukemia, a disease that until recently had no treatment. Interferon also has been found in clinical tests to fight chronic leukemia, kidney cancer, and Kaposi's sarcoma, the cancer peculiar to AIDS victims.

Another T-cell substance, interleukin, has been described by the National Cancer Institute as one of the major advances against cancer in a decade. The institute's Dr. Steven Rosenberg reported in December 1985 that, with interleukin, advanced cancers in one patient had retreated completely, and 11 patients had at least a 50 percent reduction in tumor size. "Here, really for the first time, we can use the immune system to attack a broad array of cancer," he says.

Besides interferon and interleukin, scientists have identified other powerful immune system chemicals. One, tumor necrosis factor, seems to destroy cancer cells without hurting normal cells.

Genetic Engineering

Interleukin and interferon are available in large amounts because scientists now "grow" them, using bacteria or yeast. Your white cells form interleukin, for example, under the control of your genes. A gene is another bit of chemical called DNA, containing the information the white cell needs to form interleukin. Through genetic engineering, scientists can take the gene for interleukin from a human cell and put it into a common germ. That germ grows in a vat much as yeast grows in a beer vat. Because the germ now carries that bit of human DNA, it then makes interleukin in large quantities. Scientists also are commercially manufacturing tumor necrosis fac-

tor and other T-cell substances that control the immune system.

Hybridoma

This bizarre hybrid is made up of two cells: the B cell, which provides antibodies, and a white-cell cancer called myeloma. By fusing two cells, you get a hybrid that produces antibodies and lives forever. And the hybrid can be made to produce antibodies to any virus or germ—even to a cancer. These are called monoclonal antibodies because they are specific to one particular germ or cancer. Hybridomas have produced antibodies to melanomas and colon and pancreatic cancers.

Norman J. Arnold, of Columbia, South Carolina, was diagnosed as having incurable pancreatic cancer in July 1982. He went to the Wistar Institute, a biological research institution in Philadelphia. There, the director, Dr. Hilary Koprowski, injected him with monoclonal antibodies against the cancer. His cancer receded. Mr. Arnold had no sign of the disease for 2.5 years.

"The future of immunotherapy is bright," says Dr. Koprowski. "Monoclonal antibodies are the greatest medical tools developed in the last 50 years. They are in everybody's lab."

As research into the marvelous immune system continues, every scientist I interviewed expressed the same optimism. Immunology will lift much of the burden of disease.

Is Mending Sick Genes a Miracle Cure?

GENE THERAPY. SUDDENLY, LIKE A FLAG RAISED on the horizon, these words have arrived on the medical frontier, changing the world of medicine forever.

Scientists say this new form of treatment will be able either to cure or control a score of seemingly incurable diseases. The list includes several cancers, cystic fibrosis, AIDS, a rare inherited blood disease that acts like AIDS, hemophilia, and more. In 1 week in November 1993, the American Medical Association published 150 reports on the subject, trumpeting the quickening pace of these advances.

Genes are bundles of chemicals deep in your cells that manage the vast and complex chemical factories in muscles, nerves, skin, and bones. Humans have at least 100,000 genes, each controlling a different function. Sick or missing genes can mean cancer, deformity, or early death. Repair the sick genes or install the missing ones, and, in theory, you'll have healthy cells and a healthy body. This is what gene therapists do.

On September 14, 1990, Ashanthi DeSilva, then 4, became one of the first to receive gene therapy. She suffered from a rare blood disease passed on to her by her parents, who weren't sick. Lacking a particular gene, her blood cells could not make ADA, a chemical white blood cells need to fight infection. Her parents, Raj and Van DeSilva of Avon Lake, Ohio, watched their infant develop severe chest and ear infections within 2 months of her birth. She ran high fevers, suffered from diarrhea, and failed to gain weight.

Ashanthi was 2 before her illness was diagnosed. Fortunately, a pharmaceutical company had produced a cow's blood derivative, PEG-ADA—a type of ADA that can be injected frequently enough to keep the immune system going. For Ashanthi, it was lifesaving. But, as she grew, she was kept from school for fear she would catch a germ too tough for her fragile immune system to handle.

Meanwhile, the *human* gene for making ADA had been isolated and copied, and scientists at the National Cancer Institute (NCI) and the Heart, Lung, and Blood Institute—both in Bethesda, Maryland—were developing an ADA deficiency treatment.

To get the ADA genes into Ashanthi's white blood cells, her white cells were harvested, then grown in laboratory dishes. The lab-grown ADA gene was then spliced into a harmless virus. If the theory worked, the virus with the ADA gene would enter the white cells in the dishes. The white cells, now fortified with ADA from the virus, would be injected back into Ashanthi, ready to fight off infection.

The theory was applied in 1990. It worked. At first, Ashanthi had frequent treatments; now an annual treatment suffices. And she goes to school.

Dr. R. Michael Blaese, department chairman of NCI's Metabolism Branch, led the team that prepared the new treatment. Since then, he said, he has given such therapy to more patients. Although his work looks promising, it will be a few years before the vaccine can be offered to everybody.

Dr. George D. Lundberg, chief editor of the AMA's scientific journals, predicts, "Genetic diagnoses, screening, prevention, and treatment will expand enormously, with great potential for improvement—and for generating ethical conflict. The science of genetics is now soundly based and moving at such speed that we have new discoveries daily."

Scientists already have tried gene therapy on cancers of the brain, breast, colon, and skin, and they have detected a glimmer of improvement in the cancers.

In 1989, Michelle Goldman was diagnosed as having melanoma, a lethal skin cancer that spreads to other organs. Cancer had settled into most of her body. "I was told I had 90 days to live," she says. "I didn't think anybody could help."

Then she found Dr. Steven A. Rosenberg, chief of surgery at the National Cancer Institute. At the time, Dr. Rosenberg was testing a treatment that used the patient's own white blood cells. In earlier tests, his team had found that white cells called tumor infiltrating lymphocytes (TILs) will cluster around cancers. But because cancer cells may grow faster than the TILs can reproduce, there may not be enough of them to beat back the cancer.

Dr. Rosenberg's idea was this: First, harvest a segment of the patient's cancerous tumor; next, separate the cancer cells and TILs; then grow the TILs in a lab dish, where they can multiply. By injecting billions of the patient's *own* TILs into the blood, he hoped to create a white-cell army to hunt and kill the cancer, wherever it was.

"We were looking for ways to grow more TILs or to make them more powerful," Dr. Rosenberg says. He found that the drug interleukin-2 sped up the growth of TILs. (Interleukin-2 is a hormone given off by white cells.) He considered giving each white cell the ability to make a potent poison for cancer cells. For this, he turned to tumor necrosis factor (TNF), a substance our white cells make to kill cancer cells. Our bodies seldom make enough TNF to kill off the cancer, however, and it has terrible side effects if doses are too large.

Dr. Rosenberg theorized that, because TILs cluster around cancer cells, if these lymphocytes could make tumor necrosis factor, their toxin then would poison *only* the cancer cells. The trick was to get the gene that makes TNF *into* the TILs, so they could then create their *own* TNF.

By then, the TNF gene had been isolated and copied, and scientists were able to splice almost any gene into a harmless virus. Dr. Rosenberg planned to use viruses spliced with the TNF genes to get them into the TILs, so the genes could make their cancer-killing toxin where it would be most effective—at the cancer sites.

The news that Dr. Rosenberg was preparing to apply this experiment to humans raised protests, from scientists and laypersons. They said they feared that too little would be done either to safeguard patients or to avoid an "accident" that might turn a harmless virus into a lethal one.

Dr. Rosenberg asked the permission of seven federal agencies to prepare a virus that had been spliced to a "marker" gene. It's called a marker gene because, through blood tests, scientists easily can detect the protein it makes. This helps them track the movements of the TILs.

Given the go-ahead to try his therapy on a willing patient, Dr. Rosenberg chose Michelle Goldman. "Every bit of the treatment was scary," she recalls. "I didn't know what I'd do if it didn't work." But the TILs did their job brilliantly, and her cancers melted away like butter. That was in 1989. Michelle Goldman—the patient who, at 26, was given 90 days to live—survived longer than anybody depicted. But again larger-scale studies are needed to pin down the risks and benefits of this strange treatment.

Of the nearly 100 cancer-riddled patients he has treated, Dr. Rosenberg says many stayed disease-free for months. He adds that the actual numbers would be detailed in an article he is writing for a medical journal.

Michelle Goldman was among the first persons known to have a gene injected into her body. The treatment of Ashanthi DeSilva with the ADA gene quickly followed. The floodgates have opened. Hundreds of scientists are looking to gene therapy to help cure intractable diseases, including the following:

• Cystic fibrosis. The most common deadly inherited disease among Americans, cystic fibrosis affects those who lack a gene to make the chemical that causes salt to move beneficially in and out of the cells. As a result, phlegm clogs the lungs of victims, drowning them. They often die in their teens.

At the National Institutes of Health in Bethesda, Dr. Ronald Crystal gave gene therapy to four cystic fibrosis patients in their 20s. To solve the salt problem, he used a common cold virus to carry the missing gene into their lung cells. Their condition is stable, but it's too early to tell, said Dr. Crystal, who now heads the Division of Pulmonary and Critical Care Medicine at New York Hospital. Still, he says, "This has the potential to cure cystic fibrosis."

• Familial hypercholesterolemia. This rare disease affects people who lack a gene enabling the liver to regulate and store cholesterol. As a result, cholesterol piles up, sticking to the walls of blood vessels, clogging or narrowing them, and impeding blood flow. Patients often die of heart attacks before their teens. Dr. James Wilson, director of the Institute for Gene Therapy at the University of Pennsylvania in Philadelphia, grew the liver cells of three such patients in lab dishes and sprinkled the cells with a virus spliced with the missing gene. He then injected the patients with their altered liver cells. His first subject was a woman of 26 who'd had her first heart attack at age 16. "She has had no problems since the procedure," says Dr. Wilson. "She is not totally cured but is significantly improved."

Questions have been raised. For example, if scientists found genes for intelligence and used gene therapy on early embryos to produce more intelligent children, would it be moral? "The 'designer child' is way down the road," said Arthur Caplan, director of the Center for Biomedical Ethics at the University of Minnesota. "But, in 50 years, I'd be shocked if we weren't in debate about designing our descendants."

There may be more questions than answers now, but scientists know gene therapy is giving them a handle on something earthshaking. They are not about to let it go.

How Vaccines May End Infections Forever

NO MORE INFECTIONS. NO MORE HEPATITIS. NO more pneumonia and influenza. No more venereal disease. No more children's contagions. Good-bye to malaria, meningitis, and maybe, one day, the common cold.

Before the 20th century ends, science may bid good riddance to most, if not all, diseases caused by viruses and bacteria. Spurred by the successes of vaccine treatments over the past decades, biologists and chemists are creating amazing new vaccines that stop those germs invading and growing in our bodies.

What exactly is a vaccine? Simply put, a vaccine is a dose of just enough of a particular germ to trigger your immune system but not make you sick. Into each vaccine scientists put all or part of the particular germ against which they want to protect you, but first they weaken, dismember, or kill that germ in the laboratory. Once you swallow or take shots of this altered germ, the pieces tell your body to make antigerm proteins called antibodies. The antibodies stave off the deadly germs from getting a foothold in your body.

Keep in mind that vaccines prevent infectious disease; they do not cure it. Scientists are using new technology to improve old vaccines, such as those in whooping cough and influenza, making them safer and more powerful. And they are fashioning new vaccines for diseases against which we have no protection. Vaccines for genital herpes and chicken pox, for example, are two of a dozen under development.

Elena Jenkins, 10, of Nutley, New Jersey, owes her life to the new, experimental chicken pox vaccine from Japan. Five years ago, she came down with leukemia, which doctors stopped with drugs and radiation. But, like all leukemia victims, Elena became acutely susceptible to chicken pox. In normal children, only a mild rash covers the skin; when the disease attacks a person who has had leukemia, it can kill horribly by peeling away all the skin and invading the brain.

Elena's parents, Linda and Bob Jenkins, lived in dread that Elena would catch chicken pox. "We were afraid her brother would bring the disease home from school," recalls Mrs. Jenkins.

In May 1981, Dr. Ann Gershon, then of New York University Medical Center in Manhattan injected Elena with the new vaccine, which is made from live, weakened viruses. A year later, Elena broke out in a mild case of chicken pox and survived.

Dr. Jonas Salk, who in 1955 invented the first vaccine that cut down the crippling polio virus, said that modern technology opens the way "to control more and more of the major infections and parasitic diseases." That technology includes these developments:

- Growing viruses and bacteria in test tubes to produce the raw material of vaccines
- Altering the genes of viruses and bacteria so that they cannot produce disease but can stimulate antibodies
- Isolating pieces of germs that can trigger immunity against the whole germ.

Before he died, Dr. Salk told me, "If there is a will to do so, there will be a way to develop vaccines."

This scientific know-how was slow in coming. In 1796, Edward Jenner, an English doctor, observed that milkmaids who caught cowpox from cows did not catch the deadly smallpox. Dr. Jenner got the idea that rubbing pus from the cow's pox into people's skin might somehow protect them from smallpox. Thus began vaccination, which comes from the Latin word for cow, *vacca*.

Dr. Jenner didn't know it, but the pus contained the cowpox virus, now called vaccinia. (Like all viruses, vaccinia is a tiny germ, so small that 100,000 of them can fit onto the period at the end of this sentence.) And because this cowpox virus is a weak "cousin" to the smallpox virus, the cowpox antibodies stopped the smallpox germ.

Much of vaccine technology today is based on Dr. Jenner's principle—that is, using weak "relatives" or altered germs to fight more powerful viruses and bacteria.

However, most infections do not have such close "relatives" as do cowpox and smallpox, so scientists have to weaken strong viruses in the laboratory.

The technique of injecting children with vaccines made from weakened viruses has reduced measles, mumps, and rubella (German measles) to only a few thousand cases of each a year, the lowest levels in history. (The rubella vaccine is critical for any woman of childbearing age because, if she becomes pregnant, the virus can blind, deafen, or retard her unborn child.)

Despite these successes, vaccine science is not without controversy over the relative safety of live versus killed viruses and bacteria.

Those who favor live vaccines point with pride to the success of the live Sabin polio vaccine (named for Dr. Albert Sabin), which practically wiped out polio. Made from thoroughly enfeebled, but live, viruses, it is touted today as one of the safest of the live vaccines. Nevertheless, it causes 5 to 10 cases of paralysis in the United States each year. Although it protects the vaccinated person from disease, the virus in the vaccine somehow regains its strength and may contaminate others.

Dr. Salk and other proponents of his killed virus vaccine say that it is safer and just as potent as the live Sabin vaccine. They point to another vaccine, DTP, a single vaccine that contains no living matter yet has all but obliterated three long-feared childhood diseases: diphtheria, tetanus, and whooping cough, also called pertussis. (These three infections are caused by bacteria. Bacteria are perhaps a hundred times larger than viruses, and, unlike viruses, they can reproduce outside cells. They do their damage by emitting poisons.)

But even vaccines made from killed viruses and bacteria are not without problems. From a controlled British study, it has been determined that the DTP vaccine causes brain damage in one child in 310,000. Nevertheless, without vaccination, the incidence of death by whooping cough increases by 19 times, and the likelihood of brain damage quadruples. So, its advocates insist, taking the vaccine is much safer than not taking it.

In response to the need for new vaccines—and questions about existing ones—the National Institute of Allergy and Infectious Diseases has set up a priority list of 10 inoculations against serious germ maladies. High on that list are finding a new, safer vaccine for whooping cough and winning approval from the Food and Drug Administration for the chicken pox vaccine that already has saved Elena Jenkins.

The institute also advocates a live vaccine for influenza, which kills 10,000 people a year.

Several vaccines made from killed influenza virus already exist. They particularly benefit older, chronically ill people who have lung, heart, and other health infirmities. But only 20 percent of this high-risk group takes the shots. If all such high-risk people were inoculated, says the Center for Disease Control in Atlanta, flu vaccines could save an additional 5,000 lives in the United States.

But because the flu plays tricks on scientists, the influenza virus presents its own special problem. With each flu season, several different viruses may circulate in the population, so that the old vaccine doesn't work. Health officials hope that a live vaccine will be easier to manufacture and administer than a killed one. For one thing, if a new flu virus appears on the scene, scientists can quickly tailor-make a vaccine to stop that epidemic. For another, the new vaccines may be sprayed into the nose. Researchers believe that people may be more willing to inhale a vaccine than to take shots.

Older people are also reluctant to take vaccine shots for pneumonia, which kills 50,000 Americans a year. There is a pneumonia vaccine containing pieces of 23 different forms of killed pneumococcal bacteria. Dr. Maurice Hilleman of Merck & Co., Inc., the largest manufacturer of vaccines, says the injections could protect against 90 percent of pneumococcal pneumonia.

Pioneers in vaccine research are developing inoculations to fight some of society's most virulent diseases.

In 1982, Dr. Hilleman received FDA approval for his vaccine against hepatitis B, also known as serum hepatitis. He constructed a vaccine out of partial rather than the whole hepatitis B virus. This virus infection inflames the livers of 200,000 Americans a year. At risk are blood transfusion patients, medical personnel who handle blood, and homosexuals. Hepatitis B kills a substantial number of victims with cirrhosis (or hardening) of the liver. One thousand Americans a year contract cancer of the liver. In the world today, 170 million people are infected with hepatitis B. Most of them were infected with the virus during their birth from an infected mother. Hepatitis B is largely a venereal disease: you get it from having sexual intercourse with an infected person.

"With this vaccine," says Dr. Hilleman, "we could eradicate hepatitis in a few generations, just as we did smallpox. The technology is there."

Also on the way is a vaccine against hepatitis A, known as infectious hepatitis, which you get from eating contaminated food.

Scientists are also struggling with vaccines for gonorrhea and genital herpes. The herpes virus is a particular scourge because it stays in the body for life and intermittently flares up. Dr. Bernard Roizman of Chicago has altered the herpes virus so that it does not linger in the body to infect again and again. His vaccine, now under tests, could prevent the disease but not cure it once you have been infected.

Biologists from the laboratories of the New York State Department of Health have altered the ancient cowpox virus so that it could defend against both genital and oral herpes without causing herpes.

"We've been working on it for a number of years," reported a senior research scientist, Enzo Paoletti. "We're pretty excited."

Dr. Paoletti isolated a part of the herpes virus gene and inserted it into the cowpox virus. That changed the cowpox virus so that to your body it looks like an oral herpes virus and fools the body into making antibodies against both types of herpes. The cowpox virus becomes a sheep in wolf's clothing.

Dr. Paoletti and his colleague, Dr. Dennis Panicali, also have produced hybrid vaccines for influenza and hepatitis B. But it could be several more years before a hybrid vaccine passes tests for human use.

Scientists also have begun a vaccine campaign against gonorrhea, which infects almost a million people a year and can lead to sterility in women. Scientists at the National Institute of Allergy and Infectious Diseases have isolated a protein from the outer membrane of the gonorrhea bacterium. Once injected, this protein leads to the formation of antibod-ies. It has yet to be tested to see whether it can prevent the disease in humans.

Vaccine makers are even more excited by entirely new chemical methods of creating vaccines in the test tube, without using either live or killed viruses or bacteria. Instead, they synthesize small pieces of protein that trigger immunity. They have only to make sure that the piece is identical to a protein found on the surface of a virus or bacterium. In this way, Dr. Richard A. Lerner, of the Scripps Clinic in La Jolla, California, has synthesized experimental vaccines against influenza, hepatitis B, and foot-and-mouth disease, an infection of animals.

"In the future, we won't have to rely on killed or weakened viruses," says Dr. Lerner. "We can design a piece of the virus, make it, and then give it without worrying about side effects or the weakened virus turning deadly again."

Down the line lie vaccines against malaria, infant diarrhea, croup, and meningitis, and even a rare disease called megalovirus, or CMV, which attacks 1 to 2 percent of all newborns. The disease causes mental retardation in 2,500 infants a year.

Finally, although most cancers are not caused by germs, scientists are working on revolutionary new vaccines that will stimulate the body's defenses against newly formed cancer cells and, perhaps, one day even wipe out advanced forms of cancer.

The Power of Vaccines

Disease	U.S. Cases in Peak Year (before Modern Vaccine)	In 1995 (after Vaccine)
Diphtheria	206,999 in 1921	0
Measles	481,530 in 1962	312
Mumps	152,209 in 1968	840
Polio	57,879 in 1952	0
Rubella	57,686 in 1969	146
Smallpox	632,000* in 1949	0
Tetanus	601 in 1948	34

*Worldwide figure; actual unreported cases may be 10 to 50 times higher.

Cancer

How to Save Your Skin

WE USED TO BELIEVE THAT THE SUN'S RAYS funneled health into our bodies. After all, we look healthy with a tan: the darker the tan, the more robust we appear, right? Besides, the sun puts vitamin D into our skin, right?

Wrong. Except for the part about vitamin D, we've learned that these ideas are very dangerous. The healthy "look" actually is a mirage, or a mask for illness and worse.

The relatively modern craving for a suntanned skin has in recent years ignited a worldwide epidemic of deadly melanoma, a skin cancer that experts recently have projected to kill 7,300 Americans annually—with 1 in every 105 contracting melanoma in a lifetime and facing a 1-in-5 chance of dying of it.

These figures come from Dr. Darrell Rigel, a clinical assistant professor of dermatology at New York University

---

Are You at High Risk?

Dr. Darrell Rigel, of New York University Medical School, studied 200 melanoma patients and devised this test to determine a high risk of melanoma:

1. Have you had three or more blistering sunburns before the age of 20? Yes ___ No ___
2. Do you have red or blond hair, and fair skin that burns easily? Yes ___ No ___
3. Do you have lots of freckles on your upper back?   Yes ___ No ___
4. Did anyone in your family have a melanoma?   Yes ___ No ___
5. Do you have rough red spots on parts of your body that are seldom or never exposed to the sun's rays? Yes ___ No ___
6. As a teenager, did you work at least three summers outdoors? Yes ___ No ___

If you answered yes to just three questions, your risk of developing a melanoma is 20 to 25 times higher than the general population.

Medical Center in Manhattan. He has been tracking this cancer for 11 years.

"Melanoma is increasing faster than any other cancer in the United States," says Dr. Rigel. "Ten years ago, it was unusual to see someone under 40 with melanoma. Now it is common in people in their 20s and 30s."

Dr. Rigel's figures about melanoma and the death rate seem optimistic, compared with the Environmental Protection Agency (EPA) announcement that the Earth's protective ozone layer is dwindling twice as rapidly as had been expected. Worldwide data gathered by the National Aeronautics and Space Administration's satellites moved the EPA to predict that the thinning of the atmosphere's ozone shield will admit even more of the sun's harmful ultraviolet rays and lead to as many as 12 million skin cancers and more than 200,000 skin cancer deaths in the United States in the course of the next 50 years.

The depletion of ozone worsens as you get closer to the North and South Poles. In the United States, it is worst in areas north of a line reaching from Reno, Nevada, to Denver to Philadelphia. Large parts of Europe and regions around the equator also are affected. Worst in the world, however, is the "ozone hole" detected over Antarctica during the winter months. The depletion of ozone previously was thought to cease in warmer months, but it now has been found to continue into April and May, when people start spending more time outdoors.

The chief cause for this depletion of our ozone shield is said to be chlorofluorocarbons and other chemicals that eat away the ozone. The threat of global warming worsens as the diminishing ozone layer lets in more of the sun's ultraviolet rays and our atmosphere's increasing "greenhouse" gases form a thickening blanket around the Earth and prevent its heat from escaping into space. Scientists at the National Oceanic and Atmospheric Administration predict the planet's warming will speed up in the next century.

In the last century, sun-bronzed skin signaled low social status—farmhands, construction workers, and others who labored outdoors. Pale skin marked an upper-class background, particularly in women. The reverse is often true today. A tan can denote a person with enough wealth and leisure time to pursue outdoor sports and/or bask in the sun for hours.

Australia—south of the equator, with plenty of sunshine and many fair-haired, fair-skinned citizens of Anglo-Saxon and Celtic origin who like the great outdoors—has the highest rate of skin cancer in the world. According to one survey, a third of all Australians will develop at least one skin cancer. Australia holds a yearly National Skin Cancer Awareness Week, during which literature and posters are distributed and dermatologists hold free skin cancer screenings.

Australians seem to be growing more cautious about sun exposure.

Karin Eskenazi, of Manhattan—a former sun-worshipper, blond, fair, and freckled—had a melanoma one-third the diameter of a pencil eraser removed from her left shin when she was 24 years old. Says Ms. Eskenazi, "For years, I've taken winter vacations in sunny places like Florida and Mexico. I worked outdoors one summer, and I did have a blistering sunburn when I was 12. I fit the high-risk profile."

Luckily, she had noticed the new growth on her leg and quickly consulted a dermatologist. The doctor diagnosed her cancer when it was quite new and thin—only 1/32 of an inch, as slim as a postcard. At this stage, doctors can excise the melanoma and can promise an almost 100 percent cure rate. Up to 4/32 of an inch, the survival rate drops to 50 percent. If a growth exceeds that thickness, the person's life expectancy plummets.

Clearly, getting a doctor's care promptly is a matter of life or death.

Once the cancer penetrates a couple of layers of skin, its wild cells break loose and travel the tiny canals of the body to lodge in the liver, brain, kidneys, and other sites on the skin. There they settle and form ever larger clumps, choking the organs they have invaded.

For early detection, Dr. Rigel and his colleagues have developed an "ABCD" system to help you locate a cancer or a potential cancer on your body:

- *A* stands for asymmetry, or irregularity of shape, meaning that you cannot draw a line through it to create matching halves. Noncancerous pigmented lesions usually are round and symmetrical (when cut down the middle, their halves have matching shapes), but early malignant melanomas usually are asymmetrical.

- *B* is for an irregular border—common to cancerous growths. Benign growths usually have regular margins.

- *C* is for color. A harmless growth generally is one color overall and flat. Cancerous growths, however, harbor various shades—from tan and brown to black, sometimes mixed in with pink or with red and white.

- *D* is for diameter. If the growth measures more than 6 millimeters across (about one-fourth of an inch), it is dangerous.

The Skin Cancer Foundation recommends regular self-examination of every inch of your skin—from the top of your head to the soles of your feet and between your fingers and toes. (Be sure to have a dermatologist examine you annually.) To do it yourself, stand nude with your back turned to a full-length mirror. Then look into a hand-held mirror to examine the back of your neck, torso, rump, and legs as reflected in the full-length mirror. Anything you see that doesn't clear the ABCD test requires a medical exam. Even if you find skin spots (dysplastic nevi) that almost fail the ABCD test, they may be warnings that you have a genetic predisposition to melanoma. Watch these carefully and see your doctor immediately in response to any change in them.

In addition to self-examination, all of us—black-skinned to fair—need sun protection. The sun's ultraviolet light harms our skin, including the soles of our feet and our palms. Evidence suggests that damage done during childhood and the teen years creates the greatest risk, so we must teach small children caution.

To avoid trouble, heed these pointers from the Skin Cancer Foundation:

• Avoid the sun, especially between 10 A.M. and 3 P.M.

• Wear a broad-brimmed hat to shade the face; wear long pants and long sleeves.

• If you must expose your skin to ultraviolet light, use sunscreens rated 15 or higher—it will take you 15 times longer to get a sunburn. Sunscreens do not filter out all the ultraviolet rays, however, and doubts have been raised about the toxicity of urocanic acid used in some of them. It has been found to suppress the immune system and allows tumors to grow. The Food and Drug Administration is reviewing a petition to investigate.

Most doctors agree: No tan is safe; an early tan won't prevent sunburn later; and tanning parlors won't save your skin—they use ultraviolet light for tanning, and ultraviolet light hurts skin (eyes, too).

Recently, many health food stores have offered a "natural" product that produces a "tan" if taken orally. It does color the skin orange, but it is not easily eliminated by the body, and at least one case of deadly aplastic anemia has been reported in association with it.

Once a melanoma is diagnosed, surgery usually is done around and under the cancer to make sure all of it is removed. Patients often are left with large disfiguring scars that, fortunately, can be helped by plastic surgery.

Dr. Hubert T. Greenway of the Scripps Clinic & Research Foundation in La Jolla, California, uses a less disfiguring technique—Mohs surgery—invented by Dr. Fred Mohs, retired, of the University of Wisconsin at Madison.

Dr. Greenway removes the melanoma, thin slice by thin slice, and examines each slice under the microscope to see how far the cancer has spread. Subsequent slices are wider or narrower, depending on what the microscope shows. Surgery stops after several slices no longer show cancer cells, so the smallest possible scar results. He also is testing the drug interferon, which regulates the body's system for fighting germs and cancer. Greenway estimates that he and his colleagues have injected interferon into 40 to 50 patients with widespread melanoma and that 10 to 12 of them have experienced complete disappearance of the cancer.

That is a low rate of response, but the experiment shows that a manipulation of the tumor-fighting power of the blood could, in theory, cure melanoma in more people. Also, interferon does control one kind of leukemia and, injected into other skin cancers, has cured them in 80 percent of cases.

Many labs now are searching for a vaccine to stimulate the body's immune system to battle cancer. Dr. Jean-Claude Bystryn of the New York University Kaplan Cancer Center in Manhattan has tried such a vaccine on patients who'd had a deep melanoma removed. Such a malignancy usually returns.

Dr. Bystryn's vaccine is made up of extracts from several types of melanoma cells taken from different patients. By injecting this mixture into a patient, he hopes to teach the body to react and fight the cancer. In one test, he gave the vaccine to 63 persons with melanoma. Those whose bodies reacted stayed disease-free three times longer than the others.

Says Dr. Bystryn, "We still don't know for sure whether vaccines will slow the growth of melanoma, but the results we have so far are very encouraging."

At Memorial Sloan-Kettering Cancer Center in New York, scientists are studying other antimelanoma vaccines. They are trying to mimic a substance that generally appears on cancerous tumor cells but only rarely on normal cells. By injecting this artificial substance, they hope to mobilize the immune system against the melanoma cells.

Finally, perhaps the most dramatic experiment of all: gene therapy. Dr. Steven A. Rosenberg, chief surgeon at the National Cancer Institute in Bethesda, Maryland (he excised former President Reagan's colon cancer), and his colleagues there have treated two advanced melanoma patients—a woman, 29, and a man, 42.

The patients were injected with white blood cells specially bred to hunt down cancer. These cells carried tumor necrosis factor (TNF), normally found only in tiny amounts in the blood, which kills cancer cells. But when doctors tried to inject large amounts of TNF directly into cancer patients, too many of their normal cells died.

Dr. Rosenberg transferred the gene for TNF into the patients' white cells. But the gene turned on the white cells' ability to make their own TNF. So Dr. Rosenberg grew those altered cells in test tubes in large numbers (estimated at a billion and more).

When put back into the patient, these white cells should chase the melanoma cells and dump TNF on them. Dr. Rosenberg says it's too early to tell whether the gene therapy will work, adding, "What we have here is an entirely new way of attacking cancer, but it also is still entirely experimental."

Dr. Libby Edwards, chief of dermatology at the Carolinas Medical Center in Charlotte, North Carolina, also has a new treatment: she applies tretinoin solution to skin spots to make them disappear. (Tretinoin, a vitamin A derivative, is often used to reduce wrinkling of the skin.)

One of her patients—Fred Kay, 51, a lawyer from Tucson, Arizona—had moles on his body and arms. "I never had melanoma, but my brother did," Mr. Kay says. "Dr. Edwards felt I was at risk. She gave me tretinoin. Some small moles disappeared. The skin got red and crusted."

Dr. Edwards says the tretinoin did not eliminate all the moles, but this treatment is important, she adds, because it shows there may be other drugs that could work for skin spots and melanoma.

The future is bright for those who get immediate care for melanoma, dim for patients with advanced melanomas, but anticancer work being done worldwide inspires hope. Meanwhile, it's best to stay out of the sun and examine ourselves often for the deadly growths.

For the booklet The ABCDs of Moles and Melanoma, *send a self-addressed, stamped envelope to the Skin Cancer Foundation, Box 561, New York, NY 10016.*

Breast Cancer: Is a Cure in Sight?

IN THE 40 YEARS I HAVE WRITTEN ABOUT AND explored breast cancer, never have I seen such optimism as now. Powerful new scientific evidence backs up the hopeful vision. The scientists maintain that a cure for many, but not all, now incurable breast cancers soon may be realized.

That's because several hundred incredibly courageous women are putting their lives on the line for science. They also will be doing it for the 183,000 American women stricken with breast cancer each year. The disease, which often is discovered as a lump in the breast, kills 46,000 women annually in this country.

The women volunteering to test the promising cure all have advanced breast cancer. Some already have begun to take into their systems the strongest known combination of anticancer chemicals.

And, if all goes as the scientists hope, the anticancer drugs being tested by these heroic women will rout the cancer while leaving all other organs mostly unharmed. The results will be known by 1997 or 1998.

Hazel Greaves, 39, mother of two young daughters in Delray Beach, Florida, stands on the front lines of the research. "I suppose I am a guinea pig," she says, "but I am quite happy to be one—I feel a great deal better already."

In the summer of 1989, Mrs. Greaves had lost 25 pounds for no known reason. Severe, constant fatigue laid her low. In October, physicians told her that a quickly growing cancer was spreading in her breast. The doctors sent her to the National Cancer Institute (NCI) in Bethesda, Maryland.

There, in twelve 3- to 4-week cycles, medical scientists dispensed high doses of four chemicals known to kill cancers. Mrs. Greaves, however, could not tolerate the doses needed to kill the cancer. Those same drugs also destroy the bone marrow—the soft tissue in the bones that makes blood. And without bone marrow, she soon would have no red blood cells, no protection against germs.

"In between cycles, at home in Florida, I injected what doctors called a growth factor serum with a small insulin-type syringe," she says. That growth factor, found naturally in tiny amounts in blood, safeguarded Mrs. Greaves's bone marrow. Her chemotherapy has ended; doctors have found no sign of cancer.

Dr. Andrew Dorr, senior investigator at the NCI, reports that the kind of therapy given to Mrs. Greaves also partially or completely shrank the cancers in 20 other patients with advanced breast cancer. "This is all very preliminary," Dr. Dorr says cautiously. "But this is the direction we are going in."

Dr. Paul A. Marks, president of Memorial Sloan-Kettering Cancer Center in New York City, says, "We don't need statistics to know we have the real thing, at last. Still, we do have to prove it."

Dr. Marks and I were high school classmates 45 years ago and are still friends now. I do not doubt his estimate of the future of breast cancer. He credits the latest advance to other researchers at Memorial and around the world.

In particular, Dr. Marks cites the work of Drs. Janice Gabrilove and Malcolm Moore, the Memorial scientists who first identified and purified the growth factor. Called granulocyte colony stimulating factor (G-CSF), it stimulates blood cell growth. It protected the blood system for 20 women in Dr. Dorr's care.

The next step is being planned by Dr. Larry Norton, also of Memorial Sloan-Kettering Cancer Center. He will enroll women with high-risk cases of breast cancer in a study of granulocyte macrophage CSF. The women first will get GM-CSF and high doses of anticancer drugs. Months later, half the women will get GM-CSF and anticancer drugs. The others will get drugs but no GM-CSF.

Since this was first written, however, the game plan has changed. GM-CSF has proved to be lifesaving on its own. So all the women will get GM-CSF. But Dr. Norton's patients will continue as planned. Dr. Norton is testing a one-two punch against breast cancer. That means that the women will get a big dose of combination therapy (i.e., several drugs at once). This is followed up at a later time with another treatment with a combination of different drugs.

Dr. Norton's theory is that the cancer cells that survived the first set of cancer drugs will be picked off by the second treatment. Dr. Norton told me that 82 percent of the women in this group were still alive 3 years after the one-two punch treatment.

Another study is being set up with a larger number of women receiving this treatment compared to those getting standard chemical therapy.

Participating, as these women will do, in a study to test a lifesaving drug and not knowing whether you are getting that drug yourself is a test of courage. "It is a highly motivated patient who wants to try something more than she can get in her doctor's office," says Dr. Joyce O'Shaughnessy, a senior investigator at the NCI. In a clinical trial, she adds, you get good standard therapy and take a chance at getting something even better as well.

Scientists contend that higher doses of cancer-killing drugs mean higher cure rates.

There's no proof yet, but in a couple of years they expect to know for sure. It could turn out that taking the growth factor and high-dose drugs is not best for the patient.

Large amounts of the cancer drugs could severely injure other organs, sometimes fatally. Growth factor cannot protect you against such damage.

Nearly 100 years of research have led up to this exciting moment. In the 19th century, every woman who developed breast cancer died of it. The cancer cells eventually invaded other areas of the body, choked off blood supplies, and squeezed normal cells.

In 1894, the first mastectomy—removal of the cancerous breast—was performed. Later, doctors made the surgery more radical, cutting out the lymph nodes under the arm and in the chest where, they suspected, cancer cells lurked. Some cut away the muscles as well. As a result, many women ended up with painful, swollen arms as fluid choked their tissues.

By the 1940s, doctors saw that three of four women survived at least 5 years after a radical mastectomy, and 30 percent were cured—the cancer never came back. Curiously, despite many more women having had mastectomies and despite "improvements" in the surgery, the nation's death rate from breast cancer had remained unchanged over the preceding 50 years.

In 1964, when I was science editor of the *New York Herald Tribune*, I reported this fact. I saw no change in the death rates from cancer of the breast. Despite better-trained surgeons, better drugs, and improve anesthesia, nothing changed.

My report raised a storm of protest both from doctors and patients. The doctors wanted me fired, even going so far as to circulate a petition. How dare I, a nonphysician, criticize surgeons for what they were doing to save lives?

Over thirty years later, as you will see in the rest of this report, scientific research proved me right and the doctors wrong.

I had great sympathy for the patients. I received anguished telephone calls and letters. "You are telling me that I am going to die," one weeping woman said. I thought. "Yes. We are all going to die sooner or later." I tried to reassure the woman that science is moving at great speed trying to find a solution. I don't think I was very successful.

By the 1960s, scientists began to suspect that more radical mastectomies did not mean more cures, that surgery had gone as far as it could. Studies in Scotland compared the outcomes for two groups of women—those who had had the radical method and those who had had a simple breast removal and radiation bombardment of the breast area. The death rates were identical for both groups.

In 1971, about 4,000 brave women with small cancers (less than 1 1/2 inches across) began signing up for a series of studies that would change the treatment of breast cancer forever. Dr. Bernard Fisher, professor of surgery at the University of Pittsburgh School of Medicine, got 89 hospitals in the United States and Canada to test simple versus radical surgery. At random, the women were assigned either one treatment or the other. *Both proved equally effective.*

In the years since then, studies by Dr. Fisher and his colleagues have proved the following points:

• For women with small cancers, removal of the cancer (lumpectomy) plus radiation of the breast was as effective as a simple mastectomy.

• Adding chemotherapy enhanced chances of survival for women whose cancer cells had migrated to their lymph nodes. Multiple drugs given to women whose lymph nodes were cancer-free also proved beneficial. However, when the cancer is larger than 1 1/2 inches in diameter, a total mastectomy still is recommended as safest.

In May 1988, the NCI alerted all doctors and hospitals to give anticancer chemicals or an antiestrogen drug, tamoxifen, to all women who have breast cancer. Doctors also have progressed in helping patients with advanced cancers to live longer, with greatly relieved symptoms, even when their cancers can't be cured. Tamoxifen especially helps women whose cancers thrive on estrogen.

With chemotherapy, doctors can treat a breast cancer so large that it is inoperable and shrink it down to a size where surgeons can remove it, sometimes with only a lumpectomy.

For women whose cancers are widespread, doctors are using bone marrow transplants. As with CSF, doctors give the patients high doses of anticancer drugs. But first they remove a quart of bone marrow from the patient and freeze it to preserve it. Sometimes they might treat the marrow with a lower dose of anticancer chemicals to kill any cancer.

After the chemotherapy is over, the physicians reinject patients with their own thawed marrow, so the blood system can recover. Dr. Nancy Davidson of Johns Hopkins Oncology Center in Baltimore has treated 30 patients this way. A majority seemed to have lived longer than expected. But the treatment is dangerous: One of five may die, often of infections.

Jill Gordon, 38, from Arnold, Maryland, mother of twin sons, underwent the marrow technique. In 1981, she had a mastectomy followed by chemotherapy. But the cancer returned in 1988, and she went to Johns Hopkins. "It took a long time to get my strength back," Mrs. Gordon recalls, "but I feel really good now. They don't know if the cancer is completely gone. Spots on my liver could be scars, or dormant cancer."

Though national death rates from breast cancer have remained unchanged, Lawrence Garfinkel, chief statistician for the American Cancer Society, says statistics show that the number of new cancers rose 30 percent in the 1980s.

Part of the increase comes from the awareness women now have of the need for breast self-examination and mammography, so more cases are showing up sooner. Early detection increases cures and should lower the death rate. Perhaps new treatments are just keeping pace with the higher caseload. The American Cancer Society advises having a first mammogram between ages 35 and 39, one at least every 2 years from 40 to 49, then yearly from age 50.

Zahara Davidowitz-Farkas, a 38 year-old rabbi in Queens, New York, credits the mammogram with saving her life. This simple X-ray detects tumors and other abnormalities in the breast long before a woman or her doctor can. As recommended by the American Cancer Society, Rabbi Davidowitz-Farkas had a mammogram when she was 35. The X-ray was normal, but her doctor suggested she take another test the following year because she had benign cysts, common in women.

The second mammogram was normal too. But the following year, doctors found suspicious changes in the rabbi's left breast. Cancer was discovered. Weighing her options, she chose amputation of the breast, then breast reconstruction.

"What I decided to do guaranteed my life," the rabbi says. "By having the first mammograms, to use as baseline points of reference, my doctors had two sets of X-ray films with which to compare the changes in the third."

Some doctors say results for cancer patients should be better. Certainly, the new methods are getting wider use. A report from the federal General Accounting Office says that only 23 percent of all breast cancer patients got chemotherapy in 1975, but 63.1 percent received it in 1985. Some leaders in breast cancer research suspect, however, that doctors far from the major medical centers just aren't using the new methods properly.

Dr. Vincent DeVita, Jr., former head of the NCI, maintains that many doctors are not giving enough cancer drugs to their patients because of the side effects. "The high dosage needed to kill the cancer makes the patient sick," he says. "There's nausea, weakness, hair loss. When you reduce the dose by 30 percent to 40 percent, you still get side effects and are still at risk of getting sick or dying. And that reduction in dose can result in throwing away the drug's capacity to cure the cancer. Clearly, people are losing their lives because they're not getting adequate chemotherapy."

The National Cancer Institute is planning a giant national study to find out how well doctors everywhere are applying the new knowledge about cancer treatment. What they discover could save thousands of lives.

Stepping Up the Fight against Breast Cancer

JUST A FEW YEARS AGO, CANCER EXPERTS WERE enthusiastic about the strong possibility of soon canceling out breast cancer in women. The doctors had learned to use surgery and radiation treatment more precisely to attack the wildly growing cells. They also discovered how to shower the malignancy with strong anticancer drugs. They had new medications to protect healthy tissue from the bad effects of the drugs. Scientists also expected to rout out the cause of the disease, and with that knowledge they had hoped to cure breast cancer or to prevent it, or both.

But it has not happened—yet.

The American Cancer Society reports that, with 183,000 new cases annually, breast cancer kills 46,000 women each year. A woman who lives to age 85 runs a one-in-nine chance of contracting breast cancer in her lifetime. Despite new therapies, the death rate has hardly changed in 50 years, and 70 percent of new cases are diagnosed in women who have no known risk factors for the disease.

That is dark news. Dr. Samuel Broder, director of the National Cancer Institute (NCI) in Bethesda, Maryland, maintains, "No question that we have a basis for optimism, but we should have no illusions about how difficult and formidable a problem breast cancer is. There won't be a breakthrough tomorrow morning."

Nobody knows that better than Dabney Allen, 49, a homemaker in MacLean, Virginia. Doctors first found a lump in a mammogram (a breast X-ray) of her right breast in 1990. "The biopsy showed that I had the kind of cancer that was 40 percent likely to recur," Mrs. Allen tells *Parade,* "so I had both breasts removed." After surgery, the doctors treated her with four potent drugs. "But the cancer recurred in March, under my right arm and along the scar," Mrs. Allen says. "It spread to bone and to a spot on the chest wall. So my doctors say, 'Let's treat this as a chronic disease and not a terminal one.'"

Mrs. Allen will take drugs to kill her cancer cells. It is no cure, but she hopes

---

Women at Risk for Breast Cancer

Although 70 percent of women who develop breast cancer have no known risk factors, you are particularly at risk if you:

- Have a sister, daughter, or mother who has or had the disease
- Are childless
- Had first child in your late 20s or later
- Have had frequent biopsies for "lumps"
- Started to menstruate before age 13 and reached menopause after age 55
- Have been diagnosed with "lobular carcinoma in situ"
- Have had tissue tested and found to have the genes for breast cancer

---

by this method to alleviate the pain and stay comfortable for as long as possible.

The incidence of breast cancer increased by more than 30 percent from 1980 to 1987, prompting some to call the disease an epidemic. However, the American Cancer Society and the NCI believe the increase was due to more women having mammograms, which caught their cancer early. And Dr. Vincent DeVita, Jr., former head of the NCI, notes, "There is a definite decline in the death rate among young women with breast cancer."

Still, Dr. Daniel Kopans, an associate professor of radiology at Harvard Medical School, believes that the number of new cases is increasing. Is there an epidemic? "Absolutely," says Dr. Susan Love, director of University of California at Los Angeles's Breast Center. "There are too many women dying of breast cancer, and we have to do something about it."

What about mammograms? Dr. Kopans is angry with the NCI for its recent conclusion that women aged 40 to 49 do not benefit from annual mammograms. "If you screened all the women in the U.S. aged 40 to 49, you would save 3,000 lives a year," Kopans estimates. The American Cancer Society and American Medical Association maintain that there is sufficient evidence to continue screening women in that age group.

However, several studies have shown that mammography screening provides little or no benefit for women under 50. Studies in the Netherlands, the United Kingdom, and Sweden, plus a Canadian study of 90,000 women, all showed that death rates from breast cancer for women in their 40s were the same whether or not they had screening mammograms.

"Mammography screening works great over 50," says Dr. Love. "It has never really been proved to work that well in women under 50. The answer is, We need to find something that works better, not pay for something that doesn't work as well."

When Surgery Is Needed

Once, women with breast cancer were routinely advised to have a radical mastectomy (removal of the breast and lymph nodes under the arm). But 18 years ago, Dr. Bernard Fisher of the University of Pittsburgh began a pioneering study in many hospitals simultaneously. The research compared two treatments for early cancer. One was radical mastectomy. The other combined radiation with lumpectomy (cutting out small cancers). The results, published in 1985, showed the treatments were equally effective against early-stage cancer. Women now had a choice.

In 1982, Wilma Gauthier, a secretary in San Diego, chose lumpectomy. Her doctors were against it. "They told me that if I didn't have a mastectomy, I would orphan my children," she recalls. "I did feel scared that I had made a mistake. My husband supported me. It has been 12 years, and I am cancer-free."

Still, only 20 percent of women who have early-stage cancer—and so are good candidates for lumpectomy—have that treatment. Surgeons may still be recommending mastectomy.

The issue was raised again this year after it was revealed that a Canadian doctor had committed fraud when he participated in Dr. Fisher's studies. In a complicated way, he had entered patients into the research who did not meet the qualifying guidelines.

Dr. Fisher did another analysis of the results, leaving out the Canadian data. Fortunately, the outcome remained the same: Lumpectomy with radiation is just as effective as radical mastectomy for early-stage cancer.

But Fisher waited months before revealing the fraud and announcing the new analysis. Cancer scientists and women's health advocates were infuriated. "It was a terrible thing," says Dr. Jeffrey S. Abrams, a breast cancer specialist at the NCI.

New Treatments

Despite the controversies swirling around breast cancer treatment, there's an exciting outlook as the NCI's Dr. Broder sees it. Researchers are testing new drugs given in new ways.

Dr. Larry Norton, director of breast medical oncology at Memorial Sloan-Kettering Cancer Center in New York, has tried giving a one-two punch to breast cancer growths.

"Conventionally we have been giving patients all the drugs at once," Dr. Norton explains. "Now we give one or two drugs at one time, wait a couple of weeks, and then give another drug—in high doses. These women have fewer relapses than would be expected in patients with conventional treatment. Now there's a big trial starting, to see if what we saw on a small scale will work in a large trial," adds Norton. "I think it will." That could prolong many lives.

Taxol, a drug derived from the bark of the yew tree, is one of the most powerful cancer destroyers known and is being used against advanced breast cancer. The results are promising. However, taxol is in short supply, and environmentalists have been concerned that demand would lead to the loss of entire yew forests. Scientists are working to produce the substance in the lab.

A controversial new treatment for advanced cancer patients is chemotherapy in very high doses, followed by removing the patient's bone marrow, treating it with drugs to kill cancer cells and transplanting it back into the patient. The treatment is expensive, costing up to $150,000. The research continues. The effectiveness of this treatment is unknown.

Can It Be Prevented?

Scientists are also moving to prevent breast cancer. Scientists are testing tamoxifen, a drug that suppresses cancer cells that depend on estrogen for continued growth. They will enroll 16,000 otherwise healthy women who are at higher than normal risk for breast cancer. Half will take the drug, the other half a fake pill called a placebo. Only the statisticians will know who got which treatment. The system prevents unconscious bias. After 5 years, researchers will see whether those taking the drug have a lower incidence of cancer.

A drawback is the evidence that tamoxifen may cause uterine cancer in some women. Some women's health advocates attacked the project, saying it puts healthy women at risk. Dr. Leslie Ford, chief of community oncology at the NCI, heads the experiment. "The risk appears to be in the same range as that from estrogen replacement therapy," Dr. Ford says. "The risk is minuscule compared to the benefits."

Can we find the cause? One theory on the cause of breast cancer holds that environmental toxins—both artificial and natural poisons—are, in part, to blame. However, the proof eludes scientists. A high-fat diet has been pointed to as another possible cause. Some believe that pesticides or chemicals that may be stored in the fatty tissue of meat or fish or that are otherwise ingested may be associated with increased risk. Again, no real proof. In the meantime, the NCI urges women to reduce the fat in their diets to under 30 percent of calories.

Finally, researchers are tracking the genetic factor. If they can identify the gene that causes breast cancer, it could give doctors the power to intervene and prevent it. "We know it's genetic," says UCLA's Dr. Love. "Some people are born with a screwed-up gene; others develop it. We don't know what causes the gene to change. Pesticides? Pollution? Food additives? They are all possibilities. All we know is that genes are involved. And we are very close to finding them."

In 1996, scientists announced the discovery of two breast-cancer-causing genes.

However only a small group of women—less than 5 percent—carry these cancer triggers. This discovery suggests that other breast-cancer genes exist. Scientists are looking toward the day when they can destroy or change these killer genes.

Stepping Up the Fight

Maybe the best news about breast cancer is that women have taken action. Activists from all over the country have organized to push for more funding for research. Looking at the success that AIDS activists achieved in pressuring Congress for funding for more research, women with a breast cancer concern set out to do the same. The National Breast Cancer Coalition and other grassroots groups have lobbied to increase research dollars. Their efforts have been paying off. Government funding went from $87 million in 1990 to $408 million in 1993. The fight continues.

What You Can Do

To find out more about breast cancer activist groups in your community, write to the National Breast Cancer Coalition, P.O. Box 66373, Washington, D.C. 20035.

For more information, call the American Cancer Society (800-ACS-2345) weekdays, 9 A.M. to 4:30 P.M., or the National Cancer Institute (800-4-CANCER) weekdays, 9 A.M. to 4:30 P.M. local time, for free information and literature. The Y-ME National Breast Cancer Organization hotline is staffed by breast cancer survivors. Call 800-221-2141 weekdays, 24 hours a day.

Two useful books are *Dr. Susan Love's Breast Book,* by Susan Love, M.D. (Addison-Wesley), and *The Breast Cancer Hand-book: Taking Control after You've Found a Lump,* by Joan Swirsky and Barbara Balaban (HarperPerennial). Ask your librarian to recommend others.

What Is the Best Way to Treat Prostate Cancer?

SUDDENLY, IT SEEMS, PROSTATE CANCER IS IN the news. Reports say, for example, that Michael Milken, the financier who was convicted of securities fraud, is donating $5 million annually for 5 years to support prostate research worldwide. He has the disease.

Mr. Milken, 49, reportedly is under a doctor's care, and his cancer is in remission. It was declared inoperable in 1993, having spread to his lymph nodes; surgeons could not remove or destroy it.

Sen. Robert Dole was luckier. On December 18, 1991, surgeons were able to remove his cancerous prostate gland. Afterward, doctors reported no signs that any cancer remained. At 72, he was an active presidential candidate.

The prostate is a walnut-sized gland at the base of a man's bladder. It surrounds the urethra and produces part of the fluid that makes up semen. If the prostate gland falls prey to cancer and goes untreated, it could spread beyond the gland to other organs and ultimately kill the patient.

Although controversy about surgery and other treatments for prostate cancer persists, consensus is growing that men older than 70 often can afford to wait, because prostate cancer usually is slow-growing at that age. Researchers say the patient probably will die with prostate cancer, rather than of it. For such patients, surgery seems to have fewer benefits than other options. However, men younger than 60, whose cells grow more rapidly, need swift, early diagnosis and treatment to stop the cancer before it spreads and kills.

The Importance of Early Diagnosis

Scientists are working hard to identify the cancer in younger men while it is still confined to the prostate. It is no trivial issue. This year doctors will find 317,000 cases of prostate cancer in the United States, and 41,000 will die of it. The only cancer that kills more American men is lung cancer.

"We are diagnosing the disease much earlier than before," said Dr. Patrick Craig Walsh, urology chairman at the Johns Hopkins Medical Center in Baltimore and author of *The Prostate: A Guide for Men and the Women Who Love Them.* "Up 'til 10 years ago," Dr. Walsh says, "we could detect it only by feeling the gland." His reference is to the digital rectal examination (DRE), in which a doctor inserts a gloved and lubricated finger through the patient's rectum to feel the prostate gland. If the prostate seems enlarged, hard, or bumpy, the DRE usually is followed by a biopsy, a microscopic examination of a tissue sample.

"Now," says Dr. Walsh, "we also have a blood test that alerts doctors to cases that are suspicious. To follow them up, we do a simple biopsy to rule out or identify the cancer. And if it is cancer and it has not spread, then we cut it out."

That blood test measures prostate-specific antigen (PSA), a chemical produced in the prostate gland. If cancer attacks the gland, the antigen is emitted in large amounts. A high level of PSA in such a test alerts doctors to the chance that the cancer might be growing.

Dr. Joseph E. Oesterling, formerly of the Mayo Clinic in Rochester, Minnesota, and now chief urologist at the University of Michigan Medical Center in Ann Arbor, helped develop a new test with two Scandinavian doctors. It showed that PSA exists in the blood in two forms: free, or attached to a protein molecule. If the prostate is enlarged but not cancerous, more of the free PSA is found; if cancer is present, more of the attached form is found. Dr. Oesterling recommends a yearly blood test for PSA, because a rapid rise in its level can indicate cancer growth.

Testing for PSA has doctors at odds. Some complain that the tests don't find early cancer but do trigger a sequence of expensive medical steps without prolonging lives. Others urge watchful waiting for aging patients, to spare them the risks and trauma of major surgery.

Whether—and When— to Have Surgery

Thanks to Dr. Walsh of Johns Hopkins, incontinence and impotence may no longer be the expected side effects of surgery for prostate cancer. In a brilliant series of anatomic studies, he identified the nerves affecting urinary control and sexual potency and developed a surgical method that left both functions intact.

After this development was announced in 1982, surgeons nationwide rushed to learn the Walsh technique. Some also said surgery was being performed too often.

Can doctors develop a way to identify cases that require surgery? Are many prostate glands removed unnecessarily? To find out, researchers at the Mayo Clinic developed a mathematical formula. It factored in the patient's age, the apparent rate of growth of the tumor, the malignancy of the tumor's cells, and the size of the prostate gland (the bigger the gland, the more PSA it emits).

With this formula, they systematically reviewed 339 cases of prostate cancer surgery at the clinic from 1991 to 1993. The researchers, headed by Dr. Oesterling, reported their findings in the January 24/31, 1996, issue of the *Journal of the American Medical Association*. In applying their formula, they wrote, they found only 14 cases in which the surgery probably had not been necessary. This is impressive work.

Dr. Oesterling estimates that up to 30 percent of men over 50 have undetected prostate cancer, of which only 4 percent will cause trouble and require treatment. This is because age often slows the cancer's growth. Dr. Oesterling also says that the older a man is, the more PSA he puts out. A high reading at age 70, then, holds less risk for a man than it might at 50 or even 60.

"In a man younger than 60," says Dr. Oesterling, "a big, fast-growing tumor needs to be treated quickly, or the cancer might spread and become incurable. A small, slow-growing prostate cancer in men 70 or older probably won't be life-threatening. These are the men for watchful waiting."

Also encouraging is the news that some drugs can slow the cancer's growth after it has spread beyond the prostate, even if current treatments can't stop it.

A team of physicians and statisticians at Dartmouth Medical School in Hanover, New Hampshire, studied 10,598 cases of prostate removal among Medicare patients aged 65 or older. Their cancers had been removed by radical surgery (excision of the entire gland and the pelvic lymph nodes). In the period of the study, from 1984 to 1990 (after Dr. Walsh devised his method), the rate of prostate surgery had increased sixfold.

Better science and public awareness may partially explain why. In the *Journal of the American Medical Association* in 1993, the Dartmouth team wrote, "Increased detection might be the major factor contributing to the rising rate of prostate cancer." But they concluded, "Despite increasing detection of prostate cancer and increasing instances of its surgical removal, [death rates] from prostate cancer have not decreased. . . . The therapeutic benefit of radical prostatectomy [prostate removal] for . . . cancer that was detected early has not been demonstrated."

Yet Dr. Oesterling says that 10-year follow-up studies of surgical prostate removals in four medical institutions showed an estimated 90 percent long-term survival rate for patients whose cancers stayed within the gland.

Many praise surgery. Bill E. Hahn, 66, a retired salesman and resident of suburban Kalamazoo, Michigan, had a PSA test that revealed prostate cancer. It was then removed Dr. Walsh's way on January 4, 1995, by Dr. Oesterling.

"I have no sign of cancer," Mr. Hahn said. "My PSA is negligible. I have full bladder control, and I have erections."

In December 1995, soon after having the Walsh method of surgery, Army Gen. (Ret.) Norman Schwarzkopf, 61, said on national TV, "It is so stupid that anybody should die of prostate cancer—it can be detected. . . . If you are over 50 years old, you go in every year for a checkup!"

If your family has a history of prostate cancer, however, Dr. Oesterling urges annual checkups beginning at age 40.

Some alternatives to surgery are these:

• Hormone therapy. Should the cancer turn aggressive in the patient's 80s, hormones can be given to shut down cancer cells and make them less damaging. Cost, including medications, is about $500 a month.

• Radiation. X rays may match surgery's record for helping prolong life, but poorly done evaluations make it hard to tell.

• Freezing. Dr. Peter Carroll directs the urological cancer program at the University of California at San Francisco. First, guided by ultrasound, he inserts five small tubes through the skin into the prostate. He then fills the tubes with liquid nitrogen at 180 degrees below zero. The cold theoretically kills the cancer cells (and other cells as well). Dr. Carroll said that within 3 to 6 months, no sign of cancer was found in up to 80 percent of the 150 patients studied. The method, begun in 1993, is too new to assess.

• Watch and wait. Since prostate cancer often grows slowly, especially in older men, watchfulness, through regular checkups, may be best.

Is the Answer in the Genes?

"I believe that there are young men today with curable prostate cancer who can be identified through testing and treated by surgery in time to save their lives," says Dr. Walsh. He also predicts that scientists will prevent prostate cancer by finding the gene or genes that may trigger it.

At Columbia-Presbyterian Medical Center in New York, Dr. Paul B. Fisher, an oncologist/molecular biologist, has identified PTI-1, a potential prostate cancer gene. "If we can knock it out," he says, "we may knock out the cancer at its source and prevent it from spreading."

Dr. Walsh of Johns Hopkins predicts that scientists one day will prevent prostate cancer by finding the gene or genes that may trigger the disease. You may be able to help, by participating in his study.

Do you have at least three blood relatives who have been diagnosed with prostate cancer? If so, write your full name (printed, then sign it also, please) and full address (including ZIP code) on a sheet of paper. Now, write the answers to these questions:

- How many of your blood relatives were diagnosed with prostate cancer?
- How many of these relatives are still alive?

Mail this information to The Johns Hopkins Prostate Cancer Study, Dept. P, Marburg 134, Baltimore, MD 21287-2101. You will be sent a questionnaire and may be asked to donate a small amount of blood, which will be tested free of charge. All results will be kept confidential.

Digestive Diseases

Soon, We Won't Have to Worry about Ulcers

IF YOU EVER HAVE HAD TO ENDURE THE PAIN OF a peptic ulcer attack, you will be ecstatic to hear that the odds are now 70 percent in favor of your ulcer being cured—with antibiotics. And you will have plenty of company: The nation's estimated 20 million residents who either have or are expected to develop peptic ulcers will be happy to hear it, too.

Thanks to a revolutionary discovery that a particular bacterium (a germ) causes most of these ulcers, doctors now use antibiotics to treat—and often cure—them.

The antibiotics have been added to a medical arsenal of powerful drugs that curb the stomach's production of acid. For a generation now, these drugs have relieved the pain of peptic ulcers, but they haven't cured all of them. Antibiotics kills germs, so antibiotics can cure ulcers.

Previously, doctors believed that ulcers were caused by digestive enzymes that, combined with stomach acid, ate away at the walls of the stomach or the duodenum, the pipe that connects the small intestine and the stomach. Eventually, some patients with recurrent ulcers required surgeons to cut out the affected area of the stomach.

News of the theory that a specific bacterium or germ caused ulcers came from a small hospital in Australia about 15 years ago. At first, nobody in the medical world believed it. For years, doctors had blamed ulcers on smoking, drinking, bad diet, and/or anxiety. Doctors "knew" that a high-powered business executive's ulcers came with the job, that nervous tension triggered stomach acid by the bucketful, that stomach acid caused ulcers.

Now scientific proof shows that ulcers are caused by the *Helicobacter pylori* bacteria, visible only under a microscope. The bacteria settle in the lining of the stomach, opening a wound that is then made worse by the acids and digestive juices. The result is something that resembles a flattened volcano or a white-centered, red-rimmed, painful canker sore.

By killing the bacteria with antibiotics, scientists can stop the disease. Doctors estimate that they now can cure 90 percent of the ulcers that are caused by the *H. pylori* strain. And, for the first time, medication can prevent the recurrence of ulcers.

Dr. Frank Hamilton heads the ulcer program at the National Institute of Diabetes and Digestive and Kidney Diseases in Bethesda, Maryland. Like other scientists working on ulcers, Dr. Hamilton could not suppress his excitement about the subject: "This is one of the biggest breakthroughs in gastroenterology in the last three decades. For the first time, we can say there is an organism that causes peptic ulcer disease—and we can treat it."

The leading doctors I interviewed agreed that, from now on, ulcers could become a rare disease, killing far fewer than the estimated 6,000 patients who die in the U.S. annually, according to the National Center on Health Statistics. The doctors also predict that most patients will be cured—and forget they ever had ulcers.

Jay Neitz, 41, teaches neuroscience at the Medical College of Wisconsin in Milwaukee. Since the third grade, he had suffered from peptic ulcers. "They thought it was because of worry," Mr. Neitz recalls. "I went to psychiatrists. I knew I wasn't worried. I just had a sore stomach. This went on for 30 years."

Doctors tried to control his ulcer with a bland diet and pills that neutralize stomach acid. Then, 20 years ago, scientists developed Tagamet, which reduces the production of stomach acid. "That was much better," Mr. Neitz says, "but I still had terrible symptoms: nausea, stomach cramping, burning. Sometimes, I got down on the floor and curled up in pain."

Four years ago, Mr. Neitz was treated by Dr. Amnon Sonnenberg, an associate professor of medicine, also at the Medical College of Wisconsin. The news of the antibiotic treatment of ulcers had just begun to spread. Dr. Sonnenberg gave Mr. Neitz the new antibiotic therapy.

"The amazing thing is that not only do I not have an ulcer anymore," Mr. Neitz says, "but I also don't have stomach problems—no heartburn, nothing. The pain was gone in 6 weeks. I can now drink coffee and eat spicy foods, which I love. This treatment gave me a new life."

Dr. Barry Marshall, formerly a clinical associate professor at the University of Virginia in Charlottesville, was one of the discoverers that the bacterium is the cause of ulcers. In 1981, Dr. Marshall was a young internist at the Royal Perth Hospital in Western Australia. He teamed up with Dr. Robin Warren, a pathologist who also was working there.

Both doctors had noticed a bacterial infection in the lining of the stomachs of patients in the hospital and tried to find out more about it with a simple patient questionnaire. "Out of 100 patients with various diseases," Dr. Marshall says, "65 percent were tested and found to have the infection, and half of these were found to have ulcers. My colleagues were astounded. They had been taught, as I was, that germs could not live in acid."

In 1986, in a treatment study among patients whose ulcers would not go away, Dr. Marshall gave half of them Tagamet, the acid suppressant; he gave antibiotics to the other half—Flagyl with bismuth. Among the patients treated with Tagamet only, their ulcers returned at the rate of 95 percent. Among those treated with Flagyl and bismuth, ulcers returned in only 20 percent of the cases.

"By the end of 1986," Dr. Marshall says, "we knew that all these people were better. After a month or two, the patients started eating pepperoni pizza. The patients couldn't believe it."

Because some doctors couldn't believe it either, Dr. Marshall put himself at some risk to prove his hypothesis: he infected himself by swallowing a teaspoonful of culture containing the bacteria. "I came down with gastritis [inflammation of the stomach]," he recalls. As further proof of his theory, he says, antibiotics cured him.

Dr. Marshall adds that not all patients are cured for various reasons, one of which is that sometimes the bacteria develop resistance to the antibiotics.

The new findings even may help prevent stomach cancer. Dr. Martin Blaser, director of the Division of Infectious Diseases at Vanderbilt University School of Medicine in Nashville, asserts, "Stomach cancer is the world's number two cancer killer. In the United States it ranks ninth among men and eleventh among women. But the risk is higher in blacks than in whites, and higher still in Asian Americans and Native Americans.

"The World Health Organization declared *Helicobacter pylori* a type 1 carcinogen—the most dangerous type," says Dr. Blaser. "With it, your risk for stomach cancer goes way up. Preventing infection is a goal, but a vaccine is at least 10 years away." Meanwhile, the antibiotic therapy of Dr. Marshall and careful hygiene should help control the bacterium and reduce the incidence of stomach cancer.

With antibiotics, the need for ulcer surgery also should be reduced—and so should medical costs. "We can cure 85 percent to 90 percent of patients [with ulcers caused by *H. pylori*] for $500," says Dr. Marshall. "In the U.S., with current expensive treatments, a chronic ulcer now costs about $10,000."

For more information, send a self-addressed, legal-sized envelope with 78 cents in postage to the Helicobacter Foundation, P.O. Box 7965, Charlottesville, VA 22906-7965.

The Illness No One Talks About

IT'S STILL NOT CONSIDERED A SUBJECT FOR polite conversation. Far too many people turn away at the mere mention of the topic—and risk early death from disease of the stomach and bowel.

Digestive tract ailments kill thousands of Americans each year. Few people talk about them; even fewer ask for information about them—information that could save their lives.

Now more than ever, medical science can stop the onslaught of peptic ulcers, irritable bowel, colon and rectal cancer, chronic heartburn, even piles and constipation. But doctors need help: you first have to overcome your embarrassment and tell them where you hurt.

Alice Bull, 66, of Red Bank, New Jersey, owes her life to a simple test that pinpointed a small but deadly cancer lurking in the far reaches of her large intestine. It was the same sort of test that led doctors to find and remove the cancer from President Reagan's bowel in 1985.

"I heard about the test on TV," says Mrs. Bull. "I sent for it and took it. The test revealed hidden blood in my stool. And when I had X rays, there was the cancer." Surgery removed the growth.

The test was offered in 1979 in the New York area by the American Cancer Society (ACS) in cooperation with WCBS-TV News, for which I was health and science editor (now retired). More than 60,000 people sent in $2 for the test, but only 15,000 (25 percent) returned their specimens. The others, it seems, couldn't bear to take a tiny sample of their own feces. That squeamishness probably caused more than 100 deaths: the cancers were there, waiting to be detected and treated. But the victims never knew—until it was too late.

Seven years later, after the world had learned all the details of President Reagan's bowel cancer, the ACS offered the test again. This time, 35 percent sent back specimens.

How Digestion Works

Normally, everything in the digestive tract works nicely to break down the food you eat so it can be absorbed by your blood and used for energy and body repair.

Chewed food is swallowed and drops down the food pipe, or esophagus, into the stomach. The stomach then churns and bathes it in acid and enzymes. In less than an hour, the stomach begins pushing the food through the pyloric sphincter and into the duodenum. More digestive fluids come from the liver (bile, which is stored in the gallbladder) and pancreas. From there, the food moves into the narrow, 20-foot-long small intestine, where more enzymes break down the proteins, fats, and starches into food molecules that pass into the bloodstream. Finally, the undigested food—mostly plant fiber—moves into the wider, 5-foot-long large intestine, or colon.

The conquest of heartburn? Trouble can start right in the esophagus. One American in 10 suffers daily from heartburn, so called because it generates a burning sensation in the region of the heart. Rick Tucker, 40, a car dealer in Wytheville, Virginia, had such a severe case of heartburn, he thought he was having a heart attack. "I started to get chest pains," he says, "and symptoms of a heart attack—shooting pains in my chest and left arm. Just thinking it was a heart attack made my heartburn worse."

Basically, heartburn occurs if your stomach splashes acid up into your esophagus. The bitter, acidic fluid gets past the cardioesophageal sphincter, the muscle between the stomach and the esophagus, and burns the food pipe's delicate lining. Doctors once blamed this condition on a hernia in the hiatus (opening) of the diaphragm, which leads to the stomach, but many hiatus hernia patients have no heartburn.

Dr. Richard McCallum, of the University of Virginia School of Medicine, Charlottesville, contends that many heartburn patients' stomachs empty too slowly, causing the acid to collect and rise. Drugs are being developed to treat this.

Dr. Donald O. Castell, of Wake Forest University's Bowman Gray School of Medicine, Winston-Salem, North Carolina, says heartburn has many causes, including excess stomach acid, which drugs can reduce. Doctors also now have bethanechol and metoclopramide, drugs that tighten the cardioesophageal sphincter to help keep acid out of the food pipe.

Searching through the Bowel

In April 1984, George Poydinecz, a real estate investor in Clifton, New Jersey, traveled to Georgia to watch a golf tournament. While in a restaurant, he felt weak. In the men's room he found he had passed a dark, bloody stool. "I didn't have pain," he says. "I just felt weak—my blood pressure dropped. I was bleeding inside."

Doctors tried to pinpoint the digestive tract area that was bleeding. Barium X rays and CAT scans found nothing. Then, at Mount Sinai Medical Center, Manhattan, Dr. Henry Janowitz ordered a new search.

Dr. Stanley Goldsmith, of Mount Sinai's nuclear medicine department, put radioactivity on the job. He took some blood from Mr. Poydinecz's vein, mixed it with radioactive technetium, and injected it back into his patient. The red blood cells then sent out radioactive rays. Using a special camera to detect those rays, Dr. Goldsmith tracked the circulated radioactive blood. He found a pool of blood in Mr. Poydinecz's small intestines, where a dilated vein had burst. Two days later, surgery solved the problem.

Such techniques are revealing the fundamental behavior of the entire digestive tract. By mixing radioactivity with food, scientists can see exactly how each digestive organ handles food. In some people, food is dumped quickly from the stomach, but it slows down in the small intestine. In others, it stays longer in the stomach but passes quickly through the rest of the digestive tract. Such individualized information helps doctors improve treatment for severe constipation, gas pains, and heartburn.

By linking radioactivity to cancer-seeking antibodies, chemicals that attach themselves to cancers, doctors can locate tiny cancers in the large intestine long before any symptoms show.

Finally, gastroenterologists (digestive tract specialists) use a fiber-optic tube, an instrument that enables them to see every nook and cranny of the digestive system. It consists of fine glass fibers bound together in a bundle as thick as a pencil and 9 feet long. Light travels down the tube even when it bends and moves, so the doctor can see into the twisting labyrinth.

Recently, doctors at Mount Sinai reported being able to examine the entire length of a small intestine in about 5 hours, with no damage to the patient. They could locate the kind of bleeding that afflicted George Poydinecz. Previ-

ously, physicians could use such fiber-optic tubes to explore no more than 6 feet of the intestine at a time.

Good News about the Colon

The colon is a very vulnerable site. It frequently becomes inflamed for no known reason (as in ulcerative colitis and Crohn's disease); it sometimes contracts in spasms, resulting in diarrhea or constipation; it may develop pouches that become infected (diverticulitis); and at the nether end, engorged veins may pop out (hemorrhoids).

Happily, progress has been made against these afflictions. Laser light can eliminate hemorrhoids without surgery, with little or no pain to the patient; steroids can help in the treatment of Crohn's disease and diverticulitis.

Doctors estimate that they could save 30,000 lives a year if persons older than 40 would have annual bowel exams. Each year, doctors in the United States diagnose 138,000 cases of colon or rectal cancer. About 56,000 Americans die of the disease yearly.

Colon cancer prevention includes an annual test for hidden blood in the stool plus a rectal examination and an exploration of the bowel with the fiber-optic tube. The American Cancer Society says the fiber-optic examination should be done annually in everyone at ages 50, 51, and 52. After that, if two consecutive exams prove normal, you can wait 3 to 5 years for the next one.

The doctors look for polyps—wart-like growths in the bowel, which often turn cancerous. If found, the growths are removed. The ACS says the survival rate for colorectal cancer when found early is 82 percent, which means that more than 49,000 lives could be saved each year if the cancers were detected and treated promptly.

The Irritable Bowel

Sometimes the bowel contracts spasmodically in an allergic reaction to a particular food. For many patients, elimination of that food cures the irritability; for others, a high-fiber diet quiets the intestines.

More than 2 million Americans suffer from inflamed bowels. Because victims of ulcerative colitis are prone to cancer, surgeons often remove the diseased bowel. Patients then void their wastes through an opening that brings the small intestines to the surface of the abdomen, through a procedure known as an ileostomy.

Doctors now are testing olsalazine, a drug that seems to calm the burning colon. Perhaps, one day soon, other new drugs and treatments will make surgery a rare occurrence for digestive tract disorders.

Fiber Power!

AT 57, CLARENCE DEDMON HAS LIVED UNDER the cloud of diabetes for 3 years. Every day for most of that time, Mr. Dedmon, a church custodian from Lexington, Kentucky, had injected himself with insulin. Six months ago, he began eating lots of cereals, beans, fruits, and vegetables. He has thrown away his insulin needle.

If you had visited Helena LeBow at her New Jersey home last year, you might have found her curled up like an infant, clutching a hot water bottle to her gut. She suffered the excruciating pains of an irritable bowel. A few months ago, she took up Mr. Dedmon's diet. For good measure, she dusted a tablespoon of wheat bran on her breakfast cereal. She hasn't had pain since.

John Griffin, who teaches physical education at a Toronto college, discovered a few years ago, at the age of 30, that the level of fats in his blood was five times above normal. He feared a heart attack. Mr. Griffin cut his meat and white bread intake and substituted 2 cups of beans a day. His blood fat (triglyceride) level plummeted and is now below average.

And in his laboratory at Syntex Research in Palo Alto, California, Dr. Gene Spiller had fed rats a powerful chemical that ignited cancer of the large bowel or colon. When he fed the rats pure cellulose along with the killer chemical, fewer of them developed cancer. A stringy material that is found in every plant, cellulose apparently protected the rodents from the disease.

Scientists have identified the powerful agent that may control diabetes, bowel disease, blood fat, and colon cancer. It is dietary fiber, a part of all plants, including beans, whole-grain cereals, fruits, vegetables, seeds, and nuts. Once they called it roughage, bulk, residue, or simply bran and labeled it "undigestible." They thought it worthless, possibly harmful.

Now they know that this natural plant product may protect us from numerous ailments, including heart attacks, obesity, gallstones, chronic constipation, appendicitis, varicose veins, piles, stomach ulcers, and hiatus hernia, a condition that causes severe heartburn.

That does seem unbelievable. And, indeed, many scientists caution against too much enthusiasm at this stage. But they say that if we want to benefit from fiber, we must regularly eat a variety of fruits, vegetables, beans, nuts, and cereals.

In essence, joining the fiber revolution means this:

• We will eat more legumes (peas, beans, lentils, chickpeas), potatoes, corn, other vegetables, and fruits.

• We will cut down on fatty meat—such as beef, lamb, and pork—even lean poultry, and all other excess fats and oils.

• We will look for whole-grain cereals like Grandma used to make—wheat, oats, barley, buckwheat, and rye—that were hardly touched by the miller's grindstone. We'll make whole-grain dishes and breads and forget white flour. In short, we'll triple our fiber intake to about 60 grams a day.

Dr. James W. Anderson, of the University of Kentucky College of Medicine at Lexington, creator of a high-fiber diet for controlling diabetes and lowering blood fat, says, "The movement toward fiber will have substantial health benefits for Americans."

At a cost of losing the good things to eat? Not at all, says Dr. Kent Moseley, a dentist and patient of Dr. Anderson's in Lexington. Dr. Moseley, who loves to fly his single-engine Cherokee, was in danger of losing his pilot's license because his diabetes was uncontrolled. Until he switched to a high-fiber diet.

Now, instead of a traditional American breakfast of bacon and eggs, orange juice, and white toast smothered in butter, Dr. Moseley starts each day with a serving of whole-grain cereal, fruit, milk, egg whites, and whole-wheat toast. And his blood sugar, which was above the 150-milligram range, now stays down around a normal 100 milligrams.

Scientists have recently discovered that, just as there are different vitamins, each with its own power, there also are a variety of fibers—perhaps a dozen—each performing a particular job after ingestion.

But you can think simply of two kinds of fiber, soluble and insoluble. *Soluble fiber* dissolves in water to form a kind of jelly, such as pectin, which is contained in many fruits and has been used by cooks for centuries. Other soluble fibers—such as those found in beans, oats, corn, and seeds—form gums. *Insoluble fiber* does not dissolve in water but absorbs it like a sponge. The most common of these is cellulose, an ingredient of bran. You may also hear about hemicellulose and lignin, two other insoluble fibers. The biggest source of insoluble fiber in the diet is wheat bran from whole-grain breads and breakfast cereals.

Scientists believe that the two types of fiber work together. The gels and gums control blood sugar and fat and indirectly protect you against cancer and other bowel diseases. The insoluble fibers principally protect you against bowel problems and also help control blood sugar and fat.

How does fiber work? Simply stated, it reduces sugar and fat in the bloodstream by slowing absorption. Normally, the small intestine absorbs fat, cholesterol, and bile. But both soluble and insoluble fibers trap much of these substances and carry them beyond the small intestine, so less is absorbed. The fiber and the trapped chemicals then pass out of the body.

With less fat, cholesterol, and bile, less fatty material is floating in the blood. And that, researchers say, could protect against heart attack and stroke by preventing cholesterol from clogging your arteries.

With sugar absorption, the principle is a bit different. If, for example, a diabetic eats an apple instead of apple juice, the pectin in the fruit will form a jelly with water in the stomach and tie up the apple sugar. The ball of jelly moves more slowly into the small intestine, so the diabetic doesn't get the sudden shot of sugar in his bloodstream.

Dr. Anderson says that plenty of both kinds of fiber in his prescribed diet has eliminated the insulin injections for two thirds of patients who developed diabetes late in life. For those who had diabetes since childhood, the diet cuts back insulin dosage by 25 percent, a welcome relief. Dr. Anderson also has reduced his patients' blood cholesterol by 25 percent over several months. Such a reduction for the average man, he says, could cut his risk of heart attack by half.

Fiber also moves body wastes more rapidly through the lower bowel. This confers two benefits. First, it is believed that bacteria in your gut can turn undigested fats into cancer-causing chemicals. If the undigested material speeds through the body, the bacteria have less time to do their chemical dirty work. Second, as the undigested food moves rapidly through, it is not in contact with the walls of the gut long enough to allow the cancer-causing chemicals to change normal cells into cancer.

"As you eat more fiber," says Dr. Peter Van Soest, a fiber researcher from Cornell University, "you grow more bacteria in your gut. Those are young germs, and they may bind everything, including cancer-causing chemicals and take them away from the lining of the intestines."

Helena LeBow found relief for her irritable bowel from fiber. Before, with little or no fiber in her diet, waste became hard and pressed against her strained gut, irritating it. But as she ate more fiber, wastes remained soft and moved quickly through her bowel.

"I have had this condition since I was 22," she says. "The pain is awful. I was told I had a spastic colon; I had four GI [gastrointestinal] series; I took all kinds of drugs; I eliminated foods from my diet, including wheat and milk products. Nothing helped."

She finally saw Dr. Charles Gerson, a gastroenterologist at Mount Sinai Medical Center in Manhattan, who prescribed a high-fiber diet. In a week, she felt better.

Dr. Gerson says that most gastroenterologists now treat irritable bowels with fiber. Fiber also helps a related ailment called diverticulosis, in which small pouches form in the large bowel. A high-fiber diet relieves chronic constipation.

As for appendicitis, hiatus hernia, and varicose veins, verdicts are not yet in. More research is needed.

If you join the fiber revolution, you also may expect to lose weight. Studies show that people on high-fiber diets tend to eat fewer calories—despite the large carbohydrate intake—because bulk makes them feel fuller, so they eat less.

Drawbacks? You may have more intestinal gas. And mineral deficiency is possible because fiber clutches onto metals such as iron, carrying them out of the body. But no doctor has reported this symptom in people who get fiber from whole foods.

So get your fiber from whole foods—and beware of refined wood, straw, and paper products sold as fiber fillers in foodstuffs. Processed bran and fibers also may lack vitamins and minerals. In fact, it's hard to tell whether a food that's been processed really has the amount and kind of fiber you want. Until standards are set, the best thing to do is to buy foods that are chewy—like whole-grain bread.

There's a long way to go. Much more has to be known about the fiber content of food and its impact on your body. But the fiber revolution has started.

Plastic Surgery

Can Changing Your Looks Change Your Life?

WHEN YOU LOOK IN THE MIRROR, DO YOU LIKE what you see? Too many facial wrinkles? A scar across your cheek? Pits left over from adolescent acne? Not enough hair on you head? Nose too big? Bags under your eyes? Belly hanging out? Thighs jiggling with fat?

Two million Americans each year grow tired of what their mirrors tell them. So they turn to plastic surgeons for an artistic resculpting of what nature, careless living, or accident has misformed. Most women and a growing number of men are no longer self-conscious about going for a "nose job" or a tummy tuck or having their face reshaped. Nor do they worry about spending anywhere from $2,000 to $30,000 for the repair job. American plastic surgery is now a $4 billion-a-year industry.

"I love being a grandmother," says Ila Miles, a homemaker from Tucson, Arizona. "But I don't want to look like one." Mrs. Miles spent $5,800 on nose surgery and a complete facelift.

For Timothy Rothrock, 20, a student from Lock Haven, Pennsylvania, plastic surgery totally restored his face after he was trapped in a forest fire. The worst damage, however, was to his neck: he had lost the contour—the curve from his chin line to his neck. Ugly raised scars marked the skin.

Ten operations were required to stretch, lift, and reshape Mr. Rothrock's skin back to normal. "A few people still stare, and kids can be bothersome," he says. "But now the scars are not quite as noticeable."

For people whose faces are their fortunes, plastic surgery is strictly business. The roster of those who have had "repairs" reads like the guest list at a big Hollywood bash: Carol Burnett (chin augmentation), Frank Sinatra (hair transplant), Michael Jackson and Peter O'Toole (noses reshaped), Lana Turner and Phyllis Diller (facelifts), Mariel Hemingway (breast augmentation), and Eileen Brennan (face repair after a car accident).

"I feel blessed," says Ms. Brennan, now the star of a new ABC-TV series, *Off the Rack*. "Every bone was broken in the left side of my face. I didn't think I'd ever appear before a camera again."

With the increasing demand for reshaping faces and bodies have come spectacular improvements in plastic surgery, making it safer and more daring than ever before. In addition to the facelift, which achieves only surface changes, plastic surgeons today can actually modify the bone structure below the skin through facial sculpting. New methods and materials for chin augmentation and reduction can create facial symmetry where it was lacking (as in Carol Burnett's case). Techniques for eyelifts and nose surgery have been improved, so that the end result is a less "done," less artificial look.

Along with common cosmetic repairs, the list of human sculptings now includes replacement of limbs, fingers, and hair torn from their anchors by accident; remolding to normal the faces of infants born with gargoylesque features; and redesigning noses, eyes, ears, chins, hairlines, and more to satisfy the patient's deep emotional needs.

The rush to reshape nature's work signals a fundamental change in the American outlook, says Dr. William W. Shaw, chief of plastic surgery at Bellevue Hospital in New York City. "Before the 20th century, people struggled to survive epidemics and famine," he explains. "Medicine then turned its attention to chronic diseases like cancer, heart ailments—and to death. People now want to do something for themselves against aches, pains, and deformity."

The Emotional Edge

How do you know you need plastic surgery? First, consider the distinction between reconstructive and cosmetic surgery. Some cases are clearly necessary, such as a baby born with a misshapen head or a cleft palate. Or when an accident breaks the bones of a girl's face and gouges out a chunk of flesh, leaving a deep hollow. Such victims often suffer social ostracism that warps their self-esteem.

Similarly, the psychological impact of losing a breast to cancer only now is being appreciated by doctors. Women who have had mastectomies overwhelmingly talk of losing their sense of being a woman and their sexual drive, of feeling somehow ashamed. Having the breast rebuilt by surgeons has made it easier for many of these women to cope.

Peggy Palmer, a former junior high school teacher from Tucson, at first did not want a breast reconstruction because, she says, "I had to deal with the shock of having cancer." But the prosthesis proved uncomfortable. Now, with her breast reconstructed, she wears a bathing suit with a plunging neckline. "I am so pleased," she says.

And the latest development: In some cases, doctors start breast reconstruction during the surgery that removes the organ. The surgeon leaves the nipple and enough skin and muscle so that it is easier to add either tissue or plastic implants. Any woman facing a mastectomy should ask her doctor about this.

The Vanity Factor

The quest for beauty through cosmetic surgery is fraught with psychological danger. Some plastic surgeons, therefore, send patients for a psychiatric evaluation to weed out those who seek a new life through cosmetic changes. "We may improve patients' lives," says Dr. Linton A. Whitaker, a professor of plastic surgery at the University of Pennsylvania School of Medicine. "But we usually cannot make their lives entirely different."

All plastic surgeons agree: If you decide to change a nose, your eyelids, breasts, or hairline, you must be realistic about what plastic surgery can and cannot do for you. If you tend to be sullen and mean, having your flapping ears pinned back by a plastic surgeon will not transform you into a happy person.

Microsurgery

By far, microsurgery is the most exciting new technique in plastic surgery. Working through a microscope, the surgeon operates with tiny instruments and sutures (threads). Thus, the surgeon can sew together tiny blood vessels, nerves, tendons, and ligaments.

In less than a decade, microsurgery has profoundly altered both reconstructive and cosmetic surgery. Before, surgeons often could not restore circulation or nerve connections in injured or detached body parts. Today, they successfully reattach hands, legs, and other parts severed by accident.

Microsurgery also enables the surgeon to transplant large blocks of skin, muscle, or bone from one area to another. By reconnecting the nerve and blood supply in the new location, the surgeon ensures that the transplanted tissue will survive.

Outpatient Repairs

As the costs of hospitalization mount daily, many doctors have established suites for cosmetic surgery in their own offices. They can save the patient up to $2,000—a considerable sum, because almost no cosmetic surgery is covered by hospital insurance. The American Society of Plastic and Reconstructive Surgeons inspects these suites and approves them. Going to one that's unapproved may be risky.

Responding to escalating demand, plastic surgery "factories" have sprung up across the nation, advertising in newspapers and on TV that you can be beautiful at low cost. Many of the doctors working at such places have not been fully trained to do the delicate operations. Remember: A licensed M.D. is not necessarily trained to perform plastic surgery.

So check that the doctor has been qualified by the American Board of Plastic Surgery. Also, does he or she regularly perform the procedure you desire? If the answer to both questions is yes, then you can allow the surgeon to remake that part of your body.

What Plastic Surgery Can Do For You

• Facelift. The surgeon stretches out wrinkles and sagging skin by lifting up and pulling back the skin of the face. Many doctors also tighten the underlying tissue. (This combination technique lasts 7 to 10 years, rather than the usual 5 to 7 years.) A facelift achieves only surface changes.

• Facial sculpting. By adding plastic material or natural bone—or taking bone away from the jaw, brow or, cheek—surgeons can actually change the shape of the face below the skin. Such facial contouring often is accompanied by dental reconstruction and nose reshaping, or even surgery of the eyes and ears. The total cost for reshaping can go as high as $18,000 including hospitalization, anesthesia, and the surgeon's fee.

• Nose reshaping. The doctor removes humps on the bridge of the nose, makes the tip thinner, or lifts the tip of the nose.

• Eye surgery. The surgeon reduces the bags under the eyes or the sagging puffiness on the upper lid.

• Hair transplant. Tufts of hair with skin attached are transferred from one part of the scalp to another to provide greater hair density in visible areas.

• Ear reshaping. Ears that stand out can be "pinned back." And new methods of taking cartilage from the ribs and carving it into ear shapes provide ears for victims of birth defects, accidents, and disease.

• Brow lift. This procedure raises the eyebrows and reduces brow wrinkles by adjusting the brow muscles and pulling the brow up.

• Skin repair. Small wrinkles and discolorations can be removed with a chemical peel, in which a chemical is applied that destroys the upper layer of skin and allows new skin to grow in its place. Dermabrasion, another technique, is often used to treat acne scars. The doctor applies a high-speed rotating steel brush to the skin to remove the upper layer.

• Breast augmentation. The surgeon opens the skin of the breast and inserts a bag of silicone gel or saline solution. But scar tissue often forms around these implants so that, in a few months, the breast becomes as hard as a rock.

Dr. Steven Herman of New York City has used a new implant called the Même made of polyurethane, a plastic with tiny pores, and a special "furry" surface to prevent the formation of scar tissue. He reports that 265 patients have suffered no hardening of the breasts.

However, many physicians began to report that some of the implants containing liquid silicone were leaking into the breast tissue. They said that they found many women with leaking implants were showing symptoms like arthritis. The silicone, they said, was inducing autoimmune disease. These charges were followed by massive lawsuits. The manufacturer dropped the product from its inventory. Many of the lawsuits remain unsettled.

Dr. Dicran Goulian, chairman of the plastic surgery division at New York Hospital-Cornell Medical Center, says all implants have the potential to harden.

• Breast lift. Sagging breasts are raised by tightening the skin above them.

• Breast reduction. The surgeon removes inner glandular tissue to reduce breast size.

• Tummy tuck. Skin and fat from the lower abdomen are removed, and the muscle is tightened to reduce the bulge.

• Fat suction. The doctor removes fat from the neck, legs, arms, belly, and elsewhere by placing a narrow metal tube under the skin and applying a vacuum. The suction pulls fat loose. Many plastic surgeons swear by this method, which is called *suction lipectomy*. But critics warn that the method is painful and can numb nerves and tear blood vessels, leaving permanent disabilities and scars. The counterargument is that any well-trained plastic surgeon can perform the repair without harming the patient.

• Wrinkle injections. In 1981, the Food and Drug Administration approved injections of collagen, a gummy protein substance extracted from cowhide, to get rid of acne scars, wrinkles, and other early signs of aging. The collagen raises the skin so that the furrow disappears. Almost immediately, a controversy arose. Some scientists maintained that the cowhide could produce an allergic reaction and aggravate arthritic conditions. And they said the body gradually absorbs the collagen and the wrinkle reappears.

Many dermatologists continue to inject small amounts of silicone into the body for the same effect, even though the FDA has never approved the substance. These doctors say that silicone is safe in small amounts and that, since the body does not absorb the chemical, the wrinkle treatment is permanent.

• Reconstructive surgery. This includes everything from resetting broken facial bones, to rebuilding and restoring breasts destroyed by cancer, to re-creating a new face for a child born with horrible deformities. The surgery usually involves several complex operations to reshape bone, muscle, skin.

The Total Picture

These figures, from the American Society of Plastic and Reconstructive Surgeons, include only operations performed by the society's members, who comprise 98 percent of all board-certified plastic surgeons. They do not include plastic surgery by dermatologists, oral surgeons, and other nonmembers—at least 500,000 additional operations annually.

The prices quoted are for surgeons' fees only (which amounted to $2 billion last year). Not included are hospital and operating room costs, anesthesia, and special nursing. These expenses often equal the surgeon's fee, so that the total cost of plastic surgery is closer to $4 billion a year.

Number of Operations*	Type of Operation	Surgeon's Fee
160,000	Hand	$300–$3,000
150,000	Laceration	$150–$2,000
100,000	Tumor removal	$200–$2,000
75,000	Breast augmentation	$1,500–$3,000
70,000	Industrial injury	$200–$2,000
57,000	Eyelid surgery	$1,500–$2,000
55,000	Nose surgery	$1,500–$2,000
45,000	Burn repair	$500–$1,000
45,000	Reconstruction	$500–$2,000
40,000	Facelift	$2,000–$5,000
35,000	Facial fracture	$1,000–$3,000
35,000	Breast reduction	$3,000–$5,000
25,000	Dog-bite repair	$200–$1,000
22,000	Breast reconstruction	$3,000–$7,500
17,000	Skin smoothing	$500–$2,000
17,000	Cleft lip and palate	$750–$1,500
15,000	Tummy tuck	$2,000–$3,500
14,000	Microsurgery	$1,000–$4,000
13,000	Breast lift	$2,000–$3,000
12,000	Ear reshaping	$800–$1,000

*Based on 15 percent increase over 1981 totals.

For information about plastic surgery or a referral, call the American Society of Plastic and Reconstructive Surgeons (800) 635-0635.

Another group specializes in plastic surgery of the face, head, and neck. For free brochures, send a self-addressed, stamped envelope to the American Academy of Facial Plastic and Reconstructive Surgery, Box PA, Suite 304, 1110 Vermont Ave., NW, Washington, D.C. 20005.

How Doctors Can Save Your Skin

THE MEDICAL NEWS ABOUT OUR SKIN AND hair, the most visible of our attributes, is good. Now, more than ever, medical science can reverse ugly disruptions of our skin and help us display a smooth, healthy complexion and a clean, thick head of hair.

Although dermatologists (skin doctors) cannot cure every skin affliction or grow a mop on a bald pate, they probably can do more for their patients than any other medical specialist.

Says a friend of mine, Dr. J. E. Jelinek, clinical professor of dermatology at New York University Medical Center, "Today we have deep knowledge about the skin and powerful techniques to clear up infections and imperfections. And the skin is on the outside—we can get to it."

The skin, the largest organ of your body, weighs about 6 pounds and covers an area of about 20 square feet. It guards your internal organs against invading germs and regulates your temperature by sweating and cooling. The skin also makes vitamins, hormones, and lubricants, and it stores energy.

When skin and hair are victims of the environment—sun, wind, germs, chemicals—dermatologists can offer the following help:

- Protect against cancer of the skin.
- Clear up acne in almost all cases.
- Block invasions of germs and fungus.
- Stop psoriasis, eczema, and dermatitis.
- Smooth out scars, pits, and wrinkles.
- Treat disease *through* the skin.
- Transplant hair to cover baldness.
- Grow some new hair on your head (not a lot).

The UV Gremlins Inside

Dermatologists see excessive tanning as Public Enemy Number 1 because it mars the skin with premature wrinkles, blotches, bloated blood vessels, and freckles. Worse, it can lead to cancer. Intense sunlight containing ultraviolet light penetrates deep inside your skin cells.

Thanks to a doctor's quick action, Jane Kimbrough, 48, of Dobbs Ferry, New York, sailed past melanoma, or "black cancer." In 1983, her doctor found a black dot on her big toe. Because it was promptly removed, she has less than a 1 percent chance of dying of melanoma in the next 10 years. Left to grow, that cancer kills 50 percent of its victims within 5 years.

"I had a friend who died of melanoma," Ms. Kimbrough says. "I consider myself very fortunate." The fair-skinned actress once worked at tanning but now shuns sun and regularly checks her body. (See "Cancer Check.") Her physician, Dr. Darrell S. Rigel, a dermatologist at New York University Medical Center, estimates that 22,000 Americans developed melanoma last year, and 5,500 died of it.

"The biggest advance is the development of sunscreens," says Dr. Rigel. "A number 15 sunscreen lets in only 1/15th of the rays. If people use such creams, the cancer rate will fall." And, he adds, that includes basal cell cancer (the one that attacked President Reagan's nose) and squamous cell cancer.

Acne Be Gone

Skin doctors also have special praise for Accutane, a derivative of vitamin A. Taken orally, it helps almost miraculously to dry up the great red sores of cystic acne. Dr. Alan Shalita, dermatology professor at the State University of New York Downstate Medical School in Brooklyn, says that, thanks to Accutane, "there is little reason for almost anybody to suffer with acne."

However, doctors reserve Accutane only for the most serious cases. It can cause liver problems, among others. If a woman gets pregnant while taking it, a deformed fetus might result.

Paul Smith, 23, a minister in Little Rock, Arkansas, has had acne since the seventh grade. Red sores covered his face, back, neck, and chest down to his wrists and thighs.

"I felt that my body had played a very dirty trick on me," he says.

Today, Rev. Smith keeps his skin 90 percent clear, thanks to a method devised by Dr. Kenneth L. Flandermeyer, associate clinical professor of dermatology at the University of New Mexico at Albuquerque. Dr. Flandermeyer has written about the method in *Clear Skin* (Little, Brown). Essentially, Dr. Flandermeyer asks patients to apply medicines that dry and peel the skin. Rev. Smith placed himself under Dr. Flandermeyer's supervision in 1980 and saw improvement in weeks. When Accutane became available in 1982, he tried it and found that it worked.

But four of five persons between the ages of 12 and 23 with less terrible forms of acne can fight blackheads, pimples, and sores with nonprescription medicines.

Dr. Shalita notes that over-the-counter drugs often effectively reach into hair follicles to combat germs living there. He contends that germs cause blackheads by turning natural skin oils into fatty acids that block follicle openings. Not all acne responds well to self-treatment. About 25 percent of young Americans must seek a dermatologist's help. "We still don't know why some people get acne and others do not," says Dr. Shalita. (See "Acne Myths and Truths.")

Combating Dermatitis

In another big advance, dermatologists have learned to control allergic skin inflammation, or contact dermatitis. For 14 years, Renate Charbonneau, a hairdresser in Milwaukie, Oregon, suffered unknowingly from chemicals in acid permanent-wave solutions. They caused severe eczema on her hands. Cortisone ointment relieves the pain, she says, adding, "By avoiding the acid perms and hair that has been permed, I can still work. I love my job."

Ms. Charbonneau's physician, Dr. Frances Storrs, professor of dermatology at the Oregon Health Science University at Portland, heads a committee that is studying the ingredients in cosmetics for the American Academy of Dermatology. "Many substances are irritating," says Dr. Storrs, "but allergy happens very, very rarely." Dr. Alexander Fisher, clinical professor of dermatology at New

York University, calls cosmetics far safer than they used to be.

Other Developments in Dermatology

Medical cosmetics are safer too, thanks to today's technology and new research. For example, dermatologists have new cosmetic ways of filling in skin defects and wrinkles. They inject collagen (cowhide protein) into a big wrinkle to puff it up. There is always the danger of an allergic reaction, but less if the skin is tested first. Doctors place chances at fewer than one in 5,000 that anything will go awry.

As to hair loss, in addition to hair transplants, a drug used to treat high blood pressure—Minoxidyl—if applied as a poultice, actually grows hair. Only a third of a group of men who used it had significant hair growth; an additional third had a fine blond fuzz, and the final third experienced no hair growth.

For large purple patches of skin—port wine stain—dermatologists can lighten them with a laser. They also now use powerful hormones to clear up eczema, psoriasis, and dermatitis in days rather than months.

Other help includes these treatments:

• An approach called PUVA clears the patchy, flaky skin of intractable psoriasis. The patient takes the medicine psoralen (P) and then stands naked under ultraviolet (UV) light in the A-band (A) wavelengths. This is reserved only for the worst cases; PUVA can increase your risk of skin cancer.

• The drug Etretinate, a cousin of Accutane, is under investigation here. In Europe, it's used to treat psoriasis.

• Oral drugs treat skin infected by bacteria, viruses, or fungi. Hospitalization once was the rule for patients with cellulitis—a bacterial infection of the skin and its underlayers. Now an antibiotic called cephalsporin effects a cure just days after a doctor's treatment.

• Acyclovir, taken orally or in a salve, eases herpes virus symptoms.

• Ketoconazole, a new antifungus agent taken orally, cures deep fungal infections.

Cancer Check

Find the early signs of melanoma on your own body and save your life. The American Cancer Society has developed a self-exam technique in which you should look for skin moles that have changed in color, size, elevation, surface, sensation, or consistency or whose surrounding skin has changed.

Dr. Darrell S. Rigel, of New York University Medical Center, has an ABCD rule, standing for asymmetry, border, color, and diameter. Melanomas tend to be irregular in shape (asymmetrical), their outlines (borders) are uneven, their colors are a mixture of browns, and their diameters are wider than a pencil eraser.

Seeing your doctor for regular checkups is also important.

Acne: Myths and Truths

Myth: Eating chocolate, other sweets, or greasy foods causes acne.

Truth: Several experiments prove that, generally, food doesn't affect acne.

Myth: If my mother had acne, so will I.

Truth: That could be true. Acne skin conditions might be inherited.

Myth: Putting oil on the skin helps.

Truth: Most oils promote blackheads, acne's first stage.

Myth: Too much or too little sex causes acne.

Truth: Sex has nothing to do with acne.

Myth: Stress causes acne.

Truth: The facts aren't all in. Many doctors believe there is a correlation.

Dental Health

OF THE 40 MILLION AMERICANS WHO HAVE LOST all their teeth, half make do with removable false teeth, and half are pitiable unfortunates unable to bite, chew, or gum any food whose texture is much harder than that of soggy macaroni. Their dental agony now can end.

After decades of work on tooth implantation by scientists here and abroad, you can be given new teeth as good-looking as those that once brightened your youthful smile. Dentists now can screw or tap special metal anchors into the jawbone. The bone grows onto the metal, forming a tight bond. Then the anchors—in the shape of blades, cylinders, or screws—become one piece with the bone and can be used to implant a single artificial tooth or a whole mouthful.

Even better news: Since the cost of the new procedure has been decreasing, dental implantation is becoming available to more and more Americans. Implanting a full mouth of teeth once cost between $20,000 and $40,000—and it still does in several big cities. But residents in many other areas are finding lower prices, often ranging from $3,000 to $10,000, depending on what needs to be done.

"It's the best thing I ever did—the best money I ever spent," says Earl Beer. Mr. Beer, 62, is a salesman and my fellow tennis player in New York. His implantation cost him $13,500. "My whole life has changed," he adds with a big grin.

Mr. Beer also is a gourmet chef who loves food. He remembers suffering the horrors of an upper denture that didn't fit, that slid around his mouth when he tried to eat foods like steak or hard fruits. And he recalls how the false teeth hurt and made him feel bad about himself. Four years ago, he replaced his loose upper dentures with implanted teeth.

"Look," he says, tapping his teeth with a finger. "All new—and solid as a rock. I can eat anything: apples, celery. I don't even know I have them. People say I look good, but they don't know exactly why."

Dr. Dennis Tarnow, head of the Department of Implant Dentistry at New York University in Manhattan, says, "Implantation is one of the most important dental developments of this generation or even of the 20th century. Millions of people will live better."

A healthy tooth is fixed in the jawbone by its root. The jawbone and root are held together by living tissue. If bacteria rots a tooth to the point where the dentist can make no more repairs, the tooth must be extracted. More commonly today, in a mouth that is not given good hygiene, germs attack the gums, disrupting the bonding among tooth, root, and jawbone. The root separates from the bone; the tooth loosens and may fall out. Most people lose teeth through gum disease, not through cavities. Teeth can be replaced by bridges, crowns, dentures, and now implants. Only money—not science or technology—bars the way to tooth implantation for most people.

Dentists down through the ages tried unsuccessfully to substitute animal teeth for human teeth. About 100 years ago, dentists learned how to make porcelain teeth, still popular today. For many, dentures proved their salvation; but for millions, the discomfort and pain of dentures made them a burden.

By the 1960s, dentists were searching for new ways to design false teeth that looked and functioned like real teeth but had no denture-plate problems.

In the early 1960s, Dr. Leonard I. Linkow—sometimes called the "father of implantology" in the United States—developed an implant using an anchor made of titanium, a rare but strong metal. To the anchor, Dr. Linkow found he could affix one tooth or several teeth in a bridge. With more implants, he could replace a whole mouthful. He reported 96 percent success; only four implants in 100 had to be removed because of looseness or infection.

"Before implants came out, dentistry was archaic," Dr. Linkow says. "All that dentists could do with bad teeth was to pull them out." He has performed approximately 15,000 implants.

James Bough, a retired telephone company employee in New York State, was one of Dr. Linkow's patients a dozen years ago. Mr. Bough was then 59. Though he had managed to keep some of his own teeth, he ultimately needed upper and lower dentures. "I couldn't stand the thought of a denture," he recalls. Dr. Linkow fitted him with the special titanium anchors and tooth implants. As Earl Beer found with his new teeth, Mr. Bough's implant allowed him to eat anything. "And it made my smile handsome," says Mr. Bough. "People tell me I have nice teeth."

It's hard to say why, but other American dentists lagged behind. Many had heard horror stories (mostly untrue) about implant failures ending with massive infections of the jawbone. It does happen, but rarely. Antibiotics kill most such infections. Also, the technique demands great skill both in implanting the anchors and in designing the whole system.

Thanks to a Swedish dental scientist, things began to change. In 1962, about the same time as Dr. Linkow's discovery, Dr. Per Ingvar Branemark found that bone actually grows onto the titanium anchor, creating an osseo merger—solid bone. (*Osseo* means bony.) American and Canadian dentists who had not believed Dr. Linkow's claims were moved to check Dr. Branemark's discovery. The implant worked. Dr. Linkow says he feels vindicated.

The American Association of Oral and Maxillofacial Surgeons reports that since 1986, when there was a noticeable change in the number of implants, dentists have performed the procedure on 230,000 patients in the United States. The total seems to be doubling every 3 years.

A German team, headed by Dr. Axel Kirsch of Stuttgart, devised a cylindrical anchor with a plastic ring that acts as a shock absorber. This system leads 30 others now on the market.

Which to choose is up to your needs and your dentist's abilities and diagnosis. Dr. Richard Guaccio, a dentist in Schererville, Indiana, warns, "If your dentist uses only one implant method, get another dentist." Dr. Guaccio is president of the American Board of Oral Implantology/Implant Dentistry.

All the methods generally follow this sequence: First, X rays show whether the jaw can take the anchors. Next, using anesthesia, the dentist cuts the gum and inserts the anchors. In 3 months, they tightly bond to the bone. (The old denture is used until a new one is made.) The dentist then attaches the new teeth securely to the anchors. The gum line covers the bottoms of the false teeth in a natural-looking way. Porcelain caps can achieve color variations like those of natural teeth.

The cost is $1,000 to $1,500 per anchor, $5,000 and up per denture. For both upper and lower dentures, with four anchors in each jaw, the cost would be $16,000 or more. But some dentists—using only two anchors for each jaw—charge just $800 per insertion, plus $3,500 to $4,000 for the dentures. Their low total is about $6,700. Dr. Charles A. Babbush of Mount Sinai Medical Center in Cleveland says he can do a lower jaw for $4,000 to $5,000, with two cylindrical anchors and a clip-on denture.

Barring those with no jawbone or some serious illness, most toothless persons can have successful implants. Very difficult cases require bone transplants with bone taken from the patient's hip. With shrunken or no jawbones, the failure rate is high, especially in the upper jaw.

The experts say age is no drawback. Dr. Al Guckes of the National Institute of Dental Research in Bethesda, Maryland, has been working on children 13 or older.

Despite enthusiasm for implants, insurance does not always cover them, and some dentists still urge caution. However, Dr. Bejan Iranpour, an associate professor in the Department of Clinical Dentistry at the University of Rochester in New York, says, "On balance, the advantages and benefits of implants are far greater than the risks." He adds that the benefits include comfort, the absence of denture problems, better gum hygiene, facial improvements, better chewing ability, and psychological satisfaction.

The big biological problem: lack of jawbone in 10 percent of patients. The search is on for bone stimulators, including hormones. Now being tested is Gore-Tex, a thin cloth found in all-weather sportswear. Small pieces attached to badly thinned jawbone encourage bone growth by blocking other cells from filling in missing spaces in the bone.

Improvements in implantation technique and research are increasing the number of implantations at a dizzying pace. And the prices keep dropping year by year. If you have been struggling with a toothless mouth, your time for tooth implantation may have arrived.

Please consult with your dentist or local dental association for recommendations on qualified implant dentists.

Your Smile Can Last a Lifetime

"NOBODY NEED LOSE ONE TOOTH OR TOLERATE a moment of dental discomfort." So predicts Dr. Burton Press, president of the American Dental Association (ADA). His vision of the future relies on amazing advances in dental science over the last 10 years. They could turn us into a nation whose smiles of decay-free teeth may last a lifetime.

Even now in the United States, 36 percent of all children aged 5 through 17 have never had a cavity, thanks to fluoride in toothpastes, mouthwashes, and public water supplies. In areas with fluoridated drinking water, children's cavities dropped 40 percent.

How Fluoride Works

Fluoride stops decay by working at the tooth's surface in two ways:

1. It disrupts the reproduction of *Streptococcus mutans*, the most powerful of many acid-making bacteria in the mouth. This microbe eats the sugars and starches in your mouth and turns them into enamel-burning acid. *Streptococcus mutans* also creates plaque, the gummy substance that sticks to the teeth to build a breeding ground for more bacteria.
2. Fluoride allows the acid-scarred tooth surface to heal. In the presence of fluoride, calcium and phosphorus (both part of your saliva) fill in the microscopic pits dug out by the acid. Without fluoride, the pits get wider and deeper, and the bacteria penetrate farther into the enamel.

"Fluoride proved to us that dental disease is preventable," says Dr. Press, "so now we're going for prevention."

Rinses and Washes

In the battle against decay, scientists now explore new ways to deliver fluoride to the teeth. (Many groups believe that fluoride may cause illness, but the dental community at large rejects this idea.) At the Eastman Dental Center in Rochester, New York, and at the University of Iowa, scientists have developed a mouth rinse containing fluoride, calcium, and phosphorus. While the fluoride fights bacteria, the calcium and phosphorus rebuild the enamel where the germs have drilled microscopic holes.

Some scientists want to kill germs directly with a chlorhexidine mouthwash. While most mouthwashes do not kill decay bacteria, chlorhexidine does. The chemical even gets under the gums to attack the microbes. Europeans can buy such a mouthwash; American scientists are still testing it for safety.

Vaccines

Scientists are also trying to turn on the body's own decay-fighting power. You swallow a pill that contains *Streptococcus mutans,* the chief tooth-destroying germ. The capsule passes unchanged into the small intestine, where the germs are released.

There, the body's infection-fighting white blood cells develop antibodies to battle the bacteria. The white cells then migrate to the salivary glands in your mouth and release the antibodies that attack *Streptococcus mutans* hiding among the teeth.

At the University of Alabama, scientists have tried such a vaccine on human volunteers. The vaccine did create antibodies in the mouth, but the researchers have yet to prove it stops cavities.

At the Forsyth Dental Center in Boston, scientists have gone one step further. Instead of using the whole *mutans* gene, they extracted the enzyme from the germ and put that in a pill. Animal trials there proved that the body can make antibodies to the enzyme alone. The antibodies interfere with the gum's ability to make acid and to stick to the teeth.

Sealants

As I first reported in *Parade* ("New Teeth That Really Look Real," July 3, 1983), dentists have also developed a clear plastic bonding resin to prevent decay bacteria from invading crevices in the biting surfaces of the teeth. Considered highly effective, the sealant can reduce children's cavities in those surfaces by 80 percent. (It does not, however, protect the sides of the teeth.) The method, called bonding, is just beginning to spread in the dental community.

In another experimental technique, the dentist bonds to the teeth a resin drenched in fluoride. Night and day, the mineral drains into the mouth, bathing the side enamel while the sealant protects the biting surfaces.

Effects of Food

New and surprising findings about the effects of food on teeth can give you and your children a chance to help in the battle against decay.

For example, Dr. Stephen Moss, professor of pediatric dentistry at New York University Dental School, says, "We used to talk about 'good' foods and 'bad' foods. Sugar was bad; an apple was good. We're now learning that it's not so much what you eat or how much but how often."

Research reveals that every time you eat, *Streptococcus mutans* and other bacteria start their 20-minute acid-producing cycle. So if you snack more than three or four times a day in addition to your regular meals, you are putting your teeth in danger. It doesn't matter whether you eat something with 2 percent sugar or 10 percent sugar. A snack could be anything from a piece of fruit to soda pop to a full meal. And when you drink 10 cans of sugary soda, you are snacking 10 times a day, and the bacteria are producing acid for at least 3 hours. Anything that hangs around the mouth longer than soda—and most things do—stimulates the germs to activity over a longer period.

In a surprising finding, Dr. Juan Navia of the University of Alabama showed that, in rats, crackers and wheat flakes cause more cavities than chocolate or caramels. Why? Because breadstuffs stay in the mouth longer than candy. Experiments at the University of Minnesota, at the Eastman Dental Center, and in Sweden confirmed these results in human teeth.

Dr. Moss showed me a 5-year-old child whose teeth had all rotted down to little points. The mother had allowed the boy to suck on a milk-filled bottle all day long. The constant bathing of the teeth with milk sugar gave the germs a field day.

Dr. Moss warns mothers, "Don't use the milk bottle as a pacifier," adding, "A mother who feeds a child honey, raisins, or bananas with the idea of avoiding sugar is making her child worse off than with candy, which isn't such a good idea in the first place."

Gum Disease

Despite the progress against decay, dentists have had less success against gum disease—periodontitis—which causes more tooth loss by far than caries, or decay. Again, bacteria are the villains, but dentists don't know exactly which ones.

They do know that plaque forms a haven for those bacteria under the gums. There, they attack not only the enamel but also the gums and the jawbone. Eventually, abscesses develop, the jawbone thins, teeth loosen and fall out.

You can prevent gum disease only with careful teeth cleaning with a brush and dental floss added to a once-a-year cleaning by a dentist or dental hygienist. These professionals push their scraping instruments under the gum to remove the hidden plaque.

Once you have an extensive gum infection, only a dentist can pull you out of it. Sometimes it takes surgery. The dentist, or a gum specialist called a periodontist, opens up the gum to remove the plaque and infections by sight.

Now there is controversy over a gum treatment developed by Dr. Paul Keyes, who formerly worked at the National Institute for Dental Research. Dr. Keyes tries to eliminate the bacteria of gum disease. First, he scrapes the teeth to remove plaque. Then he treats the tooth surfaces with germ-killing chemicals. He trains the patients to clean teeth with bicarbonate of soda, plain salt, and peroxide in a pulsating irrigating device.

Critics maintain that such self-help treatment can mask symptoms while the hidden infection rages. Patients may not realize that they have gum disease until their teeth fall out.

Artificial Bones

As teeth fall out, the jawbone shrinks. False teeth often lose their grip, which makes it hard for the wearer to chew. For many, dentures inflict pain and discomfort.

"I was a mess," says Joe Lesser, a retired milliner in New York City whose dentures didn't fit well at all.

Dr. Arthur Ashman of New York implanted in Mr. Lesser's jaws an artificial bone made of plastic particles called hard tissue replacement (HTR). In the months that followed, Mr. Lesser's own bone cells infiltrated the plastic and created real bone. Dr. Ashman, one of HTR's inventors, also stuffs it into the sockets of lost teeth to prevent future bone shrinkage.

Specialists insert two other materials—tricalcium phosphate and hydroxyapatite—to help build up jawbones, or else they implant metal strips under the gum to lock dentures tightly to the jawbone.

Experts disagree on the value and safety of these implants, although many patients swear by them.

As Dr. Press predicted for the future of dentistry, no one—not even those who lose a tooth—need suffer a moment of discomfort.

New Teeth That Really Look Real

IN ALLENTOWN, PENNSYLVANIA, 9-YEAR-OLD Michael Kline fell off his bike, grinding his face into the pavement like a basketball. The impact tore out his upper right front tooth (the lateral incisor) from his mouth, split the left incisor in half, and cracked two other teeth.

"I didn't want to go to school," Michael says. "I thought the other kids would make fun of me."

Today, you cannot tell that an accident had wrecked Michael's mouth. His patched-up teeth look just as good as his undamaged ones. And his extensive dental work required no needles, no painful drilling or grinding, or any costly porcelain or gold crowns.

Instead, Michael's dentist, Dr. Jerome Kaplan, used a technique called bonding to repair the boy's split, cracked teeth and to replace the knocked-out tooth (which was retrieved by an alert neighbor) in Michael's mouth.

Taking advantage of growing plastics science over the last two decades, dentists across the nation have enthusiastically latched on to bonding to restore broken, chipped, discolored or widely spaced teeth. They fuse (or "bond") a synthetic compound called bonding resin to the surface of the tooth, or whatever is left of it.

Because the resin transmits and reflects light more like enamel (some say better than porcelain caps), the dentist can match the chemical almost flawlessly to your own tooth enamel. The bonded tooth simply looks more natural—hence Michael's picture-perfect smile. Dentists are also using the resin as an adhesive to bond bridges in place, and orthodontists have found that bonded brackets make for less conspicuous braces. (No more "metal mouths" or "railroad tracks," as kids used to say.)

However it is used, bonding is quicker, easier, less painful, and cheaper than conventional methods, and treatment requires fewer office visits than conventional dentistry.

Bonding is relatively simple. To rebuild Michael's cracked teeth, Dr. Kaplan first washed them with a weak acid solution to etch microscopic pits in the surface of the enamel. (This process is called acid etching.) Next, he fitted little plastic hoods over each tooth corner and squirted the bonding resin under the hoods. When the liquid resin flowed over the pitted enamel, the fluid filled the holes and adhered to the surface, taking the shape of the tooth. To harden the resin, Dr. Kaplan blasted it with a ray of ultraviolet light for 20 seconds. Then he shaped and polished each tooth, much like an artist sculpting a creative work.

To anchor the knocked-out tooth back into Michael's jaw, Dr. Kaplan bonded it to the adjoining tooth with bonding resin.

Bonding technology is not limited to cosmetic dentistry. Researchers are looking into bonding as a cavity preventive and as a possible alternative to silver fillings and gold inlays.

The late Dr. Michael Buonocore of the Eastman Dental Center in Rochester, New York, who developed the acid etching technique, used bonding to seal children's teeth against decay. In one year-long test he found that such sealing reduced decay and cavities by 90 percent.

"After 8 years [of tests], we still get a 60 percent reduction in cavities on the biting surface," says Dr. Zia Shey of the University of Medicine and Dentistry of New Jersey, who is conducting similar tests.

Dr. Shey etches and paints the biting surface of the 16 molars, where most cavities occur. Fluoride applied to the teeth or in drinking water protects the other tooth surfaces, he says. Together, dental bonding and fluoride can almost eliminate caries or cavities.

Drs. Stanley Handelman and Dennis Leverett of the Eastman Dental Center tested bonding as a treatment for small cavities. They found that when the cavity hole was sealed, the bacteria that made the hole were trapped inside. Deprived of oxygen and nourishment, the bacteria died.

"There's no question that dental bonding is absolutely revolutionary," says Dr. Leverett. "In essence, we can repair cavities without drilling and filling."

Ruth Whittemore, a 66-year-old widow from Baltimore, Maryland, is the happy recipient of another of this new technology's advances—false teeth that are held in place by bonding.

The apparatus is called the Maryland bridge because it was developed at the University of Maryland Dental School by Drs. Gus Livaditis and Van Thompson. Dr. Thompson also devised a way to etch metal so that it can be bonded to tooth enamel. Mrs. Whittemore's bridge has metal wings attached to a porcelain tooth. Her dentist bonded those wings to her adjacent teeth. In one painless visit, the bridge was done.

Under the conventional method, the dentist grinds down the patient's healthy adjoining teeth into flat-topped pyramids and pins porcelain caps or crowns over them. Then the dentist wires a metal band with the false tooth to the caps. In addition, the dentist often kills the nerves of the healthy teeth with root canals. The process is usually painful and requires several fittings and visits.

"I have one of the old bridges in my mouth, and I can taste the metal and feel the edge of the caps with my tongue," says Mrs. Whittemore, who now has three Maryland bridges. "I cannot tell that I have the Maryland bridges. They feel like my own teeth. And people tell me that I look much better these days, but they don't know why. It's because the new teeth look like teeth."

Bonding is also the preferred treatment for people who were born with badly discolored or pitted teeth or who developed them from antibiotics they were given as children.

A dentist has three ways to restore such unsightly teeth quickly, without grinding or damaging them further. He or she can cover up the discoloration by bonding veneers of plastic (which look like false fingernails) to the patient's teeth. Or the dentist can paint the resin directly onto the etched tooth, changing the color while painting to get just the right shade, much as a manicurist applies nail polish. Or the dentist can employ the method that Dr. Kaplan used on Michael Kline, putting a hood over the tooth and filling the space between the hood and the etched tooth with resin.

Children and adults who shy away from the shiny metal "railroad tracks" of conventional braces now can request "invisible braces." The orthodontist bonds a clear, and therefore hardly noticeable, small square resin bracket to the front of the tooth. Then the restraining wire is run through the bracket.

Patricia Ritsen, 30, of Verona, New Jersey, developed a bad overbite on the right side because a tooth that she lost at 11 was never replaced.

"I was sitting in the dentist's office," she says, "and I saw another woman smiling. I didn't realize that she was wearing braces. And when I found out, I said, 'I want that.' Nobody can tell I'm wearing braces, either."

Despite such testimonials, dentists agree that bonding has its drawbacks. Bonded teeth are not as strong as crowns, and they may crack, chip, and stain. Heavy users of coffee, tea, tobacco, and curry, for example, may find it necessary to have the teeth polished every 3 months or to replace them after 3 or 4 years. And some people who have had the veneers pasted over their teeth complain of gum irritation.

Dr. Robert Binder, chairman of orthodontics at the University of Medicine and Dentistry of New Jersey, treated Ms. Ritsen. He warns that the bonded surface can bend and sometimes come off, although he says that he has not had much trouble with bonded brackets.

Says Dr. Thompson, "Bonding is not a panacea. It is for selected patients who have good, sound adjacent teeth and good, sound enamel on their teeth."

Whatever the drawbacks, bonding has roared through dentistry. Dentists, normally conservative in adopting new materials, have had to change their practices in the last few years because patients are demanding bonding treatments. True, a lot is still unknown and untested. But bonding is making a big difference, for better, and better looking, teeth.

Brush That Plaque Away

NOW THAT FLUORIDE IN TOOTHPASTE AND drinking water have cut dramatically the threat of tooth decay, dentistry is concentrating mightily on conquering plaque, the sticky film that forms on your teeth. Unless you clean off plaque regularly, it can trap harmful germs that can cause tooth decay and gum disease. In the extreme, diseased gums can loosen your teeth so that eventually they fall out.

Your weapons against plaque include toothbrushes, toothpaste, dental floss, toothpicks, and plaque-fighting mouth rinses.

"With these," says Dr. Stephen Moss, head of pediatric dentistry at the New York University College of Dentistry, "we are winning the war against plaque."

To make the plaque killers work, you have to use them correctly. Most people don't even correctly use the best weapon against plaque—the toothbrush.

"You need to brush your teeth at least one full minute," says Karen Baker, assistant professor at the Colleges of Dentistry and Pharmacy at the University of Iowa. "Most people brush for only 30 seconds."

How you can wage the war on plaque:

- Brush with soft bristles at least 60 seconds at least once a day (each time you eat is better).
- Use a toothpaste containing fluoride.
- Clean between the teeth and gums with waxed or unwaxed dental floss. Or use a Stim-U-Dent toothpick.
- At least twice a year, have your dentist or dental hygienist scrape the surfaces of your teeth to remove built-up plaque and tartar, especially under the gums.
- Limit daily meals and snacks to three each.
- Rinse with a mouthwash containing germ killers that control plaque.

Your saliva contains a substance that coats your teeth. The plaque-forming bacteria attach themselves to that coating. After you eat anything, the plaque-making process starts again.

Dr. Sebastian G. Ciancio, clinical professor and chairperson of periodontology at the State University of New York at Buffalo, notes that 24 hours after you clean your teeth, plaque has grown again. He urges that you brush and floss at least every 12 hours.

Your saliva adds calcium to plaque, which hardens into tartar. The bacteria also produce acid that causes cavities. Fluoride slows the acid production and toughens the teeth against cavities.

When the plaque invades the spaces between teeth and gums, it allows other bacteria to attack the gums, infecting and inflaming them. Once this happens, you have gingivitis—inflammation of the gingiva, the gums.

"Almost everyone has some gingivitis," says Dr. Alan Polson, chairperson of the department of periodontology at the Eastman Dental Center in Rochester, New York. The center developed a simple test using the Stim-U-Dent toothpick for cleaning plaque from between teeth and under the gum line. If gums bleed while using it, you have gingivitis.

As gingivitis progresses, pockets of infection form under the gums, which become more inflamed and increasingly shrink away from the teeth. The bacteria then harm the teeth's supporting bones, and the teeth loosen. Surgery may be needed. After age 40, more teeth are lost to gum disease than to cavities.

Dental researchers hope one day to create a vaccine against gum disease. "We are moving closer," says Dr. Robert Genco, chairperson of the Department of Oral Biology of the School of Dental Medicine, State University of New York at Buffalo. "We have found three types of germs responsible for much of gum disease."

Meanwhile, use these tools well:

• Toothbrushes: Whether manual or electric, the brush must be soft, with rounded bristles that won't hurt the gums. Place the brush at a 45-degree angle to the gum line and then jiggle it in a rotary motion. This thorough scrubbing removes plaque. Also clean your tongue with your brush. Interplak, a new electric brush, has rotating bristles that get down between the teeth.

• Toothpastes: Manufacturers of several brands say that they help loosen plaque and tartar. And they probably do. Many have American Dental Association (ADA) acceptance for fighting cavities. All contain fluoride, which fights plaque-forming germs. Many dentists say brushing with a paste of bicarbonate of soda mixed with hydrogen peroxide helps kill germs and plaque formation.

• Mouth rinses: Only two plaque-fighting mouthwashes now have the ADA seal: Peridex, available only by prescription, and Listerine, a 109-year-old, over-the-counter product. Other products are under consideration.

• Irrigators: These devices squirt pulses of water between the teeth and at the gums. None has ADA acceptance for plaque removal, but they do remove large particles of food from between the teeth.

Plaque-Fighting Weapons

The following have ADA acceptance for fighting plaque and gingivitis:

• Manual toothbrushes: Alm, Butler, Colgate, Dental N, Disney, Improve, Lactona, McDonald's, Oral-B, Pepsodent, Pepsodent Plus, Py-Co-Pay Saftex, Py-Co-Twin, Reach, Sensodyne Search.

• Electric toothbrushes: Braun, Broxodent, Interplak, Ratadent, Sears,* Sunbeam, Water Pik, Wong 2000,* Wong Orabrush.

• Hygiene aids: Butler, Dr. Flosser, Johnson & Johnson and Oral-B dental flosses, Stim-U-Dent toothpick.

No toothpaste or gel has ADA acceptance for fighting plaque, but the following accepted products (in paste and gel form) contain fluoride, which fights tooth decay:

• Toothpastes and gels: Regular and Extra-Strength Aim, Aqua Fresh, Aqua Fresh for Kids, Colgate Tartar Control Formula, Colgate with MFP, Crest, Crest Toothpaste for Kids, Crest Tartar Control Formula, Dentaguard, Macleans, Zact HP, Zact Smoker's.

*Provisional acceptance.

Eyes and Ears

Who's Afraid of Hearing Aids?

PRESIDENT REAGAN WORE A HEARING AID, AND he beamed. He seemed to be saying, "I like to hear when folks talk to me."

Not so for the 17 million Americans who need but refuse to get hearing aids—or for the other 4 million or so who have bought hearing aids but won't wear them. Unfortunately, only 4 million people in the United States actually allow themselves to benefit from today's modern hearing devices.

Result: Many of the hard-of-hearing suffer loss of human contact. They miss the punch lines of jokes and must constantly blurt out "What?" Many avoid groups, where mixed noises blur the speech they want to hear.

Jane Madell is director of audiology at the New York League for the Hard of Hearing, a clinic in Manhattan. She is an expert at detecting hearing loss, analyzing what's wrong with patients' hearing and fitting them with the right hearing aids. "Many who develop a hearing loss do nothing about it," she says. "They don't realize that the longer you go with this loss uncorrected, the more difficult it is to correct."

Dr. James B. Snow, Jr., head of the National Institute on Deafness and Other Communication Disorders in Bethesda, Maryland, says, "Hearing aids have been greatly improved and miniaturized and can help nearly all who have lost hearing."

George M. Hoherz, 73, of Traer, Iowa, waited two decades before finally seeking help for his hearing. "Before I got the hearing aids this year," he says, "I kept turning up the volume on the TV. Now, my wife asks me to turn it up."

Why did he wait so long to get help? "I probably didn't realize what I was missing," Mr. Hoherz confesses. "It was not for vanity."

Sadly, vanity is the reason many Americans don't seek help for their hearing loss. They equate hearing aids with age and infirmity.

In Washington, D.C., Professor Sam Trychin heads the Living with Hearing Loss program at Gallaudet University for the Deaf, in Washington, D.C. His studies have revealed that up to half of those who buy hearing aids don't use them. Some of the reasons: too-great expectations, too-great results (hearing aids provide too many sounds—more than the wearer can sort out), and technical troubles.

"The sounds coming through a hearing aid at first might seem tinny and mechanical," explains Dr. Trychin, a professor of psychology. "Or, after a period of not hearing well, users may find the sounds distracting. Or, because how a hearing aid works is unclear to its wearer, the sounds are inaudible.

"One man said his hearing aid didn't work," he adds, "so I opened it up. When I said, 'Where's the battery?' he actually asked, 'What battery?' Be patient—as you use the device, your ears and brain adapt; the new sound gets more 'normal.'"

For a hearing aid that fits your needs, see a medical doctor or an audiologist. An audiologist has a Ph.D. or a master's degree and has studied how to measure hearing capacity, prescribe and fit a hearing device, and counsel and train patients to make the best use of their hearing.

Hearing aids come in several styles:

• In-the-ear. Good for mild to severe hearing loss. A plastic mold with a microphone and amplifier fits in the ear canal. Tiny switches may be hard to control; molds may feel odd at first.

• Behind-the-ear. Helps mild to severe hearing loss. The microphone and amplifier rest behind the ear in a small packet. A plastic tube conducts treated sound waves into molds shaped to fit in the ear canal. Also look for devices with behind-the-ear pieces designed to fit on the ends of eyeglass frames.

• Body-assist. This kind of hearing aid helps persons with very severe to profound hearing loss. A microphone fits behind the ear; the amplifier package—the size of a deck of cards—is worn about the chest. Magnified sounds are piped into a molded earpiece.

• Cochlear implant. Excitement is high over this thumb-size system that enables many with severe hearing loss to understand sound and speech. A tiny receiver is implanted in the bone behind the ear, and 22 electrodes are inserted into the cochlea, the snail-shaped part of the inner ear. The patient later is fitted with a tiny external microphone that sits behind the ear and is wired to a small box containing a speech processor, which can be worn in one's clothing. The microphone relays sounds to the processor, which changes them into electrical impulses. These impulses are then transmitted to the nerve fibers of the cochlea, which send signals to the brain.

The Food and Drug Administration (FDA) okayed these implants for adults in 1985 and for children in 1990. So far, reportedly with good results, several thousand adults and children have had the implants.

One of those children is Caitlin Parton, now 11, of New York City. Caitlin was deafened by meningitis at age 2, yet I saw her talking with her speech therapist and her mother, Melody Parton, and it was clear that she heard their every word, even when their lips were covered. How?

As part of FDA testing before the operation was approved for other children with hearing loss—Dr. Noel Cohen of New York University Medical Center performed cochlear implant surgery on Caitlin. "Before the operation," says Mrs. Parton, "Caitlin had been losing her vocabulary and getting harder and harder to understand."

When I first met Caitlin, just after the implant, her speech was incomprehensible to me. Now she speaks clearly, goes to school with hearing children, easily learns new words and ideas, and says she loves math!

The implants do best for patients who had some speech before an accident or a disease destroyed their hearing, but they also have helped improve speech for those who were born deaf.

Since quick detection and treatment net the best results, Dr. Maurice Miller, chief of audiology at Lenox Hill Hospital in Manhattan, urges the testing of newborns. "The most rapid development of language and speech is in the first 2 years of life," he says. "A child not stimulated by sound before age 2 has lost the opportunity to communicate with other humans by speech."

The current theory explains what happens to the brain of a baby as it struggles to learn the meaning of the sounds coming into the brain. An infant is born with 100 billion nerves (neurons) in the brain. One of the great insights, first suggested by linguist Noam Chomsky, was that the infant is born with a tangle of neurons able to decipher meaning in any language. Exposed to English, the child learns English; to Chinese, Chinese; and so forth for the hundreds of languages on this planet. The brain is capable but not able until the exposure. In the process of learning, the child's brain selects the neurons that most efficiently interpret the mother tongue. Those neurons survive; neurons unstimulated by the native language die.

A deaf child's neurons are poorly tweaked if at all. There are no efficient channels left even though after the critical age—infancy to age 5—the child miraculously regains use of the ear. The brain, deprived of that early excitation, no longer has enough neurons to learn the sound and meaning of speech.

It is wise to have hearing checked at the first hint of trouble and wise to protect it, too. New evidence strongly suggests that permanent hearing damage is produced by very loud music—especially from boom boxes, powerfully amplified car radios, and high-decibel rock concerts. Some rock musicians have lost much of their hearing, and at least one rock fan has initiated a lawsuit against a music group for hearing loss.

Research shows that loud noises injure the fine hair cells inside the cochlea, which are stimulated by vibrations to send nerve impulses to the brain. The good news: In other species, the damaged cells, if left to rest, can regenerate themselves. Scientists say the search is on to find natural chemicals that trigger such regeneration in humans and perhaps restore hearing.

One great advance is the production of hearing aids with increased precision in making voices stand out from the background noises. Some other advances on the horizon:

• Computer circuits, now being tested, could be used to analyze a sound and then replay it to the patient. These might enable audiologists to cus-tom-tune hearing aids for each individual.

• Research has uncovered the gene responsible for profound deafness in some people. This could lead one day to treatment or even a cure.

• Other research indicates that deaf people can "hear" extremely high-frequency sounds. If this remarkable research is confirmed, one day the deaf might be helped to hear.

Meanwhile, hearing aids, sometimes little bigger than a peanut, are allowing those millions smart enough to use them to tune in on life again.

Saved from a Silent World

COMEDIANS HAVE MADE FUN OF THE DEAF AND the hard-of-hearing for years, but the desperate tragedy and suffering of such conditions are not funny. Without hearing, you cannot easily learn language, the essence of humanity. And without language, you lack the ability to express thoughts, needs, and feelings fully.

Approximately 28 million Americans have hearing loss. Two million with profound hearing loss remain bottled up in silence, often needlessly. In addition, 13 million are afflicted by hearing impairments of all kinds. Today, new electronic hearing aids and other devices, new medical treatments, and new training concepts help thousands of hard-of-hearing people stay in the world of sound.

Although Stephen Weitz, 33, of Queens, New York, has had severe hearing loss in both ears since birth, he has learned to read, write, and speak fluently enough to become an acoustic engineer, working on the manufacture of hearing aids.

"I have deaf friends," says Mr. Weitz, "who communicate only in sign language. They have shut themselves out of the hearing world."

His wife, Fanny, is profoundly deaf. A hearing person finds it difficult to understand her hollow, nasal-sounding voice but has no problem understanding her husband's. For Mr. Weitz, early training made the difference. Until a psychiatrist discovered that 3-year-old Stephen had suffered such a severe hearing impairment that he could not speak, many viewed him as mentally retarded. When properly diagnosed, he entered the training program at the New York League for the Hard of Hearing. Mrs. Weitz did not get to the league until age 6.

To have success, league experts maintain, it is vital to learn as early as possible whether a child has severe hearing loss. Even infants can be diagnosed by analyzing their responses to sounds projected in an acoustically controlled room.

"We can teach 90 percent of the children here with severe hearing loss to speak so clearly that you think only that they have a foreign accent," asserts Jane Madell, the league's chief audiologist, or hearing specialist, "and they understand everything you say."

However, many experts doubt that the league's success is as great as this. Still, its program is impressive.

Here are some of the weapons against silence being used nationally:

- Hearing aids that can compensate even for extremely distorted hearing
- Cued speech, a method for improving lipreading
- Equipment that allows the deaf to "talk" on the phone via teletype or computer
- Various pagers, wake-up alarms, burglar alarms, and smoke detectors that set off flashing lights and activate vibrators under a pillow; a microphone

that flashes when a child cries; flashing-light telephone ringers
- TV subtitles that appear on the screen through a special hookup

Also benefiting about 10,000 people who are beyond a hearing aid's help is an electronic device called a cochlear implant. It is placed under the skin behind the ear, with wires to stimulate the auditory nerves and help the totally deaf person "hear." The wires lead into the cochlea in the ear, which turns sound waves into electrical nerve impulses.

Dr. William House, president of the House Ear Institute in Los Angeles, pioneered the device. The first implant provided one channel, enabling most patients to hear some sound but not enough to recognize speech. Still, it enhanced lipreading ability.

Adults, primarily, have had the implants, but more and more children are getting them. Matthew Fiedor got an implant in his right ear when he was 2 years old at the House Ear Institute. His mother, Paulette, says he went from a child silenced by meningitis to one who talks intelligibly, hears, and can discriminate between voices. "He is now a loving and outgoing child," she says.

Some hearing specialists say implants should be used in children only after it is proved that other methods, such as hearing aids and training, cannot help.

Improved hearing aids, developed in the last decade, powerfully amplify sound. They can be made to fit snugly, as one piece, in the ear and are scarcely noticeable. (President Reagan's use of one triggered a huge demand for them.) These devices lead all other developments in keeping the hearing-impaired individual hearing as much as possible. They have grown in importance as scientists have become increasingly aware that not every "deaf" person is totally devoid of hearing.

The New York League for the Hard of Hearing's training program for the profoundly deaf requires that every child—even infants—be fitted with strong hearing aids to ensure that whatever hearing they do have is enhanced. The children are taught to recognize the distorted sounds without any clues, such as lipreading. In fact, the teachers cover their mouths to prevent guesswork.

The league places such children in regular classrooms with hearing children. The only difference is that the teachers wear microphones that broadcast their voices directly to the children's hearing aids. Result: Most league students can attend regular schools instead of schools for the deaf. The students can read on a par with their hearing age group, the league reports.

Most educators of the deaf support teaching children both sign language and lipreading. Such training helps a few achieve speech at a high level of intelligibility, but not most. On average, such children seldom exceed fourth- or fifth-grade reading levels.

Among those favoring sign language as the primary means of communication is Phyllis Frelich, 42, the actress who won a Tony Award in 1980 for her performance in *Children of a Lesser God*, a play about deaf persons in a hearing world. She talks only in sign language or through a signing interpreter.

"You should teach children to speak, if possible," she says, but urges, "If it becomes clear that a child cannot learn to converse through speech, admit it and teach the child sign language so that communication is possible."

Discovering that deaf children who used only sign language often read poorly disturbed Dr. R. Orin Cornett. He is professor emeritus in audiology at Gallaudet College, the world's only college for the deaf, in Washington, D.C. So he invented "cued speech," to enhance a deaf person's lipreading ability.

In cued speech, the speaking person makes a hand movement to indicate the sound being spoken. This differs from sign language, in which the signs represent general concepts rather than specific words. For example, the consonants *m, b,* and *p* look very much alike on the lips. Dr. Cornett invented a sign for the hearing-impaired that enables the lipreader to combine the information of the lips and hand and figure out in a split second that the sound uttered is, let's say, *m.*

Cornett says that the children who master cued speech improve their lipreading enormously and become able even to repeat foreign words they have never seen. They learn to speak more clearly, he adds, noting that—unlike users of sign language only—they learn to understand spoken English.

Says Dr. Cornett, "In general, deaf children don't know English, so they cannot read." He cites cases of deaf children who became avid readers after they mastered cued speech.

Dr. Cornett and Robert Beadles, of the Research Triangle Institute in Research Triangle Park, North Carolina, are developing a computerized device that employs a microphone and produces the cue signs in digital-display form. It's called an Autocuer. The two are working to so miniaturize the computer that it will fit in a pair of special eyeglasses, showing the digital cue at the mouth of the person speaking.

In the absence of cued speech or sign language on most telecasts, there is closed captioning. A special device attached to the TV produces subtitles on the screen for approximately 100 hours of captioned programming each week.

Research goes on. So does the controversy. In the deaf world—and it is a world unto itself—deafness is worn like a badge of courage. Therefore, many persons with severe deafness desire little or no benefit from the technology available. To hearing persons, this philosophy sounds strange. Few people who can hear would not want to lose that ability, and if they become hard-of-hearing, they want all the help they can get.

For more information on schools and treatment, write to the Better Hearing Institute, P.O. Box 1840, Washington, D.C. 20013, and the House Ear Institute, 256 S. Lake, Los Angeles, CA 90057.

New Devices Can Help You Hear

MEDICAL SCIENCE HAS NOW DESIGNED POWERful instruments for bringing the sounds of the outside world to people who are hard-of-hearing or profoundly deaf. Thanks to these new techniques, many are being offered the chance to communicate with those around them who have no hearing problems.

The National Institute on Deafness and Other Communication Disorders (NIDCD) reports that 28 million Americans have some difficulty hearing. Estimates are that 80 percent of the difficulties cannot be corrected, though they can be helped. But many of the profoundly deaf want no part of this brave new world of improved hearing.

Through a sign language interpreter, I interviewed two seniors at Gallaudet University for the deaf and hard-of-hearing in

Washington, D.C. Don Miller, 23, was born deaf. His major is sign communication. Jenny Lin, 21, lost her hearing at 2. She is studying communication arts. I asked each one, "Suppose science had developed a little box to be inserted in your head to give you perfect hearing. Would you take it?"

"No!" said Ms. Lin. "I don't need to hear. I have already established my identity as a deaf person. All my opportunities and all my experiences lie in the deaf community. I cannot imagine being a hearing person."

Mr. Miller agreed. "We would not use technology to feel the equivalent of a hearing person, because we already feel the equivalent of a hearing person," he said. "Their achievements differ."

Gallaudet's president, Dr. I. King Jordan, 51, echoes those sentiments. "The notion that deafness is a handicap bothers me. Deaf people should not be labeled and limited in their aspirations." Dr. Jordan, a psychologist, lost his hearing at 20 in a motorcycle accident. He wears a hearing aid, he says, to pace his speech.

Cynthia Compton, an audiologist at Gallaudet, notes that while hearing devices are controversial, some students do wear them. "There is political pressure for all students to use American Sign Language and not use auditory technologies, even if they can," she says.

The feeling that deafness is a difference, not a disability, is shared by many of the deaf and hard-of-hearing. Says Harlan Lane, a linguist and psychologist at Northeastern University, "It's very difficult for hearing people to understand, but being deaf is legitimate." He opposes the new hearing devices for children born deaf. He points out that, even with the technical advances, the distinctive tones of deaf speech can immediately be discerned by hearing people; that deaf people often have to ask for messages to be repeated; and that they frequently are unsuccessful in their attempts to speak in a hearing world.

But Jane Madell, the director of audiology at the New York League for the Hard of Hearing, says, "The deaf want it both ways. If, as they say, deafness is just a difference and not a disability, then they are not entitled to the special disability programs that deaf children now receive."

The following sections describe some of the devices now being offered to people who are deaf or hard of hearing.

The Cochlear Implant

Doctors can implant this small device directly under the skin behind the ear and into the cochlea. The cochlea is a shell-like bony chamber in the inner ear. It is shaped like a trumpet seashell. Normally, the fine hairs in the cochlea transform sound into electrical signals. The auditory nerve picks up those signals and conducts them into the hearing center of the brain. The brain unravels the electrical signals to find meaning. Profound deafness results when the cochlea no longer does its job.

The implant gets signals from a microphone behind the ear that picks up outside sounds. The microphone's electrical signals feed into a pocket-sized computer called a speech processor, which is worn on a belt around the waist. The processor changes those signals into special electrical pulses. These, in turn, activate the implant to create pulses that travel down fine wires to the auditory nerve. This nerve carries the signals into the hearing center of the brain. Even though the messages are "noisy," the brain receives enough information to pick out the meaning. About 10,000 formerly deaf children and adults can hear as a result of this implant.

An implant—and, for that matter, any hearing aid—works best when the patient has had some early experience with normal hearing or speech, because electrical waves establish speech pathways in the brain in those early days. Nevertheless, scientists are discovering that vigorous stimulation of the brain (such as that provided by an implant), even in patients born deaf or who became deaf soon after birth, slowly improves hearing. The important issue is adjusting the cochlear implant to suit each person's hearing pattern.

"The implant gives me a pretty natural sound," says Donna Sorkin, executive director of the group SHHH (Self Help for Hard of Hearing People). She began to lose her hearing in her 20s and lost it completely by 40. Ms. Sorkin had a cochlear implant 2 years ago. "I can recognize voices I had heard before," she says. "I can use the phone by plugging my speech processor into an auditory adapter on the phone. Before my implant, I had not used a conventional phone for 6 years."

Not everyone does so well, but almost every patient improves. Critics point out that there can be infections, and the implant device (which costs $15,000) is hard to replace if it stops working.

The Multichannel Auditory Brainstem Implant

The Cochlear Corporation, which makes the cochlear implant, won permission from the Food and Drug Administration (FDA) to test an implant that skips the ear altogether. This device can help people whose auditory nerve has been severed to remove a tumor. The implant uses electrodes placed in the auditory region of the brainstem that transmit sound information to the brain to be interpreted. The process happens almost instantaneously.

High-Powered Hearing Aids

Evidence suggests that early exposure to sound and speech, even for just a few days after birth, improves the deaf child's chances of developing good speech patterns with the later use of technology.

Some hearing aids employ FM radio waves to transmit sound from the mouth of a lecturer all the way across an auditorium to the ear of a wearer who is hard-of-hearing. One tiny aid the size of a small snail leans against the eardrum to produce high-quality sound reception. Another device creates clear sounds by accommodating the patient's particular hearing pattern. If, for example, the patient cannot hear high-pitched voices, the instrument automatically boosts the loudness of those weak frequencies as they enter the ear.

Molly Lubin, 10, was born deaf. At 5 weeks, she was fitted with hearing aids to boost what hearing she had. A teacher helped her become aware of sounds. Today, with the hearing aids, Molly can make phone calls. She reads lips, but she also can understand speech without lip-reading. Molly had the leading role in her class play last year. So natural was her voice that other parents did not know she was deaf.

"Some hard-of-hearing people condemn us for bringing Molly up orally," says her mother. "But why wouldn't you want your child to be oral if she could?"

As for the profoundly deaf, they take pride in a nonhearing community and culture. But new hearing research and technical advances will enable many more individuals to make deafness clearly a condition of choice.

To learn more, write to the NIDCD Information Clearinghouse, 1 Communication Ave., Bethesda, MD 20892-3456.

How Science Is Saving Our Sight

HOW MUCH IS YOUR EYESIGHT WORTH? SUZIE K. of New York City will tell you that you cannot put a price on being able to see. She lost her vision in 1976 because a doctor failed to diagnose and then treat her eye disease. She sued for malpractice and won $6 million. At the time, she said she would rather see than have the money.

A rapid increase of pressure in her eyeballs destroyed the optic nerve, blinding her. The disease that caused such damage is caused acute glaucoma, and it can be stopped if caught in time. Each year, glaucoma and a dozen other disease and injuries blind 50,000 Americans. A half million persons in the United States are now legally blind. Many could've saved their sight had they received medical help early enough to stop or slow the damage. Millions more lose vision sharpness to such treatable conditions as nearsightedness, farsightedness, and astigmatism.

Fortunately, medical scientist have discovered new ways to reverse failing eyesight and even restore lost vision:

- Lasers for delicate surgery inside the eyeball to repair the retina, the eye's "photographic plate"
- Surgery of the cornea—the window of the eye—to correct nearsightedness without spectacles
- Sound waves to detect eye cancer
- Nuclear magnetic resonance (using very high-frequency radio waves) to detect eye cancers and tissue changes
- New plastic lenses for the cornea (contact lenses) or inside of the eye to replace clouded human eyes.
- New drugs to treat glaucoma by reducing the pressure of the fluid in the eyeball

The new eye science has given Kenton Kidd, of Clovis, California, a chance to recapture some of the vision in his right eye. When a box of apples fell on him, the retina detached and a hemorrhage into the eye formed a blood clot that clouded his vision further. The result? "It was like looking through a smoke screen," he says.

Mr. Kidd found his way to Duke University in Durham, North Carolina, where Drs. Robert Machemer and Eugene de Juan take on "hopeless cases." The surgeons, successful in about half of their operations, work inside the eye through three small holes made in the side of the eye. In one hole, hardly bigger than the eye of a needle, they thread a small bundle of glass fibers. That enables them to put a light inside the eye. Into the second opening go the surgical instruments. And into the third, they feed fluids and gases to keep the eye firm.

In Mr. Kidd's case, they cut out the blood clot, removed the scar tissue at the back of his eye, and patched together and reattached pieces of undamaged retina. Now he sees a swatch of light in that eye.

On another front, new machines enable doctors to detect disease in the eye. High-frequency sound waves aimed inside the eye and reflected back can help detect cancers. At New York Hospital–Cornell Medical Center in Manhattan, doctors have been able to diagnose even this type of cancer.

Taken altogether—new methods, new machines, new drugs—science is making it possible for everyone to see better.

Remember, in school, how you took a magnifying glass and focused the sun's rays into a small circle that got so hot it could ignite a piece of paper? A laser, similarly, concentrates light onto a spot that is tinier than a pinpoint and at temperatures that are hotter than the sun. Doctors have turned that burning point of light on eyes afflicted with disease. In each case, the light beam is focused on the diseased spot. Dr. Lee M. Jampol, professor of ophthalmology at Northwestern University Medical School in

Chicago, says that eventually lasers will largely replace surgery within the eye.

Lasers—various kinds for various illnesses—have been helping conquer blinding diseases, including those discussed here.

Diabetic Retinopathy

This is a condition in which the blood vessels of the eye change because of diabetes. In diabetes, the tiny arteries that feed blood to the retina close down, killing part of the tissue. The dying retina puts out a chemical, causing blood vessels to grow in the healthy part of the retina. The arteries swell and leak fluid and blood into the eye, destroying vision. The laser beam kills the dying part of the retina, stopping the release of the growth chemicals, thus ending or slowing the destruction.

Macular Degeneration

This is the most common cause of legal blindness under age 60. For some mysterious reason, blood vessels behind the retina enlarge, leak, and bleed, forming scar tissue and destroying central vision. This can happen at a point called the macula. The laser can seal up the leaking blood vessels under the macula. But this works only for about one patient in six. The blue-green argon laser must not be directed at the center of the macula where most of these blood vessels grow, because the result would be to destroy vision.

However, Dr. Lawrence Yanuzzi, surgeon director at Manhattan Eye, Ear and Throat Hospital in New York, has a krypton laser that can get close to the macula safely. Unlike the blue-green argon laser, the krypton laser produces red light and can pass through the macula to repair the leaking blood vessels behind it.

Tom Ward, of Sedona, Arizona, a retired banker who took up painting, owes whatever sight he has to the krypton laser. Because of macular degeneration, he lost central vision in his right eye 15 years earlier. Mr. Ward's blood vessels started leaking again. Dr. Yanuzzi sealed the blood vessels with krypton light.

"I can see quite well with my left eye," says Mr. Ward, "but I cannot hit a tennis ball, because I have poor close-up vision."

Detached Retina

Sometimes the retina falls away from the back of the eye. As a result, the light coming into the eye no longer focuses on the retina. With the laser beam, a surgeon can spot-weld the filmy tissue.

Glaucoma

In the United States 2 million persons have glaucoma, with 300,000 new cases a year. Glaucoma is to blame for one out of eight cases of blindness in the United States. Ironically, this disease is easily diagnosed and arrested—if caught early. In glaucoma, the pressure of the fluid in the eye builds up, destroying the optic nerve. Sometimes, the pressure rises up because the fluid in the eye does not drain.

With a laser beam, the doctor can make the drainage holes in the iris—holes as small as the period at the end of this sentence. Laser treatments also help up to 80 percent of patients with a second form of glaucoma, in which fluid flows abnormally between the iris and cornea.

In treating glaucoma, the drug timolol and pilocarpine have had good results as well.

An early method for detecting glaucoma involved putting a drop of anesthetic on the eyeball. Then a tiny plunger was lowered onto the cornea to test for increased pressure. Newer machines blow a puff of air painlessly on the unanesthetized cornea. The deformation of the cornea indicates the pressure and the presence of the glaucoma.

Dr. M. Bruce Shields, professor of ophthalmology at Duke University, heads a group evaluating the use of a new instrument that combines a computer with light patterns to treat glaucoma. The patient sits in front of a light source that blinks on at different locations—up, down, and side to side. The patient pushes a button upon seeing the light. The computer tracks the response and maps out the patient's visual field. If glaucoma is present, the computer shows a loss of peripheral (side) vision.

Dr. Shields's group also is evaluating a small camera placed very near the eye that takes a color picture of the optic nerve. In response to pressure, the optic nerve will change its color.

Cataracts

Sometimes, after the removal of a cataract (a clouded lens in the eye), a membrane left in the eye also becomes clouded, obscuring vision. A new laser called a YAG (yttrium aluminum garnet) vaporizes the membrane.

Eye Health Checklist

If you have any of the following signs or symptoms, you may need the help of an ophthalmologist.

Blurry vision

Double vision

Dimming or sudden loss of vision

New spots or shadows

Red eye or eye pain

Discharge, crusting, or loss of side vision

Chronic, heavy tearfulness

Halos around lights

Flashes of light

Swelling of an eye

Crossed eyes

Bulging of an eye

Wandering eye

Twitching eye

Difference in eye size

Diabetes

Don't Take Your Contact Lenses for Granted

THANKS TO BATTALIONS OF CLEVER CHEMISTS, millions of Americans now just pop contact lenses into their eyes and forget about them. Sometimes they forget about them for far too long—for weeks, sometimes months. We're talking about soft pliable lenses. These plastic lenses provide normal sight. And you can scarcely feel them resting snugly against the delicate eyeball. They're called extended-wear lenses.

There are also "hard" lenses. These become uncomfortable when left in the eye too long, such as when the wearer sleeps with them in.

Contact lenses have evolved rapidly since World War II, when it was noted that fragments of the plastic canopies sometimes entered the eyes of pilots and were tolerated well. This observation led to the evolution of the modern plastic contact lens. In the 1950s, the first hard-plastic lenses were produced. Not everybody could stand those thick, stiff objects resting on their eyeballs, but many others wore them happily. By 1970, comfortable soft-plastic lenses came on the market. These are worn by half of all users of contact lenses today. Also popular are gas-permeable hard lenses, which allow oxygen through the cornea, letting the eyes "breathe." Care and cleaning are simpler too. Still, these lenses are more likely to slip or pop out. They can also become scratched or chipped and so require daily scrutiny.

In 1980, the FDA approved the extended-wear lens. The manufacturers maintained—and the FDA agreed—that wearers could safely leave these lenses in for a month. Today, the FDA recommends that the duration of use be shortened to from 1 to 7 days between overnight removals for cleaning and disinfection.

Reports indicate that the care-free attitude inspired by the dime-sized soft disks have cost too many people the sight of an eye, and hundreds more have forfeited their ability ever again to wear these comfortable lenses. All this has resulted from eye injury caused chiefly by injection or trauma. And these conditions were brought on by the wearers themselves: they simply left the lens in their eyes too long. Or they failed to clean them carefully enough, leaving germs on the lens that, when reinserted, infected the eyes.

Typically, the careless wearer has taken the lens for granted. Usually, nothing goes wrong—the lens stay in place, and the wearer enjoys the freedom from cumbersome glasses. Lenses also enable wearers to pursuer strenuous sports like tennis without having to worry about breaking their glasses.

But sometimes, if someone abuses the principles of long-term wear, a lens sticks to a cornea—the clear front window of an eye. By trying to remove the stuck lens, the wearer may tear that delicate tissue, and blindness may follow. In such cases, surgeons try restoring sight with a corneal transplant. But sometimes that doesn't work—the blindness is permanent. All in the name of comfort.

Some experts recommend that extended-wear lenses be left in the eyes for no longer than 7 days continuously without overnight rest. Only 1 in 500 users get into trouble each year, and the degree of infection varies.

But to those affected, of course, the problem is significant.

Unfortunately, too many contact lens wearers take their lenses for granted because they are so comfortable. They leave them in too long, don't clean them enough, and even use their germ-laden saliva to wet the lenses. As one expert puts it, "They behave as though they're dealing with socks. A contact lens is a medical device."

Dr. Scott MacRae, of the Oregon Health Sciences University in Portland, says if you wear such lens for 20 years, your chances of experiencing a serious problem with them in that time—all

things staying constant—can be as high as 1 in 25. However, some conservative eye doctors say that nonstop wear, even for 7 days, is dangerous.

"It was once said to be safe to wear extended-wear contacts for up to 30 days," says the corneal specialist and surgeon Dr. David Haight, chief physician for the Corneal Lens Service of the Ophthalmology Department at Manhattan Eye and Ear Hospital in New York City. "We know better now," he adds. "The maximum recommended time is 1 week, but some people should not try to wear them as long as a week at a time because their eyes are just too sensitive."

Dr. Oliver Schein and his colleges at Harvard Medical School discovered that 7 days may be too extended a time for wearing the lens. Their study showed that if you wear any soft contact lens overnight even once, you run the risk of developing a sight-threatening crater on the cornea. That risk is nine to 15 times lower for people who remove their lens daily.

Dr. Schein warns that if you don't clean your lenses properly, you may add to the danger. "Contact lenses are generally safe for everyone," he says. "But though hygiene is important, constant overnight wear appears to be a major risk factor."

If any of the nation's 20 million users of all types of contact lenses wear their lenses overnight, they imperil their eyesight. But 4 million users of extended-wear contact lenses go for days without removing them, putting their eyes into great jeopardy.

Of course, the number of people blinded by the muss of contact lenses is small. Many more suffer an allergic reaction that sometimes can doom their ability to wear contact lenses of any kind. That condition is called giant papillary conjunctivitis (GPC). Its symptoms include a cobblestone-like swelling under the upper lid, mucus secretions, redness, and irritation.

Cheryl Sacra, a writer in Hoboken, New Jersey, wore soft contacts for 10 years. "They were convenient, and I got used to them and took them for granted," she says. "But then I went to my eye doctor, because they had become so uncomfortable. My eyes were itchy, red, swollen, and sticky, and a cloudy discharge fogged the lenses. I could not see." She adds that now she can't wear the soft lens for more than a few hours.

You can develop GPC in response to chemicals in the lens itself or from the buildup of protein deposits on the lens from natural eye fluids. GPC develops not only with extended-wear lenses but also with soft and hard lenses. It is most common with soft lenses.

Rarely does GPC lead to blindness. But if you don't take care of that little piece of plastic, your eye becomes so sensitive to the lenses that you can no longer wear them. The protracted wearing of contact lenses also can cause additional blood vessels to grow into the cornea and obscure vision somewhat. These abnormally engorged vessels shrink when the lens is removed.

Three lens makers are also offering disposable extended-wear lenses. They are Johnson & Johnson's Acuvue, Bausch & Lomb's SeeQuence, and Ciba Vision's NewVues. You wear the disposable for up to a week and then throw them away. Though 7 days gives less time for the buildup of deposits from the fluids in the eye, the lens is still unhygienic. In some future brands, the lens may be made to be disposed of each day.

Dr. MacRae notes that the cornea normally swells up a little at night without a lens because the shut eye lid reduces oxygen passage by about one third. As a result of leaving the lens in, the swelling increases and the oxygen decreases all the more. With deposits on the lens, the swelling can lead to scraped corneas and infection.

Dr. Richard Lippmann, director of the FDA's Ophthalmic Devices Division in Rockville, Maryland, says, "Some problems have been identified with disposable lenses, similar to the types of problems we see with extended wear: deposits and infections."

If you take your lenses out every night and clean them, chances are you won't run into any problems. Nevertheless, too many people treat their lenses too casually. Although there are germ-free cleaning, disinfecting, and storage solutions on the market, many people use tap water (loaded with germs) for their lenses. Or they try to make their own mixtures with salt tablets. Dr. MacRae says that half the people who wear such lenses don't follow directions for cleaning and care. Most people get away with it but endlessly risk infecting their delicate eye tissues.

It's easy to avoid trouble with contact lenses—just follow directions and see your eye doctor at least once a year. If you do, you'll increase your chances of getting all the advantages and none of the troubles of contact lenses.

Sleep

TONIGHT 50 MILLION AMERICAN ADULTS WILL crawl into bed, draw up the covers, lay their heads down on their pillows, and then, try as they might, they will not be able to find restful sleep. You may very well be one of them.

Do you ever pass the whole night in the clutches of unremitting insomnia? Does it take you an hour or longer to fall asleep? Do you fall asleep but wake up at 4 A.M., then find yourself unable to get back to slumberland? Or are you the victim of recurrent nightmares and sleepwalking?

If you answered yes to any of these questions, you very likely suffer from a sleep disorder. Whatever your sleep problem, help is available.

A Too-Sleepy America

"America is not getting enough sleep," says Dr. William C. Dement, a pioneer sleep scientist from Stanford University. "I can pick a room full of 500 college students, and by just droning on, I can put 400 of them to sleep. Most adults are chronically sleepy in the daytime because they're not getting enough sleep. That means we're not alert enough during the day for efficient thinking and working."

Factors that prevent many people from getting a good night's rest include poor sleep habits (such as keeping irregular sleeping and waking hours), anxiety, depression, abuse of drugs and alcohol, illness, and physical abnormalities.

How much sleep do we really need? There is no absolute answer. The amount of sleep you need depends on your age, your physical and mental health, and your lifestyle. How long you sleep also may vary depending on illness, stress, and other factors.

The average adult, however, gets between 7 and 8 hours of sleep a night, so we view this as the norm.

Occasional Sleeplessness versus Chronic Insomnia

One adult in four has insomnia—trouble falling asleep or staying asleep. To some people, it happens once in a while; for others, it's a chronic problem that they cannot shake.

Ruth Sanborn is typical of one kind of insomniac. "Sometimes," this Chicago teacher told me, "I lie awake all night, two or three nights in a row. I get panicky and perspire so much that the sheets get damp. The next day, I find it difficult to handle any stress."

At their sleep lab at Hershey Medical Center of Pennsylvania State University, Drs. Joyce and Anthony Kales have studied hundreds of insomniacs like Ruth Sanborn, people whose sleeplessness starts with tension and anxiety, usually over some event of the day. After a night or two of troubled sleep, most resume their normal sleep patterns.

The chronic insomniac, however, finds it hard to turn off his anxiety and tension. He is the person, say the Kales, who keeps his problems to himself, who doesn't let out anger or disappointment.

Responding to the stress of the day, the chronic insomniac's racing thoughts activate his physical arousal system, making it more difficult to get to sleep. Chronic insomniacs, therefore, are physically more aroused just before bedtime. Their body temperatures and heart rate are higher, and they move around in bed more than normal sleepers do.

Night Terrors

Acute stress or a frightening, traumatic event affects some people in the form of recurrent nightmares or sleepwalking episodes. To avoid the terrifying dreams, some wake themselves early in the dream phase. Later, however, they cannot recall the nightmare or hence, why they woke up. Some sleep-inducing drugs, if not used on a long-term basis, seem to relieve the symptoms in a few patients.

The Troubled Mind

The Kales say that four of five people who consult them for long-standing insomnia have actual emotional problems (such as neurotic depression, obsessive-compulsive disorders, or anxiety states). Often, insomnia sends a sufferer to the doctor's office, where the underlying emotional problem is then diagnosed and treated.

What's the connection? Some researchers believe that emotional disorders affect changes in brain chemistry that also affect sleep.

Much of what we know about the body during sleep was discovered in sleep disorder centers—soundproof, temperature-controlled laboratories where scientists observe sleep. Today, there are about 300 such centers in the United States. Researchers there attach wires to the patient to pick up brain waves and to measure body temperature, hormone secretion, breathing, heart rate, and other body functions before, during, and after sleep.

Physical Problems and Strange Sleep

Illnesses like angina (heart pain) and asthma (breathing problems) can disturb sleep. Some biological or physical abnormalities primarily affect sleep. For example, people who sleep long enough but wake up beaten (i.e., sleep does not restore them) are now believed to suffer from brain-wave disturbances. And those who have been insomniacs since childhood may have been born with abnormal sleep-wake systems.

Cora Hipkiss, of Newark, California, suffered attacks of uncontrollable sleepiness; she cannot stay awake for more than 4 hours at a time. This mysterious sleep disorder is called narcolepsy.

"I once drove a car and fell asleep," she recalls. "A truck driver saved me by blasting his horn and waking me up."

The cause of narcolepsy is unknown. Dr. Dement suspects the chemicals that move from nerve to nerve in narcoleptics' brains. Dr. Charles Pollak of the Sleep-Wake Disorders Center at New York Hospital-Cornell Medical Center in White Plains believes that, instead of functioning within a normal 24-hour cycle, narcoleptics' body "clocks" (discussed later) regulate their lives in intervals of only a few hours. He suggests that narcoleptics take daytime naps to relieve their relentless sleepiness.

Apnea

People with this condition stop breathing (sometimes hundreds of times) during the night because their windpipes collapse. Their choking and gasps for air wake them up, so that they never get a good night's sleep. Therefore, they are unable to stay awake during the day. Treatment of the breathing problem eliminates the daytime sleepiness and restores sleep.

Because many people with apnea are grossly overweight (between 200 and 350 pounds), weight loss can get rid of the breathing problem. Some victims of apnea need a positive pressure pump to push air into their lungs during sleep.

Muscle Spasms

Doctors call body twitches that disturb sleep "sleep-related myoclonus" (*myo* meaning muscle, and *clonus,* spasm). One condition associated with myoclonus is called "restless leg." Tingly sensations trigger the leg to jerk and wake the sleeper.

The Psychological Angle

About a third of insomniacs suffer from the interaction of physical and psychological problems, says Dr. Peter J. Hauri of Dartmouth Medical School in New Hampshire. Insomnia deepens as the victim tries harder and harder to fall asleep. Soon bedroom, bed, blanket, and pillows become symbols of sleeping failure. The fear of not being able to sleep keeps the victim awake.

Such people are advised not to try to force sleep but to get out of bed and do something unexciting, staying awake as long as possible, and getting into bed only when exhausted. After two or three nights, Dr. Hauri says, the bed is a welcome place.

Some patients throw off insomnia with relaxation therapy. With the guidance of a psychologist they learn how to relax the whole body. It produces the same relaxed state as meditation. Some sleep scientists say that biofeedback also helps. In this treatment, the psychologist places several pieces of metal (electrodes) against the skin of the forehead. If a muscle is in tension, the patient can see it on a computer screen. The patient then uses various relaxation methods to relax the forehead and can watch the success or failure on the screen. Some experts say that biofeedback works faster than other relaxation treatments.

"Blue Monday"

On weekends, most of us go to bed later and sleep later the next morning, letting our inner body clocks take over. Between Friday night and Sunday morning, we may be out of step by up to 4 hours.

On Sunday night, we return to our regular bedtime of, say, 11 P.M. By then, however, our bodies are not ready for sleep until 3 A.M. So on Monday morning, when we are awakened by a 7 A.M. alarm clock, we are really in the middle of our sleep cycle. We feel sleepy and unalert. To avoid "blue Mondays," try to go to bed and arise on weekends at the same time as during the week.

The Brutality of Shift Work

Factory, postal and hospital employees, bakers, truck drivers, police, and fire fighters often rotate their work hours in three shifts: day shift (8 A.M. to 4 P.M.),

evening (4 P.M. to midnight), and night, or "graveyard" (midnight to 8 A.M.). The problem for these workers is that shifts often change weekly. This is not enough time to reset the internal body clocks.

Seventy percent of shift workers have trouble falling asleep and staying asleep; they complain of stomachaches and irritability. (One man joked that he was going to bed hungry and waking up ready for love, instead of the reverse.)

Such work schedules probably disturb the sleep and digestion of 20 million to 30 million people, says Dr. Charles Czeisler of Harvard Medical School. He devised a shift schedule for a Utah chemical company that closely followed nature's body clocks. He reports that complaints about sleep and stomach troubles dropped dramatically, and work production increased by 20 to 30 percent.

Shift workers who have trouble sleeping should go to sleep at the same time every day and should eat a similar meal at the same time each day for the duration of the work shift.

The Dangers of Pills

Most experts agree that sleeping pills should be used only for occasional sleeplessness. A conference of experts assembled by the National Institutes of Health warned against using sleeping pills of any kind for chronic insomnia, except perhaps for a month to make other treatments easier.

Rules for Better Sleep

Sleep experts have developed some simple rules for good sleep.

Rule 1. Go to bed and get up about the same time every day, weekends included. A regular routine keeps you in step with your biological rhythms.

Rule 2. Exercise regularly. Some people, however, may find exercise too physically arousing if it's done too close to bedtime.

Rule 3. Recognize that sleeping pills, alcohol, caffeine, and cigarettes may induce sleeplessness. People who drink or smoke often remain awake in bed for a long time. Sleeping pills are often successful in breaking the distorted cycle of sleep-awake. *Warning:* They should be used to change the cycle and usually not longer than a month.

Rule 4. We all have the capacity to fall asleep. It is built into us. If we don't sleep for a night or two, no harm will come unless we try too hard. So don't try to force sleep. If you cannot sleep, get out of bed. Do something boring. Don't watch TV—it may stimulate you to remain awake.

Rule 5. Find a quiet place. Noisy environments disturb sleep, even for deep sleepers.

Rule 6. Don't use the bedroom for reading, watching television, playing games. You will associate bed with activities that make the mind race. Bedrooms are only for sleep and sex.

Rule 7. Learn some kind of relaxation technique. Meditation is one, biofeedback another. You can relax by alternately tensing and relaxing your muscles.

The Body "Clocks"

How well you sleep also depends on how well synchronized your body's "clocks" are.

For example, if you go to bed at 11 P.M. and rise at 7 A.M. every day, you may find yourself becoming sleepy and waking at about those times without a mechanical clock. Your body seems to keep time. That's because humans have at least two major interior timing systems, each cycling about 25 hours. One clock is set by the light-and-dark cycle of the day. Your eyes, seeing the light of day, signal the brain that it is time to wake up.

The other clock regulates your body temperature so that it rises during the day, drops during the night, and then rises again. This "temperature" clock is reset by your routine of waking, sleeping, and maybe eating. Because we do these activities based on the day-night cycle, the two biological clocks normally run together.

For further information, write to NHLBI (National Heart, Lung, Blood Institute) Information Center, P.O. Box 30105, Bethesda, MD 20824-0105.

Could You Use More Sleep?

IF YOU WANT TO INCREASE YOUR ODDS OF having a long and lively lifetime, scientists say, work on getting an average of 7 or 8 hours of sleep a night. If you get only 6 hours or less, you stand a 70 percent chance of dying before your time. Fortunately, your brain won't let you die of a lack of sleep without a struggle. After 4 to 5 days of wakefulness, it will put you to sleep whether you wish it or not—with luck, not while you're driving your car.

Scientists are finding that if you don't get enough sleep, you are putting yourself at increased risk of heart trouble, digestive disease, fertility problems (if you are a woman), or a serious, even fatal, accident. When tired, your sight, hearing, and attention are slow to alert you to dangers, and once you are aware of them, your reactions also are slow.

Dr. H. Craig Heller, a professor of biology at Stanford University in Palo Alto, California, is one of a small army of scientists studying the reasons why many people can't sleep and awake refreshed, why the brain puts you to sleep, and why lack of sleep triggers such powerful effects.

"It's like a bank account," Dr. Heller says. "You have to keep some minimum balance. If you keep on making withdrawals without making deposits, you run up a deficit. Then the pressure builds, biologically, to 'deposit' some sleep."

He also notes that most major catastrophes have occurred in the early morning, when workers probably were drowsy from deficient sleep. He includes the explosion at the nuclear plant at Chernobyl in Ukraine, the release of toxic gas at Bhopal, India, and the nuclear accident at Three Mile Island in Pennsylvania.

Dr. William C. Dement, Dr. Heller's colleague and a pioneer sleep scientist, calls us a sleepy people in an epidemic of sleep deficit. Scientists estimate that more than 100 million Americans have sleep troubles of some kind. Getting too little sleep heads the list. As many as one American in five gets fewer than 6 hours of sleep a night. Some people can get along on 6 hours, but most of us need between 7 and 8, and children and young adults need up to 10 hours. As we age, it becomes more difficult to get enough sleep. At any age, however, we all can pile up a sleep deficit that eventually will force us to fall asleep—whether we're ready or not.

Dr. Dement says that many of the sleep-starved—who *think* their brains are working full-speed—actually are struggling to think and keep awake. A boring speaker, alcohol, soothing music, or seemingly nothing at all can lull to sleep such a person or impair judgment.

The 1992 report of the National Commission on Sleep Disorders Research, which Dr. Dement chairs, estimates that 40 million Americans suffer from some kind of *chronic* sleep sickness. About half of them are plagued by a condition called sleep apnea (from the Greek, meaning "not breathing"). Such individuals actually stop breathing while asleep. As carbon dioxide builds up in the lungs, the brain senses something gone wrong and sounds its alarm, waking the person enough to activate the chest and diaphragm muscles. With a terrible snore, the lungs suck in fresh air. Sleep ends for the moment. This can happen 500 times a night, fracturing any peaceful, restorative slumber. During the day, the afflicted person, lacking a restful night, constantly dozes off.

I. M. "Rusty" Gralnik, an engineer in Santa Clara, California, tells this story: "I would go to a ball game and, instead of going in the stadium, stayed in the parking lot to sleep in the car. I didn't know something was wrong—I just thought I was tired. I would fall asleep working at my computer or while trying to read. A year ago, my wife was complaining that I was a terrible host: I'd fall asleep in front of our guests."

People with sleep apnea inhale with high suction. It was so high in Mr. Gralnik's case that it caused his throat to close, waking him repeatedly. This happens most often to people who are greatly overweight, although Mr. Gralnik is thin. Scientists have developed a breathing machine for apnea patients that pushes air into the nose under positive pressure, expanding the windpipe and making breathing easier.

"I feel a little more alert now," Mr. Gralnik says, "but I've been down so long, it will take a while for my body to rejuvenate." For those not helped by the machine or unable to sleep while using it, surgery opens the throat.

Rusty Gralnik's apnea was diagnosed at Stanford's sleep laboratory, which boasts rooms with air and light controls, and infrared TV cameras that "see" in the dark. A microphone and wires lead from a subject's scalp to a recording machine, so doctors can see and hear the breathing, the snores, the apnea. Now 140 medical centers have such labs.

Great progress has been made in helping insomniacs—people who can't fall asleep easily. Many perceive, sometimes falsely, that they have not had enough sleep or have endured bad, non-restorative slumber. The National Commission on Sleep Disorders Research estimates that 60 million Americans have experienced some insomnia, 15 million of them severely and chronically.

Gina Braun, a Tucson, Arizona, homemaker and mother of three young children, bore the burden of chronic insomnia. Her worst wakefulness struck during her last pregnancy. In her 8th month, pills helped Mrs. Braun rest for a while, but their effectiveness faded.

She found Richard Bootzin, director of the Insomnia Clinic of the University of Arizona Sleep Disorders Center in Tucson. Says Dr. Bootzin, "People need to develop skills for falling asleep."

"Dr. Bootzin got me on a schedule," Mrs. Braun says. "Before, I'd go to bed at 9 P.M., wake up at midnight, and stay awake 'til 9 A.M., when my husband [a fireman] would come home from his 24-hour shift. I had no sleep cycle."

Dr. Bootzin used these do's and don'ts that sleep scientists have developed to break insomniacs' bad habits:

- *Do* keep a diary of your bedding-downs and waking-ups for a week, to observe your slumber pattern.
- *Do* maintain a regular schedule. Go to sleep and get up at the same time daily.
- *Don't* drink caffeine after noon or alcohol at any time.
- *Don't* nap during the day—be active.
- *Don't* go to bed until you're drowsy. If you're wide awake, staying in bed makes matters worse.
- *Do* keep your bed for sleeping and sex only. Read, sew, or watch TV elsewhere.

"Dr. Bootzin told me to get out of bed as soon as I felt anxious," says Mrs. Braun. "At first, I was out of bed 10 to 15 times a night. Now, if I can't sleep, I get out of bed and go read. I'm thankful things are so much better."

Most experts advise avoiding sleeping pills except for those emergencies when you cannot get to sleep and you must be rested for some important reason the next day. Taking pills long-term leads your system to tolerate them—they stop having an effect.

Besides being a bad habit, insomnia has many causes, including serious illness. If Dr. Bootzin's do's and don'ts are no help, go to a sleep center.

At the other end of the scale, 300,000 Americans have narcolepsy—they fall asleep without warning at any time, in any place. Says Joe Piscopo, a computer executive, "I slept through just about all of college and barely graduated in 1965 from the University of Illinois with a degree in computer science. From ages 16 to 25, I was in 15 car accidents—I fell asleep at the wheel. It was sheer luck that no one was hurt."

In 1969, doctors at the Mayo Clinic in Rochester, Minnesota, diagnosed his narcolepsy. They gave Mr. Piscopo a strong stimulant, which he still takes. It enabled him to found a successful software company and retire at age 42. He is chairman of the American Narcolepsy Association, which helps narcoleptics learn about their disease and find help.

Scientists have made rapid progress in helping the nation's 3 million or so night-shift workers, who must get their sleep during the day. Many arrive on the job at midnight and spend the next 8 hours trying to work while fighting sleep.

They can't synchronize the wall clock with their biological clock. This is dangerous and inefficient.

Dr. Charles A. Czeisler and others at Brigham and Women's Hospital in Boston have scored a major triumph: In just 4 days, using sun-bright light therapy, they actually shifted workers' biological clocks, allowing them peaceful sleep during the day and productive work at night. Light therapy possibly could solve night-shift problems forever, reducing accidents and poor work.

In 1993, Dr. Al Lewy and colleagues at the Oregon Health Sciences University in Portland achieved similar effects on volunteers by giving them capsules with an artificial form of melatonin, a chemical produced naturally in the brain's pineal gland.

It long has been known that the gland produces melatonin only in the dark at night, but when the artificial chemical was given to humans at night, it seemed to create no reaction. When Dr. Lewy's team gave it to the volunteers during the day, however, the chemical shifted their internal clocks.

Dr. Lewy says melatonin can help jet lag. It also may aid those who need to sleep in the day and stay up at night, or go to bed very early and rise at or before dawn. Once tested, melatonin also might help those with delayed- or advanced-sleep problems or those who get "winter depression" from waking up in darkness. Dr. Lewy says when melatonin is taken in the afternoon, the body behaves as if it had wakened to a bright dawn.

Because melatonin can be classified as a dietary supplement, it has hit the so-called health food stores in a big way. It's OK for Dr. Lewy to do experiments, it's another thing to offer it to the public before extensive testing has been done.

If you think melatonin may help you, you may want to ask a sleep expert before you start popping pills.

Are You Sleepy?

This is a simplified version of a test developed by Dr. William C. Dement and colleagues at the Stanford University Sleep Disorders Clinic and Research Center in Palo Alto, California. With a partner, take the test five times at 2-hour intervals during the daytime.

1. Lie on a bed in a darkened room.
2. When ready, nod to signal your partner to keep track of the time from then on.
3. Try to fall asleep.
4. As soon as you seem to be asleep, your partner should shake you to verify it.
5. Your partner should then record the time.
6. Total the minutes taken to go to sleep in the tests and divide by 5 to get an average.

How to Rate Your Average Score
Less than 10 minutes: See a doctor! (If you fall asleep before the clock even starts, you're sleep-starved.)

10 to 15 minutes: You may need to get more sleep.

15 to 20 minutes: You're OK. (If not asleep in 20 minutes, you're 100 percent alert—not sleep-deficient.)

The Environment and Your Health

Radon: Are You At Risk?

YOU COULD ALMOST IMAGINE IT AS THE BEGINning of an old sci-fi monster movie: Something invisible seeps out of the soil under a suburban house. Silently it creeps into the ground floor or basement, steals up to the living area. There, it enters the bodies of the inhabitants. And they die a horrible death.

That's the terrifying picture of the risk of radon gas drawn by the U.S. Environmental Protection Agency (EPA). It gives the strong impression that potentially everyone in the country stands in great danger of developing lung cancer from inhaling these invisible fumes.

True enough, radon is a gas found naturally in soil. It's not artificially made. It can escape from the earth under your house and enter your home's foundation through cracks and holes, then waft its way into where you and your family live.

The EPA has condemned radon as the number one environmental pollutant that causes cancer. "Thousands of people every year may die unnecessarily because of their exposure to radon," says Margo Oge, former director of the agency's radon division in Washington, D.C. "We believe that everyone should test their homes."

Officially, the EPA estimates that 22,000 Americans die each year because they lived a good part of their lives in buildings polluted by radon. Currently, the EPAs far-ranging estimates are that radon annually kills as few as 7,000 individuals and as many as 30,000.

In June 1988, Barry Solomon found that there was about as much radon in the house he was renting in Clinton, New Jersey, as there would be streaming through a uranium mine. (Fifty years ago, miners had a 50 percent chance of developing lung cancer from the gas. With improved working conditions and equipment, today's miners have a 5 to 10 percent risk of the disease.)

A contractor was employed to reduce the radon levels in Mr. Solomon's home. Engineers now know how to sweep radon from any house. The cost generally ranges from less than $300—as a do-it-yourself project—to $2,000 or $3,000, with $1,200 as the average price.

Mr. Solomon, 38, who—along with his wife, Debra, and his 13-year-old stepson, Michael—now lives in his own home in Bloomsbury, New Jersey, says he feels that so long as the radon problem was fixed, he felt OK. "But I would not want to live in a house with radon," he says. "Everyone should check the home before they buy or move in. It is crazy not to do it."

However, the EPA has outraged many scientists who have studied the problem closely. Dr. Anthony Nero, a senior physicist and an expert on indoor pollution in the research department of the Applied Science Division at the Lawrence Berkeley Laboratory in Berkeley, California, puts it most strongly.

"The Environmental Protection Agency has perpetrated a fraud," he says. "Everything is exaggerated—from the number of homes at risk to the individual's risk from radon. I feel strongly that, in this matter, the public has been led to worry about things of minor concern."

Other scientists disagree. Dr. Naomi Harley, a research professor at New York University Medical Center in New York City, says the EPA is on the right track. "This problem must be dealt with," she adds. "In the long term, we will have to identify the homes at risk. We need new building practices to lower the radon levels." Nevertheless, Dr. Harley also says

that the EPA exaggerates the danger and that mass testing of homes will produce many false and misleading results.

In the face of such disagreement, the average homeowner or renter—who may never have heard of radon before—struggles with what to do. Mystery surrounds the gas. There is fear of its radioactivity and confusion over the real risk it imposes. And no sure guidelines tell us how to best protect our families.

Dr. Bernard Cohen, professor of physics and radiation health at the University of Pittsburgh, has been working on the problem. It goes beyond radon, he says.

"People worry about the radiation from nuclear power plants, radioactive wastes, and accidents in nuclear power plants," Dr. Cohen says. "All these carry a low-level radiation risk with no direct experimental evidence. We've estimated everything."

Dr. Cohen has studied U.S. cities with high or low levels of residential radon. Surprisingly, he says, the high-dose counties had low rates of lung cancer, and the low-dose counties had high rates. He has no explanation.

Let's examine the danger of radon. Even though the risk of lung cancer from radon remains fuzzy, the New Jersey Department of Environmental Protection came up with some comparisons of annual numbers of deaths attributed to indoor radon and some other daily risks in New Jersey:

Drinking water	10
Fires	140
Home accidents	460
Indoor radon	500
Car accidents	980

So if you're the kind of person who nails down rugs at home to prevent people from tripping, or puts in a smoke detector, or fastens your car seat belt, then you'll do something about radon in your home. The EPA guesses that fewer than 5 percent of Americans have tested their homes for the presence of radon.

You can look at the risk another way by comparing the danger of cancer from radon to the cancer danger from other sources of pollution. So here's the number of annual estimated cancer cases in New Jersey from various sources. These calculations come from the state's Department of Environmental Protection:

Consumer exposure to chemicals	5
Drinking water	10
Hazardous waste dumps	35
Toxic air pollutants	60
Pesticides on foods	175
Indoor radon	500

Now isn't this a signal for you to panic, to move out of a radon-contaminated house, to run to your doctor for a cancer examination? At first glance, perhaps. But despite the EPA's figures, other data show that radon jeopardy is no greater than many other daily risks. And, most important, you can do something about radon risk.

First, let's take a closer look at radon as a substance. It comes from uranium atoms, which are found in most rocks and soils. Uranium is radioactive, which means it gives off rays and particles. As it does so, the uranium atom turns into a radium atom, also radioactive. In time, the radium atom converts into a radon atom, which floats out of the soil as a radioactive gas.

After the radon atoms are released from radium, they break down radioactively into four different atoms: lead, bismuth, and two types of polonium. These are called radon daughters. As you breathe air contaminated with radon or its daughters, the radioactive atoms stick to the linings of your lungs. They then break up, shooting out radioactive particles of helium. The helium particles crash into the cells of your lungs, changing their chemistry and triggering cancer.

So the sequence is like so:

Uranium—> Radium—> Radon—>
Radondaughter—> Cancer

Scientists measure the radon in your house in picocuries per liter of air. A liter is about a quart. A curie—named for Marie and Pierre Curie, the discoverers of radium—is the amount of radiation given off by a gram of radium. *Pico* means one-trillionth. So a picocurie is the radiation given off by a trillionth of a gram of radium. Yes, that tiny amount of radon radiation can hurt you.

The EPA says that if your living quarters have 4 picocuries of radon per liter of air, your lifetime risk of lung cancer in such a house is 1 percent. Put another way, of 100 people living in the house, one will get lung cancer from radon.

Here comes the really confusing part, the part that has stirred most of the controversy: The 1-in-100 risk estimate is based on your spending 70 years of your life in a house polluted with 4 picocuries of radon per liter of air. But the average American moves every 7 years. You have only a small chance of moving into one such radon-polluted house after another. So, if you lived only 7 years in such a house, your chances of developing lung cancer from exposure to radon would drop to 1 in 1,000, provided you were not exposed to radon before or after. But radon is nearly everywhere—the danger builds up.

One study in New Jersey did find a connection between lung cancer in women and the radon content of the homes in which they lived. Other states are trying to duplicate this study.

Then there's the question of exactly how many homes in the United States have radon levels above 4 picocuries per liter of air. The EPA says 10 percent of homes go above that level. That could mean as many as 9 million dwellings. But Anthony Nero found only 6 percent of homes above 4 picocuries. And because

people move around, he says, probably only 1 percent of the population gets the 4 picocurie exposure.

A final complicating factor is cigarette smoking. Of the 177,000 deaths from lung cancer each year in this country, experts say cigarette smoking causes about 85 percent of them—150,000. Between 7,000 and 30,000 may be radon induced. In addition, there is evidence that smoking and radon together act more powerfully than simply adding the risks of each.

If you live a long time in a house with a radon level of 4 picocuries and you smoke, you could double your risk of getting lung cancer. A two-pack-a-day smoker runs a 30 percent chance of getting the disease; in such a radon environment, the odds of getting lung cancer reach 60 percent.

This makes the analysis of radon risk devilishly difficult. No wonder figures for radon deaths vary wildly.

Dr. Harley, for example, estimates that 10,000 Americans die each year from radon, the National Academy of Sciences puts it at 13,000, and the EPA estimates swing from 7,000 to as high as 30,000. Dr. Nero says that, despite the uncertainties, the figure of 15,000 lung cancer deaths annually from radon appears to be the best guess.

Dr. Rosalyn Yalow, a Nobel Prize winner and radiation expert, says that radon is not a significant health hazard in the absence of smoking. She also says we are wasting millions of dollars on radon testing.

Nevertheless, William Belanger, radon representative for the EPA's Region III, which covers Pennsylvania, Delaware, Maryland, Virginia, and West Virginia, says, "Radon is the number two cause of lung cancer in the United States. Smoking is number one. Because more people are exposed to it, radon is a greater threat than any other pollutants."

Radon radiation, on average, far exceeds the radiation that comes from other natural sources, nuclear power plants, or medical X rays.

Nationally, the EPA has counseled that every home below the third floor be tested. Drs. Nero, Cohen, and Harley say that's nonsense. To test every house in any meaningful way would cost billions of dollars. There are more than 90 million homes in America. At $20 a test, that's $1.8 billion for the first test alone.

The cheapest method to test for radon places a can of charcoal in the basement for 3 days. It absorbs the radon gas. A special laboratory test measures the amount of gas and calculates how much radon there was in each liter of air. The canister method gives only a 3-day profile of the radon levels, which could be totally misleading: The annual average level actually could be much lower or much higher than a 3-day test would indicate. Correct readings would depend on the amount of radon in the soil, whether your house has cracks in the basement (if it even has a basement), how drafty your house is, and the climate you find yourself in (a house in a cold climate sucks in more radon than a building in a warm climate). The EPA says, however, that the short-term test gives the right answer 90 percent of the time.

The scientific community is urging the EPA to make a thorough nationwide survey to identify regions where homes are likely to have higher levels of radon. Once those areas are known, people there can test their homes thoroughly with an instrument that picks up the radioactivity over a period of several months.

Dr. Nero wants to get to those 300,000 residents of the 100,000 homes where radon levels approach or exceed the safe limits for uranium miners.

Stanley Watras lived in such a home in Boyertown, Pennsylvania. He worked as a construction engineer at the Limerick Nuclear Power Generating Station at Pottstown, Pennsylvania. Safety officers there found that Watras's clothing was contaminated with radon, though he worked nowhere near any radiation.

"I went to the radiation detection station. When I stepped into it, I blew out the monitor. Every inch of my body was contaminated. Red alert! A bulb went off in my head: I knew I had to be bringing radon from home." He took his wife and two children to a motel and then rented another house for 7 months.

"My first reactions were terror—horror—thinking about my family, what they had been living in," Mr. Watras remembers.

The Philadelphia Electric Company volunteered to measure Mr. Watras's house and found 4,400 picocuries of radon per liter of air in the cellar, 3,200 in the living room, 1,800 in the bedrooms. The Watras home was far worse than an old-time uranium mine!

The electric company agreed to take on the Watras family's house as an experiment. Contractors sealed and caulked the cracks in the basement. They laid air pipes under the concrete foundation slab and on top of the soil to suck the radon away. With fans, they decreased the air pressure in the house to keep the radon out. They lowered the levels from as high as 4,400 picocuries down to 4 picocuries, the highest level rated safe by the EPA. Mr. Watras is now in the business of inspecting and installing radon correction devices. He still lives in the house.

If you live in areas like northern New Jersey, eastern Pennsylvania, or southern Connecticut, where many houses have been found to have high radon counts, you might find it worthwhile to get a charcoal can and do the test. Your state environmental protection agency will tell you where to get a reliable test kit. Some states, like New Jersey, will retest your house if your own test reveals a high level of radon.

If you live in a high-rise apartment house, the chances of radon contamination are low. As you go higher above the ground, the radon levels drop. The EPA suggests testing all schools.

The word on the risk of radon is this: It's real, it's bigger than most other environmental risks of cancer, but probably it's not so big as the government implies.

By 1996, additional studies indicated that the radon cancer burden was not as great as the EPA said. The controversy continues. If you're worried, test your home.

For a brochure on radon and how to buy a home test kit, call (800) 505-RADON.

Wiping Out Allergies

A TINY SPECK OF DUST LANDS ON THE INSIDE lining of your nose. Within minutes, the spot flushes red and swells up. You sneeze. Your nostril pours out fluid. More dust. More sneezes. More fluid. It's hay fever. You have a full-blown allergy attack.

Something is out of kilter in your immune system. This system that fights viruses, bacteria, and fungi now overreacts to that plant particle. You suffer the misery of a runny nose, itching, red eyes, headache, and congestion. Worse, you could end up with asthma, a disease that throttles breathing.

Forty-one million Americans—one in six—suffer from allergy, a disordered immune response. They spend up to $5 billion a year warding off the ill effects of plant pollen, mold, mites, spores, foods, animal hairs, even cockroach dust.

Help is on the way: Scientists have made two basic biological discoveries that could in a decade vanquish allergies—no more sneezes, wheezes, itches, running noses, bleary eyes; no more fearful reactions to a piece of fish.

Dr. Gillian Shepherd, head of the allergy clinic at the New York Hospital–Cornell Medical Center in Manhattan, says that the new findings could one day put her out of business.

"One discovery could lead directly to drugs that interrupt the immune system's overreaction," Dr. Shepherd says. "The second finding has pinpointed natural substances that turn off that system."

Leslie Naschek, 28, an accountant in New York City, can hardly wait. "I'm allergic to dust, weeds, and grass," she says. "Two years ago, I suddenly started having a runny nose and sneezing. It's difficult, walking around with a tissue in your hand all the time. I couldn't sleep. I took antihistamines. They helped, but not a lot."

Giant drug companies are searching for those chemicals that will cut short the allergic reaction. Three compounds currently are being tested in allergic patients.

And in medical laboratories worldwide, scientists have come close to unraveling the mystery of allergy attacks.

Leslie Naschek, researchers found, fell victim to chemical reactions in her blood tissues. To take a peek at the allergic reaction, let's start with a grain of ragweed pollen. Under the microscope, it looks like a basketball with thorns.

On the ragweed pollen's surface lies a protein molecule too tiny to see, even with a microscope. It consists of long chains of thousands of atoms of carbon, oxygen, hydrogen, and nitrogen. Living things produce hundreds of such proteins, each of a different size and shape.

When that ragweed pollen lands on the nostril's lining, it finds its way to a living white blood cell, called a mast cell. The mast cell responds as if struck by an ax. It pours out a dozen chemicals, among them histamine. Histamine flows to nerve receptors, causing itching. Histamine makes blood vessels leak serum, resulting in a runny nose and teary eyes. The chemical also contracts the airways (bronchi) of your lungs, slowing airflow. A host of other proteins—such as pollens, dust particles, cat dander, insect dust—can trigger similar reactions.

More than 20 years ago, scientists realized that if they could block histamine, they could relieve the symptoms of hay fever. Chemists developed several antihistamines, which relieve the itching and liquid discharge. Nonprescription antihistamines such as Benadryl and

ChlorTrimeton are sold for a few cents a pill.

"With most antihistamines, since people develop tolerance," Dr. Shepherd notes, "they need to switch to another one with a different chemical formula."

These drugs also make people sleepy. They interfere with thinking and judgment. A few years ago, the Merrell Dow Company developed Seldane, a prescription drug. An antihistamine, Seldane doesn't reach the brain, so it cannot make you drowsy. Janssen Pharmaceutical brought out Hismanal, also a prescription antihistamine that does not cause drowsiness. It is taken once a day.

Doris Palazzo, 31, an office manager for a Manhattan allergist, gets hit hard by allergy discomfort each June. She takes Seldane. "Seldane has helped a lot," she says. "It's the one thing that doesn't make me fall asleep."

Another drug, cromolyn sodium, has given doctors a powerful tool to prevent allergic reaction. This chemical stops the pollen (and any other allergy trigger) from reaching the mast cells. It can be sprayed into the nose up to five times a day.

A few years ago, cortisone, a hormone that your body makes, was produced in spray form. "Cortisone has been a huge boon to the treatment of local allergic problems in the nose and of asthma," Dr. Shepherd says. "It is the single most effective medication. In spray form, you get it just where you need it— on the surface."

Although cortisone is not safe in pill form—it induces fluid retention, weight gain, and loss of calcium from the bone— it does not cause these side effects in spray form. The amount in the blood-stream is so small that it causes no problem.

The latest research shows how the foreign protein (such as pollen) cripples the mast cell.

When the ragweed pollen comes to rest on your nose tissue, white cells— B cells—gather around and make a protein called IgE. The IgE and the ragweed protein fit together like a key in a lock.

Here is the first of three major scientific discoveries: For every foreign protein, your body's B cells join to make a special IgE that fits only that protein. So if you're allergic to grass pollen, you have an IgE that fits grass protein.

The second discovery is that the surface of each mast cell contains thousands of protein molecules that fit the ends of the IgE molecules. These are called IgE receptors. So you have a sandwich: the IgE attaches to the mast cell, the ragweed protein to the IgE. When that happens, the histamine and other chemicals gush forth.

The third discovery: Scientists have been able to create in the test tube unlimited amounts of IgE receptors. It will be possible to find a substance that will fill the receptor so that the IgE can't attach to and cripple the mast cell. The mast cell's allergic reaction won't happen. The allergic chain of events will be stopped!

Dr. Jean-Pierre Kinet and colleagues at the National Institute of Allergy and Infectious Diseases isolated the IgE receptor. Pharmaceutical companies hope to use it, he says, "to test 50,000 different drugs to see if any could inhibit the binding of IgE to the receptor."

Scientists also have tested substances occurring naturally in the human body called alpha- and gamma-interferon. Normally, these are made in tiny amounts by white cells in the blood. Five years ago, bioengineers created them for the first time in the test tube in large quantities. These substances are able to block IgE in the lab but, so far, not in patients.

At the same time, researchers are closing in on the causes of asthma. Dr. William W. Busse, professor of medicine at the University of Wisconsin Medical School in Madison, has fixed on the common cold. "Grandma may have been right in saying, 'Johnny has too many colds, and it makes his asthma worse,'" he says.

Dr. Busse found that cold-virus infection intensifies the allergic reaction in asthma, attacking white cells that release substances that cause inflammation. It is assumed that the surfaces of the bronchi swell up, turn red, and get hot.

Scientists are beginning to hypothesize that it may be the inflammation following the allergic reaction that actually causes damage.

"I could say, 'Avoid a cold if you have asthma,'" Dr. Busse says. "But it would be empty advice—it's so hard to do. Or, 'Avoid shaking hands.' The virus is passed from hand to nose. Or, 'Keep kids out of school and out of touch with other kids.' But who would do that?"

Dr. Michael F. Mullarkey and his colleagues at Virginia Mason Clinic in Seattle, Washington, have found a new way to fight the underlying inflammation in asthma. It might even reverse the disease.

Until now, doctors would give cortisone pills to patients with severe asthma. The pills quelled the inflammation and saved their lives. The cortisone also swelled their faces and softened their bones.

By accident, Dr. Mullarkey happened on methotrexate, a drug used to treat leukemia and severe psoriasis. He was treating a patient with psoriasis who also had severe asthma. Her psoriasis improved and so did her asthma. Out of 25 patients with severe asthma who were treated for 2 years, 24 (all but one) cut their cortisone needs by at least 50 percent. Fifteen stopped taking cortisone altogether. Four have no sign of asthma.

After the treatment, Marilyn Tonstad, 54, did not have an asthma flare-up for at least 6 months. "I used to not be able to breathe at home, walking from room to room," she says. The treatment remains controversial.

Doctors also can desensitize allergic reactions in patients. One method entails giving weekly injections of the offending protein in gradually increasing amounts until the reaction to it subsides. Then shots are given monthly to prevent further allergy attacks.

There is proof that desensitization works for patients allergic to bee stings. Bee-sting allergy can kill—by stopping your breathing. And desensitization does work in hay fever and other pollen allergies, but not for everybody and not every time. Before desensitizing you, an allergist will test you, putting tiny amounts of various substances under your skin. Those that create itchy red welts are the offending allergens. Doctors also can measure IgE directly in the blood.

No other allergy test works. Some doctors have used the "cytotoxic" test for food allergies, in which a patient's white blood cells are isolated and tested for their reaction to food products in small amounts. If the cells die, the patient is pronounced allergic to those food products. The American Academy of Allergy and Immunology says the cytotoxic test has no scientific basis.

One way to control allergic reaction is to avoid the substances that trigger your allergies.

Mites are hard to avoid. The tiny pests are found everywhere. They grow in damp carpets and mattresses. And when their bodies fall to dust, their proteins get in your nose and lungs. They provoke allergic reactions, particularly in asthmatics. So do cockroaches.

Thorough housecleaning and frequent vacuuming to prevent dust accumulation can help dramatically to eliminate allergic reactions caused by these pests.

All the scientists with whom we spoke forecast a bright future for allergy and asthma sufferers. As biologists have uncovered the mysteries that cause allergy, chemists have gone to work to put those discoveries to quick use.

In a few years, an allergic reaction may be treated as easily as a headache.

They're Helping People Breathe Easier

WHEN ASTHMA ATTACKS YOUR LUNGS, YOU GET the feeling you're drowning. You open your mouth for breath, but no air seems to come in. You utter a wheezing, whistling sound and breathe faster—more than 20 times in a minute.

You can get air in, but not out. Your chest contracts with the effort. And your heart begins to pound, sometimes at double its normal rate. In an extreme case, your lips turn blue. You look and feel as though you're about to die.

Each year, 5,000 Americans die of asthma. The figure of 5,000 is small compared with the 1.5 million people in this country who yearly experience heart attacks. But with more than 13 million Americans suffering from this disease, according to an estimate by the American Lung Association and consequently missing an estimated 3 million days from work annually for people over age 18, asthma is of major concern.

At the Mayo Medical School in Rochester, Minnesota, doctors discovered a mild form of asthma that could swell by 20 percent the number of people who suffer from the disease. Dr. Edward O'Connell, professor of pediatrics, allergy, and immunology at the school, says that people with a "cough-variant asthma" cough off and on for years without realizing they have a problem. "It leads us to think that asthma is much more common than we thought," he says.

Every year, asthmatic Americans spend more than $6.9 billion on drugs, doctor visits, and hospital stays.

Asthma once ruled the family of Harold Higgins of Whitehouse, Texas. Paige, 6, and her brother Taylor, 4, both have suffered from severe asthma since infancy. "Every day," recalls their mother, Anita, "we were consumed with worry about how the children were doing. Seeing your child turn blue and unable to breathe is a very frightening experience. They knew us well at the Mother Frances Hospital emergency room."

Doctors know more about how to help parents deal with an asthmatic child. They have new drugs that open up the airways of the lungs to free patients to live normal lives. Such celebrities as Christopher Reeve, Jim "Catfish" Hunter, and Elizabeth Taylor are among the many who have achieved success despite asthma. And, most important, scientists are getting closer to discovering the biological causes of the condition.

"We used to think asthma was all in your head, that emotional problems caused it," says Dr. O'Connell. "We still don't know what causes it, but we do know what makes it worse. We are now trying to understand asthma on a molecular level."

Dr. Allan Weinstein, an asthma expert in Washington, D.C., says he became a doctor because he'd suffered from allergies and asthma. "There is no cure," he says, "but there's no reason to put up with the symptoms. We can treat them."

An understanding of asthma is rapidly increasing now. Researchers have uncovered possible causes both inside and outside the body.

To find the inside causes, doctors must examine the interiors of the nose, throat, and lungs, traveling through tubes that branch out like an upside-down tree. These tubes are called bronchi. The bronchi contain little muscles and a thin skin covers their inner walls. Normally, air travels through them to add to your blood's oxygen supply.

During an asthma attack, several frightening things can happen at once. The bronchial muscles, from your throat down, contract violently, almost closing the airway. The bronchial walls become inflamed. The skin covering the walls swells up with fluid. And a thick, sticky liquid fills the remaining space, making breathing almost impossible.

One of the factors causing this reaction may be traced to the white blood cells. White cells usually protect against germs. But, in asthma, they flock to your lungs and release a substance that severely irritates the bronchi. Some doctors are studying that substance, hoping to learn how to direct it away from the lungs. (The reaction and the thick irritating substance are not unlike the symptoms of cystic fibrosis. Scientists have discovered a chemical that liquifies that viscous discharge.)

Meanwhile, scientists have tracked down some outside sources that trigger the asthmatic response. Chief among them is allergy. Dr. Michael Kaliner headed the allergic disease research at the National Institutes of Health in Bethesda, Maryland. He reports that 90 percent of asthmatics under the age of 30 have allergies, but fewer than 50 percent of older asthmatics have allergies.

Dr. Kaliner cites hay fever—caused by allergies to ragweed, tree, and grass pollen—and sneezing fits in reaction to cat dander, mold spores, mites, and cockroaches. These all-too-common substances exist either in powder or particle form. Once inhaled, inflammation of the nose or lungs results.

Dr. Thomas Platts-Mills, professor of medicine at the University of Virginia in Charlottesville, maintains that house dust—loaded with particles of dander, spores, mites, and roaches—is a leading cause of asthma. "We are convinced," says Dr. Platts-Mills, "that at least part of the increase in sicknesses and deaths from asthma can be attributed to changes in our houses over the last 20 years." He notes that the changes create breeding grounds for the mites, which thrive in environments with the following:

- Fitted carpets that can't be cleaned (Vacuum cleaning doesn't work against mites.)
- Central heating that keeps mites warm year-round
- Airtight homes that maintain the humidity in which mites thrive
- Cool-wash detergents that allow mites to escape unscathed from your washer (Hot water kills them.)

In addition, infestations of cockroaches and mites may account for the rise of asthma cases in our inner cities, where, says Dr. Charles Reed of the Mayo Medical School, asthma is far more common than elsewhere.

Dr. Floyd J. Malveaux, of the Johns Hopkins Medical School in Baltimore, says that young African Americans with asthma are five to six times more likely to die of the disease than young whites. He says he doubts that mites and roaches account entirely for the high asthma rate in our inner cities. Another factor he cites is that African Americans get poorer medical care than whites.

Aspergillus, one particular kind of mold, accounts for severe complications in many cases of asthma. Under a microscope, this mold looks like a tiny golf-ball covered with fine hairs. It grows in dank cellars, barns, wet roof gutters, and other damp places. It sends out microscopic spores—tiny seeds—that aggravate asthma. An even more damaging aspect of *Aspergillus* is that it can grow in your lungs.

Virus infections can trigger asthma, too. Bronchitis, colds, and flulike diseases can make existing asthma cases worse. Some people have asthma symptoms only when they have a cold or other virus.

Jo LoCicero, 61, of Manhattan, nearly died after a virus infection led to an asthmatic explosion in her chest. "I tried to ignore it until it was almost too late," she recalls. "I wasn't feeling well—gasping for air when I talked—but I went to work anyway. I felt total fear that I wouldn't make it. I ended up in the hospital for 7 days."

Simply sleeping can worsen asthma symptoms. According to Dr. Robert Ballard, up to 80 percent of asthma deaths occur between midnight and 6 A.M. During these hours, the body circulates more hormones, which can cause breathing tubes to squeeze shut. Dr. Ballard studies asthmatics in a sleep lab at the National Jewish Center for Immunology and Respiratory Medicine in Denver. "I feel hopeful that we can help these patients," he says.

You also can fall prey to asthma activators at work: Wood and vegetable dusts, industrial chemicals and plastics, metal salts, animal and insect materials, drugs and enzymes—together, they may cause up to 15 percent of all asthma cases in the workplace.

Jo LoCicero may have contracted asthma from industrial products. Living in an old apartment building, she inhaled the dust from a renovation project in a neighbor's apartment. She says she never had a symptom until she started breathing in those dust particles.

If you already have asthma, be aware that certain medicines or foods can bring on an attack. Aspirin and similar compounds can aggravate asthma. Patients also need to consult their doctors about the "beta-blocking" drugs that relieve migraines and high blood pressure and also protect against heart attack.

If you eat in salad bars, you may have consumed sulfites—tasteless preservatives that prevent browning in raw vegetables and fruits. In asthmatics, such chemicals could induce a fatal attack.

One more important cause of asthma is exercise. For reasons that scientists can only guess, intense physical activity brings on contractions of the bronchial tree. Dr. Kaliner says that "exercise asthma" interferes with the school and leisure activities of most, if not all, children who have asthma.

Fortunately, in most instances, any of several medicines taken before exercise will stave off an asthmatic storm in the lungs. Breathing warm, humid air and wearing a face mask in winter also helps. The experts say that for the asthma patient who takes the necessary precautions, there's no reason not to exercise.

For example, even though exercise can trigger an asthmatic attack, treatments given just before physical exertion do prevent the gasping spasms. In the 1984 Olympic Games, Nancy Hogshead of Jacksonville, Florida, then 22, swam the 200-meter butterfly competition. In her last few strokes, powerful spasms gripped her chest. She missed the bronze medal by 0.07 seconds. That's how she discovered she had asthma. She doesn't compete in Olympic events anymore, but she does inhale albuterol before swimming. No more spasms.

World-class track and field star, and a medal-winning Olympian, Jackie Joyner-Kersee also copes with asthma. Before she takes off on a sprint, a long jump, or a javelin throw, she issues two muted coughs, and away she goes.

Today's asthma patients have plenty of medicines to help them. Doctors have prescribed some of them for 150 years. They relax the bronchial muscles when in spasm. They also clear out mucus. Modern chemistry also has created longer-lasting forms of theophylline, an old standby, that give extended relief.

But doctors now prefer the beta-adrenergic agonists—medicines that also relax the bronchial muscles and prevent spasms. Two of the best such drugs are albuterol and terbutaline.

Cromolyn, an important drug, prevents asthma attacks. It doesn't stop them while they are happening, but it definitely helps in eliminating inflammation. Inhaled, cromolyn prevents various kinds of asthma, including the types that are induced by exercise and allergy. Ketotifen, a relatively new drug that works like cromolyn, has been used abroad but is not yet approved for use in this country.

Steroid hormones in the cortisone family can ease the symptoms of asthma in all but the most severe cases. These drugs can be taken by mouth, injected, inhaled, or spread on the skin. But they can produce *many* untoward side effects unless doctors and patients treat them with caution. In high doses, the steroids taken orally can cause high blood pressure, weaken bones and muscles, and trigger diabetes.

Doctors recommend getting rid of the allergy in situations where they can pin the asthma on an allergic response. In such cases, long-term prevention of attacks is effected with small injections of the offending material—pollen, mold spores, and the like. Although many allergy specialists hold that these injections purge the allergic response, not all of the experts agree. Still, in severe cases, some doctors feel the method is worth a try.

All doctors agree that, no matter what, if an asthma patient senses an oncoming episode, he or she must act fast to stop the attack with medicine. Make no mistake: *Asthma can kill.*

Dr. R. Michael Sly of Children's Hospital, National Medical Center, in Washington, D.C., says he is appalled by the recent increase in asthma death rates among young people.

In a 1979–86 study of children and young adults, Dr. Sly found that deaths from asthma had quadrupled among 10- to 14-year-olds and more than doubled among 15- to 24-year-olds. A lightning-fast asthma attack robbed Karin Johnson of her life in 1994. The 19-year-old college student collapsed while dancing at a bar in Columbus, Ohio. Within minutes, she turned blue. Neither her friends nor paramedics could revive her.

Karin's mother, Jean Johnson, recalls, "We didn't know you could have such a severe attack so quickly. Now we realize that cigarette smoke [like that] at the bar could be the trigger."

Ms. Johnson had said at times that she felt "fed up" with her severe and lifelong case of asthma, says Mrs. Johnson. "But," she adds, "Karin loved life and was not self-destructive."

Researchers at the National Jewish Center for Immunology and Respiratory Medicine in Denver found, however, that children with severe and prolonged cases of asthma suffer psychologically as well as physically. Some become so depressed that they tire of fighting for health and make an unconscious decision to just let go. The violent discomfort of asthma may prove immensely frightening to asthmatic children, and vigilance on the part of parents and others is warranted and urged.

One medical theory is that some children may be passively committing suicide by ignoring both their medicines and their worsening respiratory symptoms. Depression is a signal.

The very real threat of death and the frightening experience of watching their asthmatic child turn blue will generate overprotective parents, says Dr. François Haas, of New York University Medical Center in Manhattan. He explains, "They tell their child, 'Don't exercise, don't run. I don't want you to have an attack!' It takes effort to deal with that and create as normal an environment as possible for the child. The parent has to become an expert on asthma."

The Asthma and Allergy Foundation of America is helping children learn more about asthma too. Through a special program, the foundation trains children to recognize the warning signs of an asthma attack. They're taught what to do if they start to wheeze or feel a tightening in the chest. And they learn how to avoid the things that trigger an attack.

Parents need to learn what to watch for—such as whether the child overuses his spray medicine or is not using it at all. And parents have to guard against being overprotective. Children can feel confused by too much concern and caution; psychological problems could result.

Videotapes taken of parent-child interactions at the National Jewish Center in Denver reveal that asthmatic youngsters get their way three fourths of the time; healthy children, only one third of the time. It is a quite human tendency, after all, to use a handicap to one's advantage. Often unconsciously, asthmatic children pick up the slightest signal of concern from their parents and learn how to manipulate them. Counseling for the children and their caregivers can be helpful here.

Happily, research is paying off handsomely with new drugs and new techniques for diagnosing asthma and training both patients and their caregivers to cope with it. Unfortunately, figures are rising on the cases of death and sickness from asthma. And the reasons why remain a mystery.

For further information, including videos and booklets for classroom use, write to the Asthma and Allergy Foundation of America, 1125 15th Street, NW, Suite 502, Washington, D.C.; or call (800) 7-ASTHMA.

Taking the Bite Out of Lyme Disease

IT BEGINS WITH THE PAINLESS BITE OF A TICK, which may be as small as a poppy seed but can swell to 100 times its weight with the blood of its victim. The bite can end in devastating arthritis, severe heart problems, and even brain inflammation. Or in no problem at all.

A tick bit Cyndi Monahan, an artist from Mount Hope, New Jersey. She wound up with hot, swollen joints in her hands, shoulder, knees, and ankles.

"I couldn't move," says Ms. Monahan, now 32. "For the next year, I was in the fetal position, with my arms locked. I couldn't walk. I lay on the couch and watched TV. I used to teach aerobics and lift weights. I could bench-press 160 pounds. After Lyme disease hit me, I was lucky to be able to lift a glass of water."

Essentially, that bite paralyzed her. The tick had injected her with a load of bacteria, which then multiplied by the millions. Her body's immune system counterattacked, creating chemicals to fight the invaders. Unhappily, those very chemicals assaulted not only the bacteria from the tick but also her joints, making them inflamed and painful.

Those ticks carried Lyme disease, an ailment unknown in the United States before 1975. Now it is spreading most rapidly through the Northeast, mid-Atlantic, upper Midwest, and Pacific Coast states. The federal Centers for Disease Control (CDC) counted more than 22,000 cases between 1982 and 1989; since then, 65,500 more cases have been reported. The tallies are still coming in.

Lyme disease—named for the Connecticut town in which it was discovered—now outranks all other human infections carried by ticks, including Rocky Mountain spotted fever.

Dr. David Dennis, who heads the CDC's Lyme disease program in Boulder, Colorado, says, "This is a very important problem. We have recorded no deaths from Lyme disease, but many of its victims become severely disabled."

Fortunately, only a small percentage of people infected with Lyme disease go on to suffer from its harshest, long-term symptoms. Exactly how many suffer from its extreme effects is unknown. Estimates range from 5 to 20 percent.

Most people—even those living in tick-infested areas—can escape the disease if they take simple steps to avoid the ticks or, if they are bitten, take powerful

antibiotics as soon as a sign of infection appears.

The history of Lyme disease reads like a detective story. It began in 1975 with Dr. Allen Steere, a young physician studying arthritis at the Yale School of Medicine in New Haven, Connecticut. He learned of an outbreak of arthritis among children and adults around Lyme and nearby towns in Connecticut.

The story includes two mothers who would not accept their doctors' diagnoses. Judith Mensch's 8-year-old daughter, Anne, had fallen ill with severe arthritis. And Polly Murray, together with her husband and three sons, also had come down with the terrible symptoms. Both called their state health department, and the Mensch family also contacted the CDC. Those calls were to have a profound impact. The agencies referred both families to Dr. Steere.

"It was unusual for children to have arthritis," says Dr. Steere. "I was interested in that."

Step by step, he gathered data on 50 more cases. They yielded these clues to put the puzzle together:

• The illness began in summer or early fall, not winter.
• The cases were in rural communities. When the disease hit more than one member of a family, it occurred in different years. That meant it was not being passed directly from one person to another. Something was carrying it.

• Some of the adults recalled a rash on a leg or an arm before the arthritis set in. They thought it was an insect bite. The rash was strange. It began as a small red spot and expanded in a large circle, up to 20 inches in diameter, with a white center like a bull's-eye of a target. Such a rash was known in Europe to be caused by a tick.

Putting it all together, Dr. Steere concluded that a tick had attached itself to his patients and injected them with the disease while sucking their blood. At that time, Dr. Steere suspected the disease was caused by a virus.

In 1977, a patient actually brought Dr. Steere the tick that had bit him. Specialists identified it as belonging to a family of ticks called Ixodes (pronounced icks-oh-deez), thousands of which were then gathered from the Lyme area.

Finally, in 1981, Dr. Willy Burgdorfer, of Rocky Mountain Laboratories in Hamilton, Montana, dissected a tick and found the species of spirochete that transmits Lyme disease. Other spirochetes (spiral-shaped bacteria) cause syphilis, relapsing fevers, and trench mouth.

The spirochete that transmits Lyme disease is named for Dr. Burgdorfer: *Borrelia burgdorferi*. Soon Dr. Steere—later with the New England Medical Center, Tufts School of Medicine in Boston—and others isolated this spirochete from the blood of a Lyme disease patient. In rare cases, unborn children get it from their mothers, but humans generally don't pass Lyme disease to each other.

Dr. Raymond Dattwyler, director of the Lyme disease center at the State University of New York at Stony Brook, has become an expert on the disease. He says it has different phases.

In many victims, the disease starts with the rash, caused by the invasion and movement of the spirochetes. This is followed by flulike symptoms—headaches, chills, fever, achiness. Some have the flulike symptoms but not rash. In the next phase, the spirochetes spread through the blood to many organs and can cause memory loss, brain inflammation, even heart or liver problems.

Tony Gwiazdowski, 38, of Hillsborough, New Jersey, almost died of Lyme disease. He went for weeks, nearly passing out from fatigue. Finally, his physician, Dr. Joseph Smith, had him hospitalized and implanted with a pacemaker for 9 days to boost his heart rate.

"Tony had a heart rate that was so slow it was incompatible with life," Dr. Smith recalls. When he learned that Mr. Gwiazdowski previously had had a rash, he thought of Lyme disease and quickly gave him massive doses of antibiotics. In a few days, the patient's heart resumed its normal rate.

"I guess I was lucky," Mr. Gwiazdowski says.

In the later phase of Lyme disease, some patients are stricken with mild to severe arthritis. Treatment now consists of powerful antibiotics—doxycycline and amoxicillin for early infection, ceftriaxone for the chronic condition. Experts agree that if Lyme disease is treated early, most of its severe ills rarely arise.

"We have had not treatment failures in the early stages," Dr. Dattwyler reports. "In late treatment, we cure the majority. Occasionally, people have a really bad time of it. Some have permanent damage, if they wait too long to get medical care." If symptoms persist after treatment, doctors are not sure whether they are due to Lyme disease or a secondary cause.

The antibiotics did not appear to help Cyndi Monahan, even when given intravenously. Through the patient grapevine, she heard about a theory of Dr. Henry Heimlich of Cincinnati, who also invented the now-famous Heimlich maneuver for rescuing a person choking on food.

Dr. Heimlich was impressed with the similarities between syphilis and Lyme disease. Both were caused by spirochetes and produced a similar variety of symptoms in several organs. In a letter to the *New England Journal of Medicine*, he suggested malaria treatment for stubborn Lyme cases. Injection of malaria-infected blood had been a treatment for syphilis before the discovery of penicillin.

So Ms. Monahan went to a lab in Mexico, where they are studying mild malaria. She was injected with blood from a malaria patient. "In 2 days," she says, "I got the fevers. They got up to 106 degrees. The fevers kept coming and lasted 5 to 10 hours a day. In 3 weeks, I noticed a difference. The joint swellings went down."

Later that year, the CDC in Atlanta, Georgia, issued a bulletin saying malaria can kill, and patients taking malaria therapy run the risk of contracting undetected secondary infections from the blood they're given. The malaria treatment is no longer recommended.

Controversy also exists over Lyme disease diagnoses. Some "Lyme doctors"—physicians who specialize in treating the disease—reportedly give the diagnosis of Lyme disease to almost any patient showing some of its symptoms. Dr. Steere reports that at the Robert Wood Johnson University Hospital in New Brunswick, New Jersey, doctors carefully examined the first 100 patients said to have Lyme disease and found that only 37 actually did have it.

Current blood tests are inaccurate. They measure the antibodies that your immune system makes to attack the Lyme disease spirochetes. For example, persons with trench mouth will test positive for Lyme disease even if they don't have it. Dr. Dattwyler and his colleagues are developing a far more accurate test, and the CDC is evaluating existing tests.

For now, a person could register positive with the antibody test but *not* have the disease or test negative yet *have* it.

Dr. Dattwyler says, to be safe, see your own doctor first. He or she will refer you to a specialist if Lyme disease is suspected.

"See someone whose practice doesn't consist mostly of Lyme disease patients," he cautions.

You also can protect yourself by avoiding areas that your health department says are tick infested. To keep out ticks, wear long pants and a long-sleeved shirt. Tuck your pants legs into your socks and tape shut the openings around the tops of the socks. Keep your collar buttoned, and tape the sleeves shut around your wrists.

Each day, inspect your body for the tick. It might look like a poppy seed—or a small, plump raisin, if it is engorged with blood—hanging on your skin. Don't mash it. Remove it with tweezers, pulling steadily. Inspect your children, your spouse, and any others who live with you, for either the tick or signs of its bite. Have someone check you over, too. Fast medical treatment is the best remedy. Also check your pets for ticks.

You can use tick-repellent chemicals on your skin and clothing. The best contain a chemical ingredient called DEET, but it may be dangerous for some adults in large concentrations and quite dangerous for small children. Permethrin, which kills ticks, is sold in some states for use on clothing.

Ticks generally are most dangerous in summer and fall, but in the northern Midwest the peak season for bites spans November to June. The tick starts as an egg laid by an adult in the spring. In summer, it hatches a larva. The larva feeds once in the summer by sucking blood from a small mammal, such as a mouse. If the mouse carries the Lyme-disease spirochetes—and in some areas, half of them do—the larva carries the spirochetes too. The larva winters over in the ground. The following spring, it becomes a nymph infected with the spirochetes. It too feeds once in the summer on birds and mammals—dogs, deer, mice, and people. By fall, adult ticks attach themselves to the same group of creatures, mating if possible. Females survive the winter and lay eggs in the spring.

Several laboratories are working on a vaccine to fight the spirochetes. It would stimulate your body's immune system, causing your blood to attack and kill the invading bacteria. But that won't be available for at least 2 years.

Dr. Steere says, "I feel as if I have been on a journey with this disease for 15 years. Piece by piece, more comes to be known. We still have more to learn, but the journey has been rewarding."

For the rest of us the lesson is simple: You *can* avoid the disease. Even in the most infected areas, only one person in 1,000 gets it and is nearly always cured. And to those who are not cured, research promises a brighter future.

For more information, send a stamped, self-addressed envelope to the Lyme Disease Foundation, 1 Financial Plaza, Hartford, CT 06103; or call (800) 886-LYME.

How Safe Is Your Home?

EACH YEAR, 7 MILLION AMERICANS HURT themselves—not in the wilds, either, but in or around their homes. Most of those injuries are avoidable; the injured might have prevented their falls, burns, poisonings, and other mishaps.

Because we often can control our safety, Dr. Joseph Greensher says he wants the word *accident* banned.

Dr. Greensher headed the National Committee on Accident and Poison Prevention of the American Academy of Pediatrics. "My dictionary defines an accident as something that happens by chance or without intention," he says. "Most injuries, particularly at home, have causes within our control."

About 26,000 Americans are killed annually by home injuries, and approximately 80,000 are permanently disabled each year.

Those statistics are grim, but the good news is that Americans are learning simple rules to prevent home injury. Death rates have fallen steadily for 70 years. In 1912, home mishaps killed 28,000 persons in the United States; by 1983, with more than twice the population, victims totaled less than 20,000.

In this report, we reveal some murderous traps at home and tell what you can do about them.

The following statistics, compiled by the National Safety Council in 1994, give a brief but stark picture of the deaths from home injuries.

Falls—Total Deaths: 8,500

More than two thirds of those who die from falls are elderly. Ten percent of those falls occur on a level area. Victims commonly trip on loose carpets, wires, or toys; lose their footing on spilled liquids or foods; or slip in the tub.

Fires—Total Deaths: 3,900

The very young and very old are fire's most frequent victims. More children die by fire than from any other home disaster. Like the very old, they are the most easily trapped.

Suffocation—Total Deaths: 2,100

These traps look innocent, but most infants get caught in the bed linens or hung up in their cribs. (Some infant sleepwear makes bedding unnecessary and furniture can be fixed so that baby's head can't get stuck.) Older people often die when they choke after swallowing something—a piece of food, a hearing aid battery, a pin.

Poisoning—Total Deaths: 6,400

Our homes are filled with toxic materials—medicines, cleaners, cosmetics, weed and insect killers, to which children are most vulnerable. (Ask your Poison

Control Center how to store these.) Also included in this category: drug overdoses.

Firearms—Total Deaths: 900
Lock up your guns and teach proper handling. Americans are said to possess more privately owned guns than any other people in the world. It is no surprise that firearms "accidentally" kill 900 of us each year.

Drowning—Total Deaths: 900
The backyard pool is increasingly the scene of tragedies. Keep pools fenced and locked; remove ladders; practice safety drills.

All Other Accidents—
Total Deaths: 3,500
Killers here include electric current (cover unused outlets), flammables and explosives (cap them tightly and store them far from pilot lights and electric switches), hot substances (keep cups and bowls containing them out of children's reach), and corrosive liquids.

Save the Children

If a doctor told you that your child had leukemia, you would move heaven and earth to get your youngster the best medical care, while hoping for a cure. Yet a home injury that could be prevented is much more likely than leukemia to kill a child under the age of 15.

Dr. Greensher tells of a little girl whose face was badly burned when she pulled a pot of hot soup down off the gas range. "I guess she's been too lucky up to now," the mother said. "It was just her turn."

The mother blamed "luck" to turn the blame away from herself. Had she turned the pot handles toward the center of the stove or used back burners only, her daughter couldn't have reached them, so no "accident" would have happened. Parents must teach themselves and their children to spot and avoid hazards.

Dr. Greensher lists three risk factors for children:

1. Personality. At high risk are curious toddlers, retarded children, and stubborn, hot-tempered, overly aggressive boys and girls.

2. Unsafe objects. Obviously dangerous are matches, guns, and fireplaces. Easily overlooked but also potentially lethal are these: too-small (swallowable), sharp-edged, or toxic toys; boiling-hot water from a faucet; medicines and poisons. Learn first aid—the wrong care can kill—and post your Poison Control Center's number near all phones.

3. The social environment—the family. A caring person must watch a child's every move. Mary Parker of Wantagh, New York, learned just how quick her 10-month-old daughter, Nicole, could be when the infant suddenly fell down the

basement stairs. "All I could think was 'Please, God, let her be alright,'" says Mrs. Parker. Nicole sustained only cuts and bruises.

When we're under stress, watchfulness declines. Dr. Greensher cites studies showing that risk rises with:

- hunger and fatigue in child or parent,
- tension either in one parent or between parents,
- a mother's illness or pregnancy or a family death,
- a change in the child's caretaker or living quarters, and
- preoccupation with personal matters or too much housework or child care.

To help prevent child injuries, the American Academy of Pediatrics has designed TIPP (The Injury Prevention Program), which shows pediatricians how to guide parents with these questions.

For Newborns to Age 1
- Do you leave the baby home alone? Bad idea. A baby cannot deal with dogs, strangers, or fires.
- Do you use smoke or fire detectors? Great idea. The alarm gives you precious minutes to escape.
- Do you leave the child unattended on tables or beds? Babies can roll over and sustain injuries as they fall to the floor.

For Toddlers through High School
- Do you check for safety hazards in other homes where your child may play? You had better do so. A child cannot be counted on to detect and correct high-risk situations.
- Do you have safety caps on all bottles of medicine? Good idea. Children can swallow lethal pills thinking they are candy. When your child visits Grandma and Grandpa, the chances are that their home is a veritable drugstore with easy-to-open caps because grandparents often have arthritis and cannot manage the safety caps.
- Do you let a child bathe alone? It takes 2 to 3 minutes for a baby to drown in a bathtub.

The general rule is this: If a child can be hurt by something, a child will be hurt. Parents should try to keep dangerous objects locked away, and their eyes locked on their children.

Protect the Elderly

For people older than 65, the home is a minefield.

Nearly half of all home injury deaths come from this age group. At advanced ages, we grow weaker, less sure-footed, and far more vulnerable.

A U.S. Consumer Product Safety Commission booklet, *Safety for Older*

Consumers, runs a checklist, including these problems:

Cause of Injury	Solution
Falls on loose rugs	Slip-resistant tape
Falls on stairs	Light switches top and bottom; hand-rails on both sides
Falls while bathing, showering	Slip-resistant surface; grab bars
Falls while reaching toward shelves	Step stool with handrails
Fire (smoke)	Smoke detectors
Fire (burns)	Electric lines not overloaded
Scalds	Water heater set at 120 Fahrenheit
Electric shock	Ground-fault circuit interrupters

Surviving Fires

Tremendous progress has been made in the reduction of home fire fatalities as a result, in large part, of the widespread installation of smoke detectors in homes. In 1977, only one household in five had them; today, that figure has risen to 13 of 14 homes, or 93 percent of households. Fire deaths fell from 7,400 in 1977 to 4,300 in 1994.

The National Fire Protection Association, in its Learn Not to Burn program, suggests the following protective measures:

- Have an escape plan and practice it with your family. But take it easy. Make it somewhat of a game. Such a drill can frighten young children.
- Get outside first; then call the fire department.
- Crawl low in clean air if you get trapped in smoke.
- Get a fire extinguisher and smoke detectors. Train the family to use them. Again, caution is advised with young children.
- Keep doors closed and close them as you escape a fire.
- Stop, drop, and roll if your clothes catch fire.

Tabatha Alcala, 8, of Phoenix, Arizona, heard most of these ideas from Tiller the Clown. Tiller, an actor trained by the fire department, spoke to her second-grade class. Tabatha, on her own, saved her baby sister and a young cousin by leading them to safety when, with her parents gone, a kitchen grease fire broke out. She followed the rules. Surely, we can too.

Find Those Traps—and Fix Them

Lock up firearms, out of sight.

Keep medicines capped, securely stored.

Use smoke detectors.

Keep pots on stove out of tots' reach.

Stairs: place handrails on both sides, and add light switches.

Carefully store gasoline and other flammables.

Avoid scalds: Set the hot-water heater at 120 degrees Fahrenheit.

Lock up poisons and chemicals—follow labels' directions.

Loose rugs? Tape them to the floor.

Don't know wattage limits? Use bulbs of 60 watts or less to avoid fires.

Cap unused wall outlets.

Watchfulness is a small price to pay for your child's or elderly parents' lives. Remember: accidents do not happen; they are mostly caused by human beings.

For more information, send a self-addressed, stamped envelope to Home Fire Safety Tips, c/o National Fire Protection Association Office of Public Affairs. Also write to the Home Safety Checklist for Older Consumers, CPSC, Washington, D.C. 20207.

How You Can Make Your Home Safe

DANGER LURKS ALMOST EVERYWHERE IN THE home. Fire can burn and kill. Electricity can shock, hot water can scald, and ice can trip you up. Burglars might enter and assault you and your family.

Now engineers and inventors have teamed up to produce a host of gadgets that will help keep you safe both from hidden and obvious dangers in your home. They range from simple nonskid strips in the bathtub to high-tech "smart houses" that are centrally wired to protect you from fire, burglary, gas leaks, and electrical accidents.

Says Carol Dawson, former head of the Federal Consumer Product Safety Commission, "New technology has pro-

vided a new world of safety devices. We encourage consumers to use them and use them properly."

The inventions could save a great many of the 26,000 Americans killed each year by mishaps in their homes. Altogether, 7 million Americans annually suffer debilitating injuries at home.

Some of the new technology requires professional installation and could cost from hundreds to thousands of dollars. But many devices are sold at neighborhood hardware stores for a few dollars.

Several ingenious safety tools and where to get them are discussed in *The Doable Renewable Home: Making Your Home Fit Your Needs.* For a free copy write to the American Association of Retired Persons, AARP Fulfillment, EEO 1053, 601 E Street NW, Washington, DC 20049. Ask for stock number 012476; or call (800) 424-3410.

Fire Protection Devices

Among the many fire safety items available, smoke alarms head the list. Nearly 95 percent of U.S. homes have these inexpensive boxes that squeal at the first taste of smoke. And since their widespread installation nationally, residential fire deaths have declined. Unfortunately, too few smoke alarms are used in most homes. Some people remove or fail to replace the batteries. One mother hated the alarm's noise when she cooked, so she took out its batteries. Her son later died in a fire in their home.

Newer smoke detector systems send radio signals to remote-operated alarms, making it possible to see or hear the alarm even from your garage or outdoors.

Sprinkler systems for your home can reduce the risk of loss of life or property, but they are expensive—$1,200 and up. They detect fire and then douse it with water. If your town's building codes permit plastic pipes, the costs are less.

Fireproof face masks, such as LIFE-AIR 5 ($225) and LIFEAIR 10 ($325), protect the face from burns, keep out smoke and toxic fumes, and provide oxygen for 5 or 10 minutes, respectively. They use compressed air and can be re-filled at most hospitals and firehouses. They are available from Mark Promotions, 532 W. Lake Street, Elmhurst, IL 60126.

New shock protectors replace standard wall outlets to prevent shocks from short circuits. Called ground-fault circuit interrupters, they perform much like a circuit breaker or fuse but are far more sensitive. Able to detect electrical leaks and shut off the circuit, they're mandatory in many hotel bathrooms. Ask your electrician or hardware store manager.

Surge protectors plugged into electrical outlets protect your appliances from abnormal jolts of electricity (as from a lightning bolt) and can prevent fire.

A remote switch turns lamps and appliances on and off. Similar to a garage door opener, a pushed button sends a signal to an outlet, and the electricity flows. You won't have to stumble through a dark room to find the light switch. There also are sound-activated switches: Clap hands, and the light goes on. Others respond to a hand waved directly in front of them.

An antenna discharge unit prevents bolts of lightning from coming into the house through your TV antenna. It functions as a lightning rod.

A new electrical outlet guard really stops kids from putting such things as pins and nails into outlets, protecting them from shock. Adults turn a dial that blocks or permits access to the wall sockets.

A security power-failure light, sold at hardware stores, goes on when electric power fails. Keep it plugged into your wall outlet to charge up its batteries. If your power is interrupted, the light goes on and stays on for 1 1/2 hours.

Various Safety Gadgets

Keep a whistle in each room to summon help quickly from a family member. Also consider the following:

• Ice grippers, pieces of metal that strap to shoes, prevent slipping on ice.

• A gas detector, placed near a gas furnace, senses leaks and sounds an alarm.

• Stepstools with handrails right up to the top step help prevent falls while climbing to get something from a high shelf. Make sure the collapsible type is fully opened and stable. Tighten screws and braces periodically.

• Nonslip mats on floors, stairs, and the legs of tables and chairs can prevent falls—the most frequent cause of home injuries and fatalities, particularly among older persons. They're sold at hardware stores, as are bathtub safety treads, which are easily glued to the bottom of a bathtub, shower, or tile floor.

• A plumbing fixture with a "pressure equalizer" prevents scalding. A sudden surge of hot water—caused by a toilet flush or cold water running elsewhere in the house—can scald. The Consumer Products Safety Commission reports that each year 75,000 to 100,000 Americans bathing in tubs and showers are scalded in this way badly enough to require hospitalization. Up to 100 victims die from the accidents—primarily those under 6 or over 60. This device equalizes the hot and cold, and it costs little more than a regular two-handled faucet. Sudden temperature changes in bath or shower water shock the bather and often cause slips and falls as well, increasing the risk of further injury.

The Safe, Smart House

Engineers are working to transform today's accident trap into a home of the future where the very walls do the safe thinking for you. They call it the "Smart House."

"The Smart House will help elderly people stay independent," says David MacFadyen, president of the National Association of Home Builders (NAHB) Research Foundation, which has encouraged the project's development. "And it will make life more comfortable and convenient for people of any age or physical condition."

The Smart House uses microchips to operate new safety gadgets, new wiring, and new materials. Still under development, Smart House could be the next building innovation. Parts of it already exist in some homes.

Our residences usually have electrical, telephone, thermostat, and doorbell wiring, water pipes, and heating and cooling systems. Some have gas delivered by pipe for heating and cooking. A growing number have television cables, anti-burglar systems, and fire alarms.

All these systems traditionally are independent of one another. The Smart House, however, has a central system designed at the request of the NAHB.

The Smart House will use one cable to carry electrical power, video, and audio signals and communications systems. If you use an electric iron with a shorted circuit, the Smart House will detect the "short" and shut off power to that appliance. If you turn on your stove with nothing on it or in it to cook and leave it unattended, the system will turn off the stove. Or if the oven is about to burn the cookies, the system will lower the heat or turn it off.

The system will turn lights on or off when you enter or leave a room, if that's the setting you select, or adjust the lighting to your taste. You may be able to give voice commands to the system: "Smart House, send heat to the upstairs bedroom."

With the fire and burglar systems interconnected, you'll get very early warnings of danger and be able to take quick action. If you are not home, the Smart House will telephone for help. Or it may respond to a special setting and turn on lights in response to a sudden noise.

David MacFadyen says the Smart House will cost the same as a regular house. Although the Smart House idea seems attractive it has not yet caught on with a wide public.

For more information, write to Smart House, L.P., 401-J Prince Georges Blvd., Upper Marlboro, MD 20774-7430; or call (800) 759-3344.

The Safety Button

Victoria Comstock-Mills, 46, a poet living in Reading, Massachusetts, suffers from severe diabetes. At least once a month she goes into insulin shock.

"Suddenly I can't see. I feel as though someone is shining a bright light in my eyes," says Ms. Comstock-Mills. "It's a frightening feeling, especially since I live alone."

But she is not entirely without help. On a chain around her neck is a button. Whenever she feels a reaction coming on, she presses the button. This summons paramedics, who arrive in an ambulance to take her to the hospital.

The pressed button activates the Lifeline. It sends a radio signal to a box attached to Ms. Comstock-Mills' telephone, which then automatically dials Choate-Symmes Hospital in nearby Arlington. If she does not answer a return call from the hospital's staff, the paramedics are dispatched.

Lifeline serves 500,000 Americans—generally old, infirm, sick, and living alone for most of the day. Each year the system responded to more than 10,000 calls a day, only 5 percent of which are calls for assistance. Most people just call for reassurance. Since Lifeline began, at least a dozen other companies have entered the field.

Andrew Dibner, 60, a psychologist and expert on aging, founded Lifeline Systems. "I feel very fulfilled," he says, "because I was able to come up with an idea that turns out to be so helpful to people."

A government-supported study has shown that Lifeline reduces anxiety about living alone, enables individuals to live at home rather than in nursing homes, reduces the number of days spent in a hospital, and saves communities $7 for every $1 they invest in the emergency service.

For more information, write to Lifeline, 640 Memorial Dr., Cambridge, MA 02139-4851; or call (800) 642-0045.

The Business of Health

Help! I'm Drowning in Insurance Forms

I'VE SURVIVED TWO HEART OPERATIONS, A HEART probe (an angiogram), a prostate operation, four spinal surgeries, and several diagnostic tests (some at $1,000 each).

My squadron of doctors also prescribed a sandbox-size collection of pills. I take nine different chemicals a day. They include wonderful medicines for my Parkinson's disease that work so well it's hard to tell I have the disease.

I am struggling with sciatica, a leg condition that still hurts despite surgeries, painkillers, and a shower of bills.

For all these maladies, I was treated by a dozen specialists, three physical therapists, and four hospitals. All sent me their bills—at least 100 of them. I sent the bills to my insurer. It has been a daunting experience.

Please understand: I acknowledge that high-tech medicine added years to my life. I feel almost as good now as I did before my afflictions began. The medical treatment I got deserves at least a standing ovation. I'm glad, too, that doctors,

nurses, and medical technologists have more expertise than most of the medical bill collectors and the health insurance companies that pay them.

Bill paying takes lots of time. And strength. And perseverance. I had to fill out claim forms, make calls, and do research to find missing or inaccurate bills.

It took me 6 months and four letters from my physicians to settle one bill worth $6,000. After a while, it's not the amount but the principle of fair treatment one fights for. And it is a fight. Ask a few of the millions who are buried yearly under the medical bill avalanche.

My insurance company sends me a single yellow sheet, printed front and back, to claim payment for each service. I have to submit a piece of paper even for a $10 prescription. Each form has mostly the same blanks requiring the same information. That includes my name, address, employer, my birthdate, my wife's birth date, my Social Security number (and my wife's), my wife's place of employment, and marital status for both of us. Including research to learn whether a particular bill already has been paid, it takes at least 10 minutes to complete one claim. I've spent hours slogging through more than 100 forms. No credit card system could work this way.

Then I got a bright idea: Make copies of both sides of one yellow sheet with the name, address, and other blanks already filled in. I'll only need to supply the required new information and signatures. Now 10 forms will take just 20 minutes!

The insurer slapped me down: "Not our form," they told me in a note.

I telephoned to ask, "What's the difference?"

They answered, "Our form is yellow!" Yellow! It takes three phone calls and a vice president to alter that idiocy.

Friends tell me I am not the only poor patient struggling with this medical bill blitz. But many just give up and pay up. Could it be that the insurance companies count on that reaction?

I sense that most of the millions who reportedly have overpaid their bills did so because they did not know what else to do or lacked the strength or will to do it.

Not so for Esther Milstein, 56, a real estate broker in San Jose, California. In February 1995, she hurt her kneecap preparing for a marathon run. Six weeks later, she had recovered. Milstein balked when her insurer only would pay $70 on her doctor's bill of $180.

"It took four phone calls just to get my doctor's billing clerk," she said. "The clerk promised to talk to the insurer. But I kept getting billed." Ten months later, the doctor cut his fee by $15. She paid $95, and the insurer paid $70.

What happens when an insurer says a doctor's bill exceeds "prevailing fees" and cuts the amount of its payment? For me, at first it meant I had to pay $400 more. The bill for my heart treatments at a large Manhattan hospital surpassed $10,000. The doctor's fee was nearly $2,000. But initially the insurer paid the doctor only $1,600. I think I prevailed through diligence. Here, for example, is how I phoned the insurer:

Me: "How do you set a 'prevailing fee'?"

Them: "We figure an average of the fees of other institutions in the same ZIP code."

Me: "My hospital is the only one in its ZIP. Which code did you use?" (They cited a New Jersey ZIP. I got the Manhattan hospital's billing manager on the line, via my three-way calling.)

He: "That ZIP is our billing drop, not our service location."

Them: "Sorry." (The insurer paid.)

Even experts give up, as in the case of Uwe Reinhardt, a professor of economics and public policy at Princeton University renowned for his knowledge of health care. "I had a regular checkup at a major hospital," he said. "We sent the $800 bill to the insurer. They sat on it. In 6 weeks, I got a letter from the hospital, saying, 'Pay up or else!' We paid, then sent a claim form to the insurer. The insurer sent me a check for 80 percent of $500 [the reduced amount Prof. Reinhardt should have been billed by the hospital as a faculty member]. I gave up."

Some say botched billings cost consumers about $40 billion a year. Prof. Reinhardt said that figure is low, because it doesn't include the time consumers must spend haggling. Ironically, the complex billing rules designed to stop false claims seem to have mutated into a maniacal billing system that may have added to the huge costs of U.S. health care. To wit: You get bills from different hospitals, different departments within the same hospital and private practitioners. Your insurer (sometimes) will pay you, the hospital, or the doctor; or it will deny payment—in full or in part—which means a fight with the insurer and/or the provider.

When I was getting duplicate bills almost daily, I'd send them to the insurer, using my copied claim forms. The reply: "This charge has been processed." Meaning what? Had the insurer (1) paid the provider? (2) Sent me a check? (3) Denied payment? Or (4) paid less than billed on charges exceeding "prevailing fees"?

I got a hospital bill for $389 printed in flaming red. The words *final notice* came with a threat to send the bill to a collection agency. I replied that my insurer won't pay a bill that does not include the service, date of service, provider, and diagnosis, along with the fee. I wrote, "Please send a bill with this information." I wrote it again when I got a second final notice. A third final notice invited me to phone. I did, and I waited 20 minutes; only a machine answered.

I wrote to the president of the hospital via fax. Within an hour, the chief billing officer called to say, "The $389 was for emergency room services, which normally are included in charges to Blue Cross. You shouldn't have been sent this bill."

I wondered, Do hospitals try to evoke payment after they provoke fear or pique?

Surely millions, weak with illness, fall at the medical billing front. Blue Cross once fined me $100 because I'd failed to tell them within 48 hours that I'd been admitted to a hospital. "But," I said, "what if I'd been unconscious? How, being sick, could I know what to do, how to do it?"

"Oh," said the phone voice, "that's printed on the back of your Blue Cross card."

Reader, stick to your guns! Seek help from experts in both camps—billers and payers—and, if you must, from the state. I cringe to think that, as a journalist, I might get more privileges than most people do. I hope this article shakes things up.

Five Ways to Lower Your Medical Bills

1. Ask your doctor or the hospital how much your surgery or other procedures will cost. If it's more than you can afford, ask for a reduced-payment plan.
2. If patient advocates are on the hospital staff, ask them to help you work things out.
3. Ask your insurer, "Is my doctor's billing form acceptable?" If not, ask them to explain exactly what they want. Also ask whether there is a cost limit for the treatment you are about to get. Discuss limits and payments with your doctor or health care institution.
4. No medical insurance? That's big trouble, especially for a family. You might find an affordable plan with fraternal, social, religious, alumni, or school groups.
5. Shop for a policy with a high deductible (the amount you must pay before insurance kicks in). It's easier to get than a low-deductible policy, the premium is less, and you're still covered for huge health care costs.

Stymied by medical bills and payments? Write your political representative or your state's department of health.

When a Life Is in Your Hands

YOU ARE IN A HOSPITAL. THE NURSE CHECKS carefully and adjusts your respirator tube. You hear the incessant beep, beep of a heart monitor. You wonder, "Is it mine?" You try to speak. You cannot. Nor can you move your arms or legs. Hour after hour, day after day, you stare at the ceiling. And you endure.

Are you dying? Probably not. But you may wish you were or wish that someone would "pull the plug" and grant you a merciful, easy death: euthanasia.

Physicians, patients, clergy, and philosophers told us their views on this issue as it confronts people today. Here is a look at many sides of euthanasia and life-sustaining high-tech medicine.

Chances are, if you fall deathly ill, modern science and the machines surrounding your hospital bed will keep you alive. In time you will mend, leave the hospital, and resume your normal life. But the man in the bed next to you is not so lucky. He will not recover, but he will endure, because those same machines can sustain his life functions indefinitely.

Doctors today are being asked—even begged—to turn off those life-sustaining machines. And dealing with such requests is not easy. Physicians are faced with legal and ethical decisions and with questions to which there are no simple "right" or "wrong" answers.

Doctors take an oath—the Hippocratic oath—and swear to protect life. They are professionally and morally bound to do so. For a physician to act to end a life is morally and ethically questionable at the very least. And yet Dr. James H. Sammons, executive vice president of the American Medical Association, says, "We must give those patients a way out. There comes the time that the physician must step back and, at the patient's or the family's request, allow the patient to die with dignity."

Danny Delio of Little Neck, New York, finally died with dignity after a year-long court battle waged by his persevering wife, Julie. At 33, Mr. Delio had earned a Ph.D. in exercise physiology and was a marathon runner. And then he emerged from minor surgery permanently unconscious. Doctors put a feeding tube through his nose and down into his stomach, allowing him to "live."

"It wasn't life," says Mrs. Delio. "Danny's father had been in a coma, and doctors tried to revive him until he died. That made a mark on Danny, and he made me promise never to let him exist even one day in a vegetative state."

She won her court case and had her husband admitted to another hospital, where he was not fed through a tube. He died 10 days later. Mrs. Delio says, "All that happened here is that a man who was already dead was *allowed* to die."

In this country, nearly all of us agree that *active* euthanasia is morally wrong. It almost always is illegal. It is illegal, for example, to shoot and kill your incurably sick wife. Roswell Gilbert did so in Florida in 1985, and he is serving a life sentence in prison. It is illegal to give a suffering person a lethal dose of drug such as morphine. And it is illegal to do anything to hasten or bring about a person's demise (e.g., by, leaving a gun or a jar of poison at the bedside).

Dr. Peter Rosier, a Florida pathologist, stood by as his wife, Patricia, incurably ill with cancer, took 20 sleeping pills in January 1986. When the pills failed, Dr. Rosier gave her a massive shot of morphine. When that also failed, Mrs. Rosier's stepfather, Vincent Delman, smothered her. Prosecutors gave Mr. Delman immunity from trial before they knew what he had done. Dr. Rosier, tried before a jury, was acquitted.

For doctors, the issue of helping a patient die cuts deep. Yet distraught patients and their families do ask doctors to help end suffering. Respondents to a survey by the Hemlock Society, which advocates assisted suicide for the terminally ill, included 79 California doctors who admitted taking the lives of patients who had asked to die. Derek Humphry founded the society after he supplied his cancer-ridden wife with lethal drugs. She later committed suicide, dying in his arms. The First Amendment, which guarantees freedom of speech and the press, also protects the society's right to hand out data on the type and quantity of drugs and where to get them.

"Many doctors interpret the Hippocratic oath to mean that if you let the patient die in a disgusting manner or in agony, *that* is doing harm," Mr. Humphry says. The Hemlock Society sponsored a referendum to allow active euthanasia in California, but too few signed the petition to get it on the ballot. Says Arthur Caplan, a philosopher and director of the Center for Biomedical Ethics at the University of Minnesota in Minneapolis, "I don't think doctors should kill. Active euthanasia is easy to abuse and misuse. It sows distrust between doctor and patient."

Such distrust is evident in Holland, according to an article by Richard Fenigsen, a Dutch heart doctor. Dr. Fenigsen writes that under new lenient attitudes by the courts, Dutch general practitioners annually kill at least 5,000 patients who allegedly desire voluntary active euthanasia. He adds that *involuntary* active euthanasia cases are growing in Holland. In these cases, patients don't want to die, but doctors kill them "for their own good" (perhaps they are suffering) or "for the good of society" (the patients are too expensive to maintain). Essentially, Dr. Fenigsen says, euthanasia has got out of hand in Holland.

The controversy deepens over *passive* euthanasia. That's when the doctor withdraws treatment. Patients have the right to refuse medical treatment of any kind, even if refusal means that life will soon end. That is a right by common law and by nearly every religion's teaching. In most states, your family can exercise your right of medical refusal if you are unable. The late Karen Ann Quinlan, a young New Jersey woman who sank into a coma after mixing tranquilizers and alcohol, continued to breathe unaided for 9 years after her parents had gained permission to shut off her respirator.

In New York, doctors and the courts may choose to honor a patient's wishes to avoid life-sustaining methods. However, if a patient falls unconscious before declaring those wishes, doctors are at risk if they don't continue treatment until death occurs.

All 50 states recognize the "living will" status as a legal document. It specifies your wishes, should you become unable to decide or to tell others what you want done. In one form of such a will, you can ask that, facing little hope of recovery, you be allowed to die and not be kept alive by medications, artificial means, or "heroic measures."

Arthur Caplan cites these problems with living wills: They may not exactly fit the situation when the time comes. The family and the doctor may not know about your will. In many instances, family members may disregard your will and order the doctor to follow their wishes rather than yours.

The New York State Legislature will be asked by the New York Task Force on Life and the Law to consider legislation that permits a person to appoint a health agent to make all decisions about medical treatment in the event he or she cannot. Mr. Caplan defines medical treatment, including tube feeding, as something only a doctor, nurse, or licensed technician can do for you.

Says J. Robert Nelson, a Methodist minister and director of the Institute of Religion at the Texas Medical Center in Houston, "I think the medical and moral duty of all of us is to keep the patient comfortable until death." Father Richard McCormick, professor of theology at the University of Notre Dame in South Bend, Indiana, agrees and adds, "Given a reasonably certain diagnosis that the person won't return to a cognitive state, I believe that artificial nutrition can be withheld, because the patient cannot get any benefit."

Doctors and laypeople alike have debated the definitions of "life" and "death." They often argue about such points as these: When is a patient dead? Can a particular comatose patient recover? In most states, doctors declare a person dead if the heart and breathing have stopped. If the heart continues to beat but the patient can breathe only with the aid of a machine and the brain is dead, the person usually is legally dead.

Dr. Matthew E. Fink heads the neurological intensive care unit at Columbia-Presbyterian Medical Center in New York City. "The most truly frightening thing," he says, "is that doctors and nurses make many mistakes about the conditions of their patients. A patient may be in a paralytic state and not in a coma."

Dr. Fink tells of an 18-year-old who was hospitalized with a severely injured head and declared comatose after 6 weeks. After examining him, however, Dr. Fink found that the patient was wide awake but able to move only his eyelids.

"I told him to blink once for yes, twice for no," Dr. Fink says, "and I asked him if his name were Bob. He blinked no. When I gave him his true name, he blinked yes. He was alive. He was thinking. He recovered in a year."

A person in a coma is not responsive and often cannot breathe unaided. Dr. Fink says that in 90 percent of such cases, he can predict whether the patient will live or die or will convert to a vegetative state. In a vegetative state, many reflexes—such as coughing, blinking and breathing—return, but the patient does not respond to outside stimuli. After 30 days, Dr. Fink says, he is almost certain that a coma victim will never wake. If, in a rare case, a victim does regain consciousness after 6 months or so, Dr. Fink asserts that he or she probably was not comatose. To avoid misdiagnosing a condition and then withholding treatment from someone who otherwise might recover, he recommends that the patient be examined by an experienced neurologist at a large, well-equipped medical center.

Though drugs can ease those with incurable and painful diseases, many

Americans often opt for passive euthanasia (ending treatment). That choice is open only to those who are competent and able to state their wishes.

Laws governing the enforcement of patients' living wills vary from state to state, and the acceptance of such wills varies from hospital to hospital and physician to physician.

To obtain a copy of your state's living will and medical power of attorney forms, write to Choice in Dying, 200 Varick Street, 10th floor, New York, NY 10014. Send a check for $3.50. To order by phone call (800) 989-WILL. You can download the forms free if you visit the website http://www.choices.org.

Talk Back to Your Doctor

A FRIEND OF MINE, A WOMAN OF 25, VISITS AN ear specialist for the first time and asks, "Doctor, what is the medication you've prescribed for my ear?" He replies, "Why should *you* want to know? From which university were you awarded *your* medical degree?"

His arrogance heightens her pain and the anxiety she feels about having an unfamiliar illness treated by an unknown doctor. She silently writes a check, vowing never to see him again.

She is right to cross such a doctor off her list (happily, his sort is becoming rarer) and to find one of the many physicians willing to treat patients as partners. As a patient, your life and health depend on talking freely to your doctor.

Many patients, fearful of learning the worst, don't want to ask about their health problems. Others, awed by the physician, are afraid to challenge medical authority. More than half of all patients who don't speak up just don't understand the medical lingo and are too embarrassed to say so. Or they feel guilty, sure that they've brought the disease on themselves. If the illness is sexual, shame silences them.

The Bonuses of Being a Partner in Your Own Medical Care

In this age of high-tech medicine, too often the physician squeezes you, the patient, out of the medical process. You're left in the dark. You don't know enough to question the doctor's move, and he or she won't explain it. The results could be fatal. On the other hand, talking with your doctor could pay lifesaving dividends.

Patients who ask questions motivate doctors and nurses to give them more information, and they are perceived as more intelligent and involved in their own care than patients who keep silent, says Dr. Debra L. Roter, professor of health policy and management at Johns Hopkins University School of Hygiene and Public Health in Baltimore. She and Judith A. Hall, professor of psychology at Northeastern University in Boston, wrote the book *Doctors Talking with Patients, Patients Talking with Doctors* (Auburn House).

By expressing yourself, you make it clear that you take yourself seriously and expect others to do so. Asking for the best care indicates that you probably will refuse treatment that seems not beneficial and are informed and alert enough to notice. Such patient awareness can be crucial in the case of medications; in some hospitals, drug errors run as high as 10 percent.

I know one diabetic who kept a nurse from injecting him with a double dose of insulin. If he hadn't known his correct dosage, he couldn't have spotted and objected to the nurse's error. Coma and death could have resulted.

What Should You Tell Your Doctor?

Nearly everything! Generally, tell your doubts, fears, likes, and dislikes about treatments. Specifically, discuss these points:

- All past illnesses
- Every drug you take regularly—prescription (don't overlook psychiatric

medications) and over-the-counter, including aspirin. Some doctors ask you to come to their offices with all your medicines *in their containers* to make sure you're getting the right doses and that drugs don't interact badly. It's always a good idea to have the doctor see all the medicines you take laid out in one place, and it's crucial for women who are pregnant or planning to become pregnant. Don't wait for an invitation—show the doctor your medicines.

What to Ask Your Doctor about Drugs

Medicines top the list of critical topics to discuss with your doctor. In fact, former First Lady Barbara Bush thought this issue so important that she spoke out on it for the National Council on Patient Information and Education. In a public service TV announcement, she urged, "Ask your doctor or pharmacist about any new medicine. Ask how and when to take it, about side effects and precautions. And ask whether it will work with other medicines you take."

More Questions about Drugs
- What is the name of the drug?
- Does it come in a cheaper, generic form? Is the brand-name drug better, or is the generic compound just as good? (The generic version often is cheaper, but it also may be less effective.)

• What should the medicine do for me? If you don't understand what the doctor says, ask for further explanation until you do. You *must* understand what drugs do. Your life may depend on it.

• What are the possible side effects? They might include fever, rashes, drowsiness, dry mouth, dizziness, and blood problems. Most medicines do elicit reactions of one sort or another in patients.

• What foods, drinks, or medicines should I avoid—or seek out? With some antibiotics, the doctor may tell you to ingest live-culture buttermilk or yogurt, which replenishes the good bacteria in the bowel that some medications destroy. Taking the good bacteria could also prevent yeast infection.

Questions to Ask Every Time

• Always ask, "Why?" For instance, a doctor says, "Avoid air travel," when you have a head cold or inflamed sinuses, assuming you already know why. People who've ignored a doctor's urgings to avoid plane travel have said, "I thought the doctor was just saying, 'Take it easy.' Then I learned why not to fly with a head cold—the hard way." During swings in the plane's cabin pressure, these people experience excruciating ear pain; some even suffer inner-ear damage. Remember this when you hear infants crying bitterly on airplanes.

• Always ask about money. Financial questions are best settled before the physician starts any complex treatment.

Even if you're insured, you need to know the cost. Not all health policies cover every procedure. And you will want a second opinion for a high-priced treatment.

Questions to Ask Your Surgeon

• Ask how many times the surgeon has performed the operation planned for you. How many did he or she do last year? A skilled surgeon in a large city may have done a commonly needed operation 100 times a year or more; a small-town doctor may have performed fewer. Clearly, the fewer surgeries a doctor performs, the greater the opportunity for error.

In New York, the state health department keeps track of coronary-bypass operations. In Pennsylvania, the state Health Care Cost Containment Council records and furnishes such data.

• Ask about anesthesia. If the doctor plans to put you to sleep with general anesthesia, find out whether the operation can be done with local or regional pain control instead. These are safer for some people and leave them feeling better at the end.

More Questions to Ask

• Ask about your illness. Once your disease is diagnosed, ask how you contracted it, if you inherited it (important information for your children), and what it means for your future.

• Ask how the doctor *knows* this proposed treatment works. If based on wide scientific evidence, fine. But if the doctor says, "In my experience . . . ," be wary!

• Ask _why_ diagnostic tests are needed. Some can be very costly and even damaging. Persist. Get a full explanation.

It's a Team Effort

Some doctors still tell patients, "Leave it to me and the nurses. We're trained to do this work." This approach dismisses patients, who might then consider dismissing _them._ The physician, the nurse, and the technician work for _you,_ so you can "fire" them.

Dr. Nancy Dickey, a trustee of the American Medical Association, reports, "New doctors are being formally trained to see patients as partners." To join the team, ask your health care providers how you can help. Here are other suggestions:

• Bring to the doctor's office a list of questions and either paper and pen or a small tape recorder for the answers. (If asked why, explain that you can't recall the doctor's words otherwise and that the better you understand, the more closely you'll follow the doctor's plan.) If the plan is too complex, ask, "What three or four things _must_ I do?"

• Reread the doctor's diagnosis of your illness, then ask for any explanations you still need. Consult books at the public library, such as _The American Medical Association's Encyclopedia of Medicine._ Ask your doctor for other titles. Ask your pharmacist for the "drug insert" that comes with your medication, which tells its side effects and how it works. But keep in mind that, by Food and Drug Administration order, pharmaceutical companies must list even rare side effects; this can exaggerate the medical dangers.

Traits of Good Doctors, Good Patients

A good doctor places you on the healing team, keeps you informed, answers your questions, and encourages you to learn more about what ails you. Failure to communicate with the patient is a failure of treatment by the doctor. If this doctor won't talk to you, find one of the many who will. You, the patient, have responsibilities, too. A good patient answers the doctor's questions as honestly and thoroughly as possible.

Marshall H. Becker, associate dean of the School of Public Health at the University of Michigan at Ann Arbor, tracked studies on patients who rejected their doctor-prescribed treatments. He found that 75 percent of such patients failed to follow prescriptions. (For example, they missed taking a medication so often as to weaken or cancel its therapeutic value.) More than half failed to follow medically advised behavioral changes, such as dieting, physical therapy, exercise, and stopping smoking.

A Personal Story

The important point I want to make is that patients who fail to follow doctors' orders are throwing away 50 years of exquisite medical research that has cut our death and sickness rates almost by one third. Don't shortchange yourself.

Several years ago I contracted pneumonia and was treated at a large, metropolitan, top-class hospital. At that time, I also was afflicted with benign prostate hypertrophy, which means that my prostate was very big but not cancerous. I had been popping pills to prevent a shutdown in the urinary tract. They worked quite well. But I had to take the medicine at least three times a day.

Hospitals generally do not like patients to bring their own medication, and nurses will not dispense a drug without a doctor's written orders. The nurse gave me one of my pills. I said, "I need two more to avoid urinary shutdown."

"I'll get doctor to prescribe it," she said. She never did.

At about 2 A.M., the feared event occurred. I could not urinate. Liquid was piling up in my bladder. I'll skip the nauseating details; the agony was unbearable. It was as if I swallowed a basketball.

The pills, even if they arrived at this time, could no longer stop the pain. The resident physician (still in training) arrived at 3 A.M. Although I was seriously failing, he failed to examine me or ask me a single question. He did talk to the nurse so quietly that I could not hear him or her.

(I later learned that he asked her if I had been urinating. She pointed to the plastic urine bottle which was about one-quarter full. Of course, if he had bothered to ask me, I would have told him that that urine was deposited before I had urinary shutoff.)

Then followed the most excruciating 4 hours in my life. It was made worse for me because I knew the consequences of shutdown: a burst bladder, kidney destruction from the bladder's back pressure, and death.

I begged and shouted and cried for help from the nurses. To no avail. Without a doctor's orders they said they could do nothing. "But it's an emergency!" No response.

Finally, at 7:45 A.M. my doctor showed up. He is a professor of medicine. He took one look at me, knew what had happened, and sprang to the telephone. In what seemed like a microsecond, the urological resident arrived to empty my bladder with a small tube called a catheter. More than a quart of fluid came out.

Moral: Yell and scream if you think you're in danger. You could save your life.

Experts urge doctors to explain why such behavioral changes are needed. Understanding the need, the experts say, makes it easier for a patient to stick with the prescribed treatment. An informal quiz on the reasons for that treatment might help. When a patient follows doctor's orders, it's called adherence. Less than 100 percent adherence could mean trouble. Dr. Becker advises doctors, "Just asking a patient *in the right way* about adherence has a good effect. A doctor might say, 'We all have troubles and miss some doses. Do you?' This nonthreatening, nonjudgmental tone increases the patient's adherence."

Dr. Roter of Johns Hopkins University studied the patients of doctors trained to handle emotional distress. When she compared them with the patients of physicians not so trained, she found that "patients of trained doctors had a greater reduction in their emotional distress . . . a better quality of life."

You Have a Right to Know

Dr. Becker suggests that a patient who does not want a certain treatment should say so and give a reason. ("I am afraid" is a good enough reason.) He says the doctor then can try to convince the patient that the treatment is worthwhile.

If a patient feels so intimidated that he or she can't say no, a second-opinion doctor from a *different* hospital with no financial interest beyond a consulting fee might be able to say no for the patient.

Thousands of hospitals nationwide now post the Patient's Bill of Rights. Its second paragraph says you have a right to get from any caregiver "relevant, current, and understandable" information about your case.

So take yourself in hand and help your doctor help you: Ask for details on your proper medication and care. Knowing the details about your treatment can help you spot and avoid errors—and may very well save your life.

When Should a Doctor Pay for a Mistake?

ALTHOUGH IT OCCURRED 11 YEARS AGO, DR. Richard Roski, a neurosurgeon, vividly remembers the scene in his operating room at Mercy Hospital in Davenport, Iowa. He was performing a standard spine surgery to relieve the herniated disc of a woman in her 50s, to cure her back pain.

Forty-five minutes into surgery, with the spine cut open, the anesthesiologist reported no blood pressure. Dr. Roski realized that he had inadvertently cut an artery on the other side of the spine, causing blood to pour into the woman's abdomen, unseen by him. The patient was on the verge of dying.

"The people in the operating room responded very quickly," Dr. Roski recalls. "We immediately knew what to do. I sewed her up in seconds to minutes. The general surgeon arrived and opened her abdomen to repair the blood vessel."

Two years after the surgery, the patient filed a malpractice suit against Dr. Roski. A jury decided that the injury to the blood vessel was a rare but not unexpected complication and cleared Dr. Roski of any wrongdoing.

Out of Control

Medical lawsuits like this one—whether the doctor is found guilty of malpractice or only of error—have increased dramatically over the last three decades in every state. In New York, for instance, in 1960, there was one malpractice lawsuit a year for each 100 doctors working. By 1995, the number per 100 doctors had jumped to 6 lawsuits—a sixfold increase! And patients were winning more and higher awards each year.

As a result, medical liability costs in the United States shot up from $15 billion a year in 1970 to $45 billion in 1993. That money goes to patients and their lawyers, but the costs are passed along the system to each of us in the form of higher fees and "defensive medicine" (i.e., when a patient is given medical care that is not necessary, such as extra tests, solely to avoid malpractice claims). According to the American Medical Association, defensive medicine added as much as $25 billion to the U.S. health care bill in 1991.

No other nation in the industrialized world is in this predicament. In Europe and Japan, *all* liabilities, including medical, are no higher than 0.5 percent of the gross national product. In the United States, the liabilities constitute 2.5 percent of the budget—five times more.

Doctors' insurance premiums in some states have risen to record heights. For example, obstetricians in Michigan have to shell out $141,880 a year to protect themselves; in Florida, $130,626; in New York, $85,827. Doctors believe that such premiums are pushing many obstetricians out of the field.

Indeed, 17 counties in Michigan have no specialist obstetrical care. Half the doctors in urban counties in Florida don't carry medical malpractice insurance. That leaves both the patient and the doctor completely unprotected.

What has caused the bloat of malpractice? American doctors complain that ambulance-chasing lawyers have opened up a vein of gold for themselves. They charge that malpractice attorneys often collect more money than the patients. The lawyers shoot back that too many ill-trained, money-hungry physicians are in practice.

Both sides hold some truth. Not all doctors are incompetent. Not all lawyers are crooks.

When Medical Treatment Kills

A 5-year study of malpractice in New York state came up with disturbing findings. The team of doctors, lawyers, economists, and statisticians was headed by Dr. Howard H. Hiatt, a professor of medicine at Harvard Medical School. The researchers examined 31,000 medical records of patients discharged in 1984 from New York hospitals, then applied the results to all 2.6 million patients discharged that year.

They learned that medical treatment had injured almost 100,000 patients, inflicting disability or extending the time they spent in the hospital. Not all injuries caused in a hospital are due to negligence. But close to a third of the cases studied—27,000—showed patients hurt by the *negligent* acts of doctors, nurses, and others. In all, 14,000 people died of injuries inflicted in the hospital—half of them because of negligence. In other words, their deaths could have been avoided.

Projected nationwide, medical malpractice kills 70,000 people a year, twice the deaths in auto accidents. Dr. Hiatt maintains, however, that many of the patients would have died of their disease anyhow, though a little later.

What Is Malpractice?

Malpractice occurs when doctors or other medical personnel fail to follow the usual practice in their own medical community. For example, if a doctor prescribes penicillin for a sore throat and you have a bad reaction, that's unavoidable medical injury. But if, 6 months later, the doctor gives you penicillin again without asking you or checking your record and you have a bad reaction, that's malpractice.

The following also constitute medical neglect:

- Ignorance—The medical staff don't know what the problem is and don't admit it.
- Lack of skill—They are not well trained and act as though they are.
- Alcohol or drug abuse while treating the patient
- Failure to tell the patient of the risks
- Lack of needed equipment, medicines, or staff

"If everybody who was negligently injured sued, the costs could be 10 times greater than now," says Dr. Hiatt. "When we looked at insurance records, we found that fewer than 10 percent of negligently injured people sued. But no more than one third of patients who did sue were injured."

The system is inefficient, he says. It doesn't identify most bad practitioners. It doesn't compensate most negligently injured patients.

Controlling Malpractice Costs by Legislation

In 1975, malpractice threatened to shut down the California medical system, because doctors could not afford insurance to protect them against suits by injured patients. In response, the state legislature passed a bill known as MICRA (Medical Injury Compensation Reform Act) to reform the law. The legislation involves the following measures:

• It set a $250,000 limit on the amount of money a patient could collect for "pain and suffering."
• It created a sliding scale of attorney's fees. It starts at 40 percent for awards up to $50,000. It goes down to 15 percent for awards over $600,000.
• It let juries know whether somebody already has paid for the injury, preventing double payment.
• It allowed installment payments for any awards over $50,000 to help patients preserve their income.

Jay Michael is president of Californians Allied for Patient Protection, a group fighting to prevent changes in the law that would remove these protections. "From 1975 to 1991," he says, "malpractice pre-

miums dropped from $18,000 to $7,000 [in California]. The insurance companies began to offer doctors protection. Lawyers are tough and highly organized, and they fight these laws."

Nine states have passed similar laws with similar results. On the other hand, Harvey Weitz, a lawyer with a large practice winning settlements for injured patients, complains that California's system no longer is fair to victims of doctors' mistakes. He says the law has made it difficult for patients, especially poor ones, to get their day in court.

A coalition of consumer advocates led by Public Citizen, which was founded by Ralph Nader, agrees that the California act has failed. Prevention of errors is a better way, they argue. They want stricter rules governing doctors' behavior and their punishment, as well as increases in the premiums of chronically bad doctors.

Other Solutions

Some doctors see no-fault insurance as the answer, which means that the patient is paid for the injury, regardless of whether the medical team was at fault. Although this approach would lower administrative costs, no-fault provides no incentive for doctors to be careful.

Dr. Hiatt suggests a modification: make the *institution* liable. Then it will pinpoint the reasons for the treatment errors and correct them. The study he headed showed that up to 90 percent of errors were preventable.

What You Can Do

Become involved in your own treatment. Be informed. Know what drugs you're taking and how much of each. Learn their color and shape. Demand full explanations of any treatment. Don't let anybody do anything to you that the doctor hasn't ordered or explained. It could cost you your life.

What It Will Take to Fix Health Care

JANE WYRICK, 46, HAD A CANCER REMOVED from her breast 5 years ago. At that time, she managed an orthodontist's office in Knoxville, Tennessee. "After my surgery, my insurance premiums rose drastically," she recalls. "Ten months later, I lost my job. I paid the premium myself for 9 months. Then I looked into a state plan, which cost $880 a quarter. I couldn't afford it, so now I am uninsured.

"It was a rude awakening. I thought I'd have my job—and my insurance—forever."

Thirty-five million Americans (most of them employed) have no medical insurance. Neither they nor their employers, mostly small-business owners, can afford the premium. When these workers or their families get sick, they delay seeking treatment, hoping the symptoms will go away. Many end up in hospital emergency rooms. The charges mount. Some of these patients die unnecessarily—maybe because hospitals give the uninsured less service than the insured.

If you look at what can happen to hardworking, honest people who have fallen into the medical trap, you can see why a new health care system is needed. The current one not only isn't serving many Americans who need it; it also is tottering on the brink of bankruptcy.

Americans spend more than $800 billion a year on doctors, dentists, hospitals, drugs, and medical machinery. Yet, for all that money, we're buying waste and abuse.

True, America's high-tech medicine keeps a lot of people healthy longer. But it is only the very rich, the very poor (who get benefits through Medicaid, a federal health plan), and the insured who benefit. Many of those without insurance cannot afford $50,000 heart transplants or $25,000 coronary bypasses.

Such expensive procedures are one reason the insurance payment system is out of control. Insurers typically reimburse patients for all services rendered by doctors, whether needed or not. Insurers have no control over which doctors the patients choose, and the patients, who pay only a small part of their bills themselves, are not always attentive to costs. The repercussions affect all of us.

Most Americans agree that an overhaul of the present system is necessary. Even the health insurance industry, long an opponent to change, recently called for a new federal law that would require coverage for all Americans, define a basic set of benefits, and contain costs.

President Bill Clinton and Congress face the awesome task of reining in the medical monster. They'll have to create a plan that meets several important standards. Here are what experts agree is needed and some ideas you'll be hearing about:

• A new health care system should be universal. No patient should be denied care because he or she has no way of paying for it. Nobody should be left out—no matter what the medical condition. And you should never lose your insurance if you're sick or out of work.

• It should be affordable for governments at the national and local levels and for the patient. The burden of payment should fall fairly on rich and poor alike.

• It should cover most diseases or conditions. The plan might include preventive measures, such as diet counseling, and long-term care, such as in-home services.

• It should reduce costs or at least hold them to the current level of the Con-sumer Price Index. It should offer incentives for providers to work at the lowest cost.

• It has to make drastic reductions in paperwork for patients and providers. Some say this paperwork costs $100 billion a year, to say nothing of the waste of time for the medical community.

• It must find ways of checking the quality of care. At best, many medical procedures do nothing for the patient's health or comfort; at worst, they are dangerous.

• It should support the morale of doctors and other medical workers by canceling many of the heavy regulations that waste time and do little for the patient.

The Canadian Model

There are as many cost-cutting schemes as there are experts. One that has been widely discussed is the Canadian plan, which provides health care at 40 percent less cost than that in the United States. That's a $1,000 difference per person per year—a potential savings of $240 billion a year. Half of the savings could come from the elimination of the huge U.S. apparatus for billing and paying claims.

Here's how the Canadian plan works. Each province designs and administers a health plan, setting its own budget. Aided by a central-government grant based on the number of patients, each province pays doctors, hospitals, and other providers without spending more than the agreed-on budget. Taxes pay for the system.

Each citizen carries a plastic health card, which he or she presents when visiting the doctor or going to the hospital. There are no claim forms to fill out—the doctor sends a single form once a month, eliminating the huge administrative costs that plague the United States. The system also virtually has eliminated the insurance companies.

Dr. Nancy Dickey, a trustee of the American Medical Association (AMA), is wary of the Canadian plan. "When you set a budget for health care and the need for services outstrips the budget, you let your patients wait," she says. "We at the AMA don't think people want to queue up."

Managed Competition and Managed Care

Many experts see these two ideas as offering the best way to reform the U.S. system. President Clinton has called for changes that include them.

Managed competition means that medical "sponsors"—large cooperatives, each representing hundreds of thousands of people—negotiate favorable deals with hospitals, doctors, and insurers, then compete for customers on the basis of price and services. (Congress would define a basic service package.)

Managed care is an umbrella term for health maintenance organizations (HMOs) and other providers who try to organize the delivery of health care in cost-effective ways. HMOs keep costs down by eliminating all claim forms; you pay one amount per person for the year, no matter what happens. You may not use the HMO at all, or you may need a $100,000 bone marrow transplant. You pay the same fee. A primary physician guides you through the system if you need specialists. Doctors (who may be salaried or have other fee arrangements with the HMO) keep costs down in their own financial interests.

Critics say that this approach can lead to too little service. Also, your choice of doctor is limited to the HMO panel, although you can go outside the HMO if you pay for it.

How would managed competition and managed care work? A group of high-powered academics and industry leaders who have been meeting yearly at Jackson Hole, Wyoming, have offered a plan for employee groups in which each employee chooses one of several HMO plans. Employers pay an amount equal to 80 percent of the premium of the lowest-cost program; the employee pays the difference—which will be higher, of course, with the more expensive plans.

The plan puts small businesses into giant pools, so they can get the benefit of low administrative costs. Nongovernment agencies monitor quality. The government pays premiums for the poor.

A Health Tax?

How to spread the financial risk will be a key issue in the coming battle over the new system. Will it take more taxes, or just a restructuring of the system to cut costs, or some combination of the two? Most experts say taxes will have to pay at least a part.

Uwe E. Reinhardt, a professor of political economy at Princeton University, has a tax-based plan to pay for the costs of universal health care. Rates start at 0 percent of income for the very poor and rise to 12 percent for the very rich. In effect, the federal government would provide insurance to anybody who needs it. The money would go to the states, based on population. Each state would create its own fail-safe plan to which everyone could subscribe. The system would bring the poor, who would pay no taxes, into the mainstream. People earning good money would be allowed to buy private insurance and not pay the tax. Competition would occur when the price of private insurance exceeded the tax a family would pay; the family could fall back on the government plan. And a tax pool would bring the government insurance to the poor.

Other experts say that employers should pay for the whole insurance premium. But that approach could crush small businesses and lead employers to offer less and less coverage.

Making Hospitals— and Doctors—Cut Costs

At the bottom of the medical chaos lies a principle doctors have defended for cen-turies: *fee for service.* That means that the doctor, or the hospital, bills you for each service. Since the doctor's fee is paid by insurance, neither doctor nor patient cares how much work is done, how many tests are taken, how many X rays are snapped. Their primary interest is in finding a cure for what ails the patient.

Actually, the more tests doctors order, the more money they and the hospital make. Some studies indicate that 50 percent of cesarean operations are unnecessary, as is 14 percent of heart surgery. Those often dangerous procedures waste billions of dollars. Billions more could be saved if doctors cut back on procedures like $800 magnetic pictures, $6,000 hysterectomies, and $10,000 spine operations.

Because hospitals get 38 cents of the health care dollar, government at all levels has been trying to pressure them to give up inefficient methods. New York state, for example, has cut hospital costs by paying a fixed amount for each procedure. This practice forces hospital doctors to think carefully before ordering a test or keeping the patient for a longer stay. Hospital schedules, often concocted for the convenience of doctors, have left high-tech equipment unused for days. Scheduling to increase use would make even the most expensive machines affordable.

One plan would put all hospital doctors on salary, leaving them without a financial interest in recommending procedures. Some argue that salaried doctors don't perform as well as those in fee-for-service practices. Tell that to the Mayo Clinic and Memorial Sloan-Kettering Cancer Center, whose salaried doctors deliver high-quality care at less cost than unsalaried doctors at big teaching hospitals.

Another way of disposing of unnecessary procedures is to ration medical care. Should a 91-year-old get coronary bypass surgery? Probably not, because the odds are he won't live long enough to enjoy the benefits. In Oregon, officials are trying a complex rationing system based on their estimates of the treatment's effects. It's still experimental.

HMOs, which offer coverage by a fixed panel of doctors for prepaid premiums, would have far more control in regulating fees charged by doctors and hospitals, while increased competition between plans would offer further incentive to cut costs.

Insurance for All?

Insurance companies could be barred from discriminating against sick people. Over the years, the industry has spent billions to capture the healthy population. With fewer claims, it can lower the premium and outbid Blue Cross–Blue Shield, which, as a nonprofit organization, tries to cover people of all ages. And reducing the number of insurance claims (U.S. doctors and hospitals fill out more than 400 varieties of the same basic form) would save time and money for doctors, patients, and people in the insurance office.

President Clinton and his advisers now face the heavy task of designing a plan that will please most people and meet the basic standards without bankrupting the nation. It will be interesting to watch, especially since your life and mine depend on it.

Aging

AS THE PRESSURE BUILT AND PAIN SPREAD rapidly through her pelvic region, Zona Bailey, 74, ran as fast as she could to the restroom door, so far away. If only she could get inside in time.

But she was too late. Embarrassed and feeling betrayed by her own body, she wondered, Had anyone seen her?

"It would happen when I went grocery shopping," Mrs. Bailey recalls. "It's a huge store, and if I was at the other end, far from the restroom, I'd be leaking before I got there. It was a nightmare."

A retired public-health nurse from Muskegon, Michigan, Mrs. Bailey was one of the approximately 10 million American men and women with urinary incontinence—the inability to control their urinary stream. Cost of treatment is estimated at $10 billion yearly.

Statistics show that 85 percent of patients with urinary incontinence are women and that, on average, a woman will wait a year before telling anyone, much less a doctor, of the problem.

I am happy to report that doctors now can cure or relieve up to 90 percent of all men and women affected by urinary incontinence. Treatments include medications to ease the condition and ex-ercises to strengthen the bladder muscles. Surgery is a last resort.

Mrs. Bailey endured her incontinence for 15 years before seeking treatment. She regrets the wait but is overjoyed by the results. "I used to have to go to the bathroom every 10 to 15 minutes," she says. "It was becoming a way of life." Her problem was a "dropped bladder," which could not empty properly and allowed bacteria to thrive in the fluid it retained. As a result, she suffered from many infections.

Finally, in 1994, Mrs. Bailey visited a urologist, who corrected the bladder's position. Her ordeal ended. "Now," she says, "I can have 4 to 5 hours between bathroom trips, and at night I never have to get up. It is wonderful!"

Dr. Victor Nitti, a specialist in neuro-urology and female urology at New York University, is enthusiastic about the effectiveness of treatments to help patients control urination. He said that many older patients wrongly accept incontinence as an inevitable condition of aging.

Dr. Nitti objects to that attitude, asserting, "Ads on TV for adult diapers support the idea that it's OK simply to wear a diaper. That's ridiculous. Most patients can be significantly improved with treatment. Rarely do we find a patient who cannot be helped." This is not, of course, to discount the usefulness of such products.

To help you understand three basic types of incontinence—stress, urge, and overflow incontinence—we offer this brief anatomy lesson: Your kidneys cleanse your blood of waste products, which travel in liquid form down two pipes, called ureters, to the bladder. When the bladder contracts, the urine moves into a narrow pipe, the urethra, which conducts it outside the body. Tiny, valvelike muscles called sphincters open and close to control the urine flow.

• **Stress incontinence.** This is chiefly a problem of women in or nearing menopause. They are producing less estrogen, a female hormone that helps keep the sphincters in good condition. A laugh, a cough, or a sneeze can cause the involuntary opening of the weakened valve. About 40 percent of cases are diagnosed as stress incontinence.

Doctor-prescribed replacement estrogen is one treatment used to strengthen weakened sphincters. A newer treatment is surgically implanted collagen (a fibrous material extracted from cow tissue), which reinforces a weak sphincter, so it requires less strength to shut.

Dr. Steven A. Kaplan, a professor of urology at Columbia University College of Physicians & Surgeons in New York City, uses this technique. "It's a quick and simple procedure," he says. Patients usually go home in a day.

Cathy Bainbridge, 33, is a bookkeeper in Germantown, Maryland. In May 1994, a doctor gave her a collagen implant. "The results were immediate," Mrs. Bainbridge says. "Now I can run after my 4-year-old son—and keep up with him!"

Some men who have had their prostate removed may develop severe stress incontinence because their sphincters were damaged by the procedure. Surgeons can correct the damage by implanting an inflatable cuff around the urethra.

Behavioral therapy also helps patients cope with stress incontinence. This approach teaches the patient to contract the sphincters or the muscles of the pelvis, or both. It includes bladder training—teaching patients to urinate on schedule. Doctors report cures for 12 percent of stress-incontinence patients who use this method, as well as marked improvement for an additional 75 percent.

• **Urge incontinence.** In about 40 percent of all incontinence cases, the patient senses an urge to urinate and cannot stop it. The methods and medicines used in treating stress incontinence often can correct urge incontinence. But when all simple methods fail, surgeons can enlarge the bladder, using an 8-inch length of the patient's own intestine. This operation, says Dr. Nitti of NYU, is reserved only for cases resistant to other treatments.

Dennis Smith, 43, of Bayside, New York, suffered from urge incontinence. "I had to go to the bathroom every 10 minutes," he recalls. "Now I'm taking Ditropan, a medicine that helps control the sphincter. It's a wonder drug. It's saving my life."

• **Overflow incontinence.** If the weakened bladder cannot force the urine out, the bladder can accumulate up to a quart of liquid, which causes it to overflow. Such an environment triggers the development of urinary stones and infections. Fewer than 10 percent of all incontinence patients have this diagnosis.

Frequently, surgery can reposition and strengthen the bladder muscle, as it did for Zona Bailey. Drugs can help, too, and exercises can fortify the bladder muscle and muscles of the pelvic support system. (The exercise consists of bearing down on the bladder and then at the point of urination quickly shutting down the sphincter. Many people have used this method with good results. A urologist can help you learn the technique.)

The outlook for urinary incontinence is promising for patients who seek help. Remember: The longer you wait to see a doctor, the more difficult and chancy the treatment becomes. And the more embarrassing things will become.

For more information on urinary incontinence, write to the Simon Foundation for Continence, P.O. Box 835, Wilmette, IL 60091. The organization offers books, videotapes, referrals, and support groups.

We Can Age Successfully

WILL YOU BE PLAYING YOUR FAVORITE SPORT AT 80? Working productively at 100? Some people are, and scientists are learning why.

Few relish the idea of growing old. Do you feel that old age awaits you on some distant shore? Do you rigorously avoid pondering how healthy you'll be when you reach that dim coast? Then you're missing out on a chance to control your future.

Fortunately for all of us, an army of scientists has targeted old age for detailed study. They know that old age brings with it disease and deterioration. But they have much good news too. It boils down to this: You can age successfully, and keep your body young and your mind alert into your 90s. Most of us know at least one octogenarian who still enjoys good health and good times.

Let me introduce you to Lou Berkley. Lou and I played tennis twice a month. Usually, he beat me—not that I was all that hard to beat—but he races around that court like a man 20 years his junior. (I am 20 years his junior.)

His brain is in great shape too. He still works for a national drugstore chain, making intricate deals for store locations. He headed the company's real estate department for years.

Lou celebrated his 87th birthday in 1996.

"I really don't know how I got here," he says with a shy smile. "I'm a little overweight. I do exercise and always have. I've kept up with the tennis. I stopped smoking 30 years ago. I didn't do anything special."

That is successful aging. He has given up tennis for a while because he has a sore arm. He'll be back.

Dr. John Rowe, president of Mount Sinai Medical Center in New York, has studied aging for two decades. He says the latest scientific studies give the same promising message: Disease and decline are not inevitable; only death is. Do the right things, and you could stay healthy and functional for decades.

"In the past," Dr. Rowe says, "we focused too much on disease among the aged. True, as a group, seniors suffer more disease and disability than younger people. But we always find, in every age group, many men and women whose bodies and minds are the equal of the healthy younger population."

A standout for successful aging in my mind is Dr. Michael Heidelberger, a pioneer in the field of immunology, who died in 1991 at the age of 103. Until he hit 100, Dr. Heidelberger took two buses every day to work at his lab at New York University. When he reached 100, his colleagues finally persuaded him to take taxis. Each year, he published several scientific papers. At his 100th birthday party, this thin, sprightly little man gave a rousing and funny thank-you speech. Ingredients for successful aging include lifelong, high-level mental and physical activity; an adequate, low-fat diet; emotional stability; and good luck, especially with heredity. You can't control inheriting tendencies for such illnesses as diabetes, heart disease, Alzheimer's, cancer, or mental depression. But you can protect yourself against some of them and lower your risk. And you have more biological reserve than you think.

When Dr. William Evans of Tufts University in Boston trained healthy men in their 60s in a weight-lifting program, most of the trainees doubled their strength. In a study of men over 60, aerobics exercise restored their heart power to that of 30-year-olds.

At Harvard, Dr. Maria Fiatarone trained frail women and men aged 80 to 100 to lift weights. "We have gotten a 100 percent increase in strength after 10 weeks," Dr. Fiatarone says, "We can increase their ability to climb stairs, to get out of their chairs faster."

One trainee, Sadie Halperin, was 86 at the time. For 11 months, she worked out at the Hebrew Rehabilitation Center for the Aged in Boston. She lifted weights and pedaled a stationary bike. "Before I started," she says, "I found everything hard—shopping, cooking, walking. I felt wobbly; I held onto a wall when I walked. Now I walk down the center of hallways. I feel wonderful!"

Her story is typical: At first, Mrs. Halperin could lift 15 pounds with both legs; later she lifted 30 pounds. At first, she pushed 20 pounds off her chest; later, 50 pounds. Such exercise increases muscle and helps battle osteoporosis by slowing the calcium loss from bones. Calcium-depleted bones can lead to deadly fractures of the hip and spine.

Usually, we lose organ function to disease, disuse, or natural aging. But here's great news: Barring disease, many bodily powers decline very slowly if maintained with proper diet, exercise, brain stimulation, and good social support. And the aerobic study shows that lost function can be recovered.

The National Institute on Aging (NIA) in Baltimore has been studying the aging process in 1,150 men and women for 34 years. Dr. James Fozard, who heads the research, notes that each organ ages in its own way, discounting disease. For example:

Lungs. Capacity drops 40 percent between ages 20 and 80, Dr. Fozard says, even without disease. Lungs lose elasticity, the chest shrinks, and the diaphragm weakens. But you can improve lung function with diaphragm-strengthening exercises. "Opera singers, who exercise their diaphragms, had much better pulmonary function than those who don't," Fozard reports.

Heart. "It was once thought that cardiac output—the amount of blood the heart pumps—declined with age even in healthy people," says Fozard. But, when heart disease is absent, the amount of blood pumped is the same, independent of age. In fact, the healthy heart seems to get stronger, and, unlike the lungs, capacity seems to increase with age.

Blood pressure. In the past, a 60-year-old with a blood-pressure reading of 160/90 would have been told, "For your age, it's normal." The upper number tells how hard the heart is working when the lower part contracts; the lower number reflects the strength of the heart muscle when it relaxes.

Now, for a pressure of 160/90 medication might be prescribed. Dr. Edward S. Lakatta, chief of the Laboratory of Cardiovascular Science at the NIA, says consistent blood pressures of 160/90 and above must be treated. In this way, you reduce risk of such deadly events as heart attack, kidney disease, or stroke. Blood pressure may rise with age because of illness, obesity, anxiety, or stiffening of blood vessels. The longer any of these factors persist, the worse the pressure gets.

Brain. Exciting news: The aging brain retains great power despite nerve loss. Past studies showed large losses of reasoning ability with old age. But in recent years, scientists have measured thinking among elderly persons of the same education. For those free of brain-hampering disease, the age factor all but vanished. "We have built up myths about the aging brain," says the NIA researcher Zaven Khachaturian. "In persons without such disease, we find no dramatic losses of thinking ability from aging by itself."

Dr. Gene Cohen, a researcher at the NIA, specializes in creativity in aging. He reminds us that two of the greatest scientists of all time had their masterworks published late in life: Copernicus at 70, Galileo at 68. Dr. Cohen urges us to develop activities to do alone and with groups: "Those who negotiate later life well have a developed variety of interests."

Memory. Aging often makes it harder to remember names and nouns, but those without Alzheimer's can achieve significant memory improvement. Reports suggest that nerve cells grow new contacts when stimulated intellectually. In France, clinics offer puzzles and games for "mental calisthenics."

"Healthy older men and women show the same emotional and personality characteristics, the same ways of coping, that younger people do," says Paul Costa, Jr., head of the NIA's Laboratory of Personality and Cognition. "Personality itself may contribute to successful aging." Usually that means an optimistic, friendly outlook. Young or old, crabbiness undercuts your ability to cope with life's problems.

Genes. Genes are bits of chemicals that control the chemistry of the cells of your body. You inherit your genes from your parents. By controlling your biochemistry, genes set the color of your eyes and your height, among other features.

Researchers hope to identify genes that lead to disease, then to change them and prevent early death. They also are hunting for the genes that produce normal aging.

James Smith and Olivia Pereira-Smith, husband-and-wife researchers at Baylor College of Medicine in Houston, have proved the presence of aging genes in human cells and pinpointed one such gene. James Smith says as few as 100 genes affect cellular aging, but he adds, "That's a lot, and they are carefully balanced."

If scientists find those genes and learn how they work, say the Smiths, they can intervene in age-related diseases. But that lies on a distant shore.

Take-Charge Questions You Should Ask

DO YOU WORRY THAT, AFTER A DECADE OR two, you will have to get used to being worn out, mentally dull, emotionally distressed, and the easy prey of diseases?

Scientists say it needn't be that way. Experts helped us answer some of the most-asked, most-worried-about questions people have concerning aging. Their replies include the latest scientific findings and tell how you can use them to take charge of your life.

I want to live long only if I can feel and look good and be mentally sharp. Can I?

The short answer is yes. It takes hard work, but the benefits far outweigh the difficulties. Aging makes organs weak and less efficient, naturally. You can't change that very much. But cumulatively, research shows, disease and disuse or abuse wreak far more havoc on your body than aging does. And yet—if you take charge of your body and your mind—you can protect yourself. Here are two surefire ways:

1. Exercise your muscles and your brain regularly, and do so with the goal of recapturing powers you may have lost.
2. Quit the abuses—smoking, drinking, high-fat foods, drugs and high-risk activities (such as motorcycling).

An ounce of prevention is still worth a pound of cure. The progress science has made in treating the illnesses of our later years has been amazing. However, at best, medicines only ease or postpone aging's symptoms. We'd do ourselves a great favor by using our youthful years to prepare for a great old age.

My habits weren't always healthy. Does this mean I will be sick when I'm old?

The answer depends on how old you are now and how "unhealthy" your habits were. Research shows it's never too late to change, and the time to start is now. In your 20s, 30s and 40s, build a pattern of diet and exercise: it will protect you against diseases of the heart and circulatory system, which kill a million citizens a year.

National health organizations endorse a diet of low-fat, low-calorie, high-fiber foods, with several daily portions of vegetables, fruits, and starches and only two 3-ounce portions of meat a day. All dairy foods should have a skim-milk base. One rule: Learn your ideal weight and eat only enough calories to maintain that weight. Control obesity, and you control high blood pressure and diabetes. Both are killers.

A woman's diet should provide more calcium as she gets older, to prevent osteoporosis, the thinning of the bones. Women lose calcium rapidly after menopause. This could result in broken bones—perhaps broken hips and spines. Younger women need to replace the iron lost in menstruation.

The low-fat and low-calorie diet, for one thing, helps you lower your blood cholesterol to a level below 200. This prevents a cholesterol pileup in your arteries. If your diet fails to help you do this, new medicines can take cholesterol out of the blood and even prevent your liver from making it. (See a doctor who treats cholesterol.) Some scientists say a low-fat diet also may protect against cancers of the breast and colon.

Studies show how 90-year-olds benefited from lifting light weights. Some of them, who formerly used wheelchairs, actually got up and took walks on their own.

A good, lifelong exercise pattern protects you against heart disease and helps control obesity, high blood pressure, diabetes, and high cholesterol levels. Recommended is a three-way program of working with weights, flexibility training, and aerobics—exercise that sets your heart pounding and lungs inhaling oxygen quickly and deeply.

Michael O'Shea, *Parade*'s fitness expert, says a daily walking program is the easiest way to start. "At least 30 minutes of brisk walking every day will launch your exercise schedule. It's safe and effective. You'll be encouraged to do more," he says. The three-pronged daily exercise schedule builds enough stamina and strength to play high-energy sports like tennis, basketball, swimming, and running. And it keeps you strong enough to play well and pleasurably into your 70s and 80s.

Smoking, drinking, and fooling around? How bad can they really be?

Pretty bad. (And we mean fatal, not naughty.) Evidence shows that cigarette smoking, taking more than two drinks a day, and engaging in risky behaviors cause hundreds of thousands of early deaths in the United States every year.

These risky behaviors figure highly in early deaths and severe injuries:

- Drinking and driving contribute to about 20,000 deaths a year.
- Smoking-related diseases—heart disease, lung and throat cancers, and emphysema took 434,000 lives in 1988 alone.
- Riding without wearing seat belts is dangerous. Belts have saved 25,000 lives since 1983, and you're three times more likely to need hospitalization without them.
- Unprotected sex, especially with many partners, can result in AIDS.
- Excessive sunbathing can lead to melanoma.

So, everything your mother told you not to do is risky. Mama was right!

Heart attacks run in my family—so what good could it possibly do me to change my lifestyle?

Plenty. Heredity and environment do limit you, certainly. But you can do much to increase your odds for a long life and good health. I know: My father died of a heart attack at age 44. Two of my three brothers had heart attacks in their 30s. Working as a science editor, I saw early findings on preventing heart attacks, and years ago I began to practice what they preached. So far, I've outlived my father by 20 years.

Since 1970, thanks to new findings about diseases of the heart and circulation, death rates in this country have fallen 55 percent from strokes and 34 percent from heart disease. Researchers credit this decline to improved lifestyles—eating less fat, quitting smoking, aggressively treating high blood pressure—and the surgical replacement of clogged arteries.

I hear a lot about "silent diseases." How do I find out if I have one?

There are many tests to detect many kinds of diseases—from certain cancers before they surface, to high blood pressure and high blood cholesterol. Although tests do uncover diseases, they rarely detect them during our healthiest years—age 40 or younger. Two exceptions are tuberculosis and AIDS. A skin test will tell whether you are infected by TB. Caught early, it can be treated easily with drugs. AIDS strikes young people too. If you or your partner have had unprotected sex with a person whose sexual or drug history is unknown, there is a chance the deadly virus may have infected you. Test results can ease your worry or permit you to get early treatment and protect your partner.

The following tests help you and your doctor spot, prevent, and treat illnesses:

- Pap smears—once women become sexually active, or no later than age 18, to detect cervical cancer

- Mammograms—for women 40 and over, to detect early breast cancer
- Prostate exams—for men 40 and over, to prevent cancer
- Rectal exams—for both sexes from age 40 on, to prevent cancer
- Skin cancer (melanoma) exams—for sunbathers at high risk, such as those who are fair-skinned or live near the equator

Vaccines help prevent illnesses, too:

- Pneumonia vaccine—Receive it only once, at 65 or older, for lifelong defense against 23 types of deadly lung bacteria.
- Flu shots—Get them annually, from age 65 on. Surprisingly few people get the pneumonia vaccine. Not enough older people are getting the vaccine to defend themselves against influenza, which can lead to pneumonia. Pneumonia is the nation's sixth leading killer. Together with influenza, it claims 75,000 American lives yearly.

Sometimes, elderly people can't seem to think or remember. Can I avoid that?

You can do a lot to keep mentally sharp at every age. Research shows that stimulation by learning adds to our brain power.

Leonard Giambra, a research psychologist at the National Institute on Aging, says, "Learning is like any skill—you have to practice it. Older people take longer to learn things. We don't know why, but what the older person lacks in speed, he or she makes up in experience and wisdom."

A Harvard University study of 4,000 persons from 1982 to 1989 found that those with a lower level of education were more likely to have memory decline and Alzheimer's with aging than those with a higher level of education. Marilyn Albert, an associate professor of psychiatry at Harvard, says, "We need to be as mentally active as possible—engaged, not isolated, from interesting and challenging ideas." Such findings encourage us to break from routine and take on a difficult mental task: a new, challenging game (bridge, chess); a new subject, such as history, computers, math, languages (I study French); or new ways to do daily work.

When I'm old, I don't want to be cranky and set in my ways. How can I not be that way?

Dr. Paul T. Costa, Jr., of the National Institute on Aging reports that most of us keep our early personality traits: a cranky (or happy) 30-year-old is that way at 60. But, at any age, negative feelings can kill. New evidence links heart disease to hostility. And hostility does not draw others to us.

Dr. Redford Williams, professor of psychiatry at Duke University, says, "If you have companionship, chances are you will live longer, free of disease or emotional distress, than those who don't." For example, Dr. Williams's research reveals this finding about survivors of heart attacks: Those who were unmarried and had no one to confide in had only a 5-year survival rate of 50%. The 5-year survival rate was 82% for patients who were married or had a confidant.

Medical research also reveals this about healthful changes in lifestyle: At whatever age you start to make them, you benefit immediately.

How to Prepare for Old Age

WORRIED ABOUT GETTING OLD?

The latest studies prove that the years after 65, 75, even 85 need not be a monotonous round of physical infirmities, mental feebleness, and dark thoughts of impending death. In fact, millions of people over 65 are living in varied stages of health, dis-

ability, and happiness. And, researchers say, closer attention to diet and mental as well as physical exercise may help improve your odds for a better, healthier, and longer life, regardless of how old you are now.

Gerontologists (people who study old age) have discovered that old people are more different from each other physically, mentally, and emotionally than are the members of any other age group.

For example, every morning and evening, 79-year-old Albert Baer briskly walks the 2.5 miles between his house and his Manhattan office, where he is chairman of the board of a worldwide cutlery business.

"Come hell or high water, I walk 5 miles," he says proudly. He does 15 minutes of push-ups a day, reads intensively, loves opera, and is happily married.

Gladys Goodman is only 64. But she cannot speak; she can barely walk; and she has trouble recognizing Norton, 65, her husband of 32 years, who must tend to her every need at their New York home.

Eli Milstein, 78, is neither as sickly as Mrs. Goodman nor as fit as Mr. Baer. A retired plumber, widowed for 11 years, Mr. Milstein lives alone in his house in Denver. He has aches and pains from bursitis and arthritis. He suffers from high blood pressure. Yet not one of these chronic health problems interferes with his puttering around the house or socializing with his friends.

Biologically, old people also differ from younger adults as much as children do. Geriatricians (doctors who specialize in diseases of the elderly) report that aging bodies respond to foods, drugs, and exercise differently. Studies show dramatic differences in liver and hormone functions from those of younger people.

"That variety also tells us a lot about how we can prepare for old age."

A population explosion of old people has led gerontologists to make a distinction between "young-old" (people between 65 and 75) and the "old-old" (those over 75). The experts are still divided, however, about how much disability there will be as we live longer.

Drs. Ernest M. Gruenberg and Morton Kramer of Johns Hopkins University point out that as doctors prolong the lives of even the chronically ill, many more old people will become disabled.

Dr. James F. Fries, of Stanford University, on the other hand, believes that sickness will decline as we approach the upper limit of life span, which he puts at 100 to 110 years.

Nutrition

Young people thinking ahead to old age should eat a diet that is about 20 percent fat, and most of that from vegetable rather than animal sources. This may cut the risk of arteriosclerosis, more commonly known as hardening of the arteries, which is the main affliction of old age and the culprit behind strokes, heart disease, circulatory ailments, and senility. Many experts credit the increase in life expectancy partly to a change in the nation's diet to more low-fat foods.

Growing proof indicates that vitamins, minerals, or other supplements prolong life, says Dr. Jeffrey Blumberg, director of the Human Nutrition Research

Center on Aging at Tufts University in Boston.

However, the role of these supplements is not without controversy. Several large-scale studies fed the experimental subjects vitamins A, C, E, and beta-carotene or any of these vitamins alone or in combination. The outcomes are confusing. Some research showed no health effect at all. Others found that vitamins E and C both protected the heart from further damage by clogged heart arteries. And still others—designed to protect smokers and asbestos workers from lung cancer—actually increased the risk of lung cancer, arteriosclerosis, and early death.

Like children, all adults need calcium. But over the age of 60, this need increases sharply—some experts say up to 1,500 milligrams a day. Calcium "leaks out" of the bones of old people. And the loss of this important bone mineral leads to fractures of the hip and spine, two conditions that can cripple and lead to death.

Menopausal women in particular may need to take calcium supplements. Now fairly conclusive evidence suggests that for women, estrogen, by pill or by patch, decreases calcium leakage from bones and the rate of hip and spine fractures.

Some are concerned that estrogen will increase the incidence of breast and ovarian cancer. So now doctors prescribe estrogen plus progestin to protect women against cancer. In any case, the estrogen also reduces the risk of heart disease to such an extent that the lifesaving is so great as to overshadow the risk of cancer. In short, estrogen gives women many more extra years.

While it is best for young people to be lean, people 65 and over can carry about 20 percent more weight than what is recommended for them on standard weight charts, says Dr. Reubin Andres of the National Institute on Aging. In other words, if you were a trim 150-pound male at age 19, you can afford to weigh 180 when you are 64, according to Dr. Andres. Most geriatricians, however, advocate maintaining the slimmer line throughout life.

Exercise

Several new studies indicate that we may never be too old to benefit from regular exercise. In Goteborg, Sweden, Prof. Alvar Svanborg has discovered that old people have fewer so-called fast-twitch muscle fibers, the tiny muscles that contract quickly and make us more agile. With exercise, the old people in Professor Svanborg's study regained most of their fast-twitch fibers.

Dr. James Hagberg, of Washington University in St. Louis, put volunteers of average age 63 through an intensive program of walking and running. Within 6 months, they regained some of their lost heart-lung efficiency, and their blood-fat levels dropped after a year.

Dr. Everett I. Smith, of the Biogerontology Laboratory at the University of

Wisconsin in Madison, proved the benefits of even light exercise for the elderly through his work with two groups of 80-year-old women in a nursing home. One group regularly moved their arms and legs while seated. After 3 years, the women who exercised had gained calcium phosphate, while the sedentary group had lost the bone minerals. (Exercise also can prevent the loss of calcium in younger men and women.)

Regardless of when it is begun, a regular, sustained exercise program may lead to a healthier, longer life apparently by protecting you against heart disease, the nation's number one killer. Exercise also reduces a danger of respiratory illness. A study of 17,000 Harvard University alumni by Dr. Ralph S. Paffenbarger revealed that ex-varsity athletes who stopped exercising were at high risk for heart disease, while former sedentary students who began exercise later in life acquired a low-risk status.

Keeping Mentally Alert

You can't teach an old dog new tricks, the saying goes, meaning that the elderly cannot learn anything new. Not so, say researchers. The latest studies show that old people can learn a great deal though not as quickly as young people. But their accumulated experience often gives them an edge. They have seen it all before and know what to do.

Other changes in mental ability occur as well. At Harvard University, Dr. Marylin Albert examined old people's thinking abilities and found that the main problem was remembering names. "They know what something is and how to use it and they know a person, but they cannot call up the name," she says. "It seems to be a naming problem."

Dr. Albert also discovered that the elderly have more trouble than young people doing two things at once. But this doesn't interfere with their doing a good job if they organize their work so that they tackle only one task at a time.

With strong mental abilities intact, many old people are going back to school. One program, Elderhostel, arranges summer vacations for old people at American universities. They study everything from mathematics to music.

Robert Fleming, 73, a retired phone company accountant from Little Rock, went to the University of Arkansas in Fayetteville to study computer science, piano, and European politics. "It gets you interested in other things," he says. "It gets the cobwebs out of your mind."

Correctable Problems

Whether you are now young or old (or young-old or old-old), no illness should go untreated. However, not all of the physical and emotional discomforts of old age are caused by disease alone.

Here, Dr. John Rowe lists 10 of the most common impairments of old age that often can be corrected by proper diagnosis and treatment:

1. Memory loss. The patient may be ill with kidney disease, suffering a nutritional deficiency, or simply taking too many medicines.

2. Hearing loss. Many old people are poorly fitted with hearing aids. Unlike glasses, which can be purchased only with a doctor's prescription, hearing aids can be had for cash in stores where salespeople may not be properly trained to fit them. You have to learn whether the seller has been trained by asking *where* he or she was trained. If it's the company that makes the hearing aid, beware.

3. Visual impairments. Modern surgery removes cataracts, drugs relieve glaucoma (pressure in the eyeball), and lasers can sometimes repair degeneration of the retina.

4. Unsteady gait or falling down. This condition may indicate low blood pressure.

5. Mental depression. Feeling helpless, sad, disoriented, and confused may come from taking too many drugs. Sometimes the patient is understimulated and needs more conversation and attention from caretakers.

6. Weight loss. The simplest but often overlooked cause is that the patient is not eating; the reason may be loneliness, poor teeth, depression, or the fact that no one is available to prepare the food.

7. Chest pain. An irregular heart rhythm may be at fault. If so, it can be corrected by a pacemaker.

8. Fainting. This is another sign of irregular heart rhythm that may necessitate a pacemaker.

9. Incontinence. The inability to control urination may result from weak pelvic muscles. Women can sometimes correct this problem with special exercises. In men, the prostrate gland is usually at fault, and surgical removal may be the answer.

10. Painful joints. The Arthritis Foundation recommends mild exercise to combat this classic symptom of arthritis.

"Everyone wants to live forever, but nobody wants to grow old," says Dr. Jeffrey Blumberg.

Perhaps the best way to combat the inevitable, or to feel as if we have, is to plan our later years around the advice of Dr. Robert Butler, chairman of the Department of Geriatrics at Mount Sinai Medical Center in New York City. He says one of the most important things for old people is to have a goal in life.

It's important, he says, to build into your life various activities, no matter what they are. The list is endless: gardening, bridge, reading, tutoring, working for a local charity or political organization, being a Big Brother, taking care of other old people, creating art, playing music.

"We find that people with a purpose and goal and an organized daily life live longer, are healthier and happier than those who wander aimlessly through their old age," says Dr. Butler.

It is sound advice for all.

How to Beat the Odds

JUST BECAUSE THEY RUN IN YOUR FAMILY doesn't mean you can't do plenty to beat the odds of having a heart attack, cancer, stroke, and other diseases.

You'll find new treatments, drugs, and surgery to help you claim a long, healthy life. Thanks to medical progress and increased public awareness, more than half the patients who would have died of our most fatal diseases 30 years ago are alive today.

For example, from 1960 to 1990, government statistics show, the death rate fell 47 percent for cardiovascular disease and 20 percent for diabetes. Also for that period, the American Cancer Society booklet *Cancer Facts & Figures* for 1994 lists drops in the death rates for these cancers: stomach, down 61 percent for men and 65 percent for women; rectal, down 50 percent for men and 63 percent for women; ovarian, down 10 percent; and cervical, down 68 percent.

Heart Disease

Happily, the news about heart disease is getting better. But the facts are grim: Every day in the United States, 2,500 men and women die of cardiovascular disease. The American Heart Association's statistics show that in 1990 the disease killed 447,900 men in the United States. The fatalities for women totaled 478,000.

The great news is that lifestyle changes really can be lifesaving. That was proved in a study by Dr. Dean Ornish, president and director of the Preventive Medicine Research Institute in Sausalito, California. His patients with severe coronary heart disease cleared their arteries after a full year on a very special regimen. They combined a very low-fat diet (only 10 percent fat) with no smoking, regular exercise, and relaxation training. Average Americans, who have high rates of heart disease, eat a diet that is 40 percent fat—mostly animal fat that stimulates the liver to make more cholesterol.

In time, X rays of their coronary arteries revealed that previously blocked blood vessels were now open. Oxygen-rich blood flowed freely into the heart muscle itself. Without this experiment, we had only statistical studies of large groups of people whose lifestyle seemed to lower their risk of heart disease.

Help yourself, and physicians can help, too. They have medicines that lower cholesterol in your blood. Excess cholesterol is clearly linked to blocked coronary arteries. Doctors now prescribe such medications as Colestipol or Questran, plastic powders that trap cholesterol and safely remove it from your body. (With a low-fat diet, exercise, and Questran, my level fell from 285 to 220. Subsequently, when Mevacor came on the market, I brought my cholesterol level down to 150. As a result, the atherosclerosis has slowed down dramatically.)

Other prescriptions might include large doses of niacin (vitamin B_3), which interferes with the making of excess cholesterol. Some physicians order Gemfibrozil or Probucol, which cuts cholesterol in the blood in some unknown way. But the star of the cholesterol medicines may be Mevacor and its sister drugs.

High Blood Pressure

More patients than ever are beating this killer disease by combining one of the many effective drugs for blood pressure with diet and exercise. To prevent or control high blood pressure, you must take medication as directed. But an estimated 50 percent fail to do so. One terrible result of this very avoidable failure is stroke, a brain-damaging hemorrhage in the skull.

Doctors prescribe heart-saving exercise for you, and the payoffs—if you do it—are great. Regular body movement maintains good blood circulation. It also lowers your blood pressure, which indirectly lowers your cholesterol production. Regular exercise also conserves calcium, which keeps your bones dense and strong. Note: Good nutrition for infants is crucial. Having dense bones by

age 2 means you probably won't develop osteoporosis.

Cancer

Again, we're scoring victories against all forms of this disease, but it remains a formidable foe. In 1990, there were 505,322 cancer deaths in the United States.

Dr. Harmon Eyre, chief medical officer of the American Cancer Society, urges you to learn your family medical history and to share it with your physician. He says knowing that a patient's relatives had cancer helps doctors diagnose, prevent, treat, or cure it. The search is on for a treatment to overcome both the inherited and the habitual tendencies of families that develop cancers. Environmental pollution containing cancer-causing chemicals may also be an important factor.

An exciting discovery in 1996 revealed that at least two genes make a woman susceptible to breast cancer and, possibly, ovarian cancer as well. However, only a small minority of women who develop breast cancer also harbor these genes. Other as yet undiscovered genes may be involved not only in breast cancer but other cancers also.

(Genes are bits of chemicals that control your body's chemical system. The genes are found in almost all cells in your body. You inherit genes from your parents. There are good genes—they make you more likely to live longer—and bad genes—they make you more likely to contract a disease.)

Colon Cancer

This cancer killed 24,385 men and 23,325 women in 1990. "We think perhaps 30 percent of colon cancer patients have a special gene," Dr. Eyre says. A low-fat, high-fiber diet is thought to be of help in preventing or slowing its onset.

If colon cancer is found promptly, surgery can remove it, and its recurrence can be prevented. If your relatives have or had colon or rectal cancer, be sure to undergo periodic exams.

Your doctor will check your stool for blood and will use special instruments to probe deep into your colon in search of polyps (small wartlike growths). Sometimes polyps turn cancerous. They can be removed and checked for cancerous cells. It is undetected colon cancer that kills, so it is vital to be tested regularly. Periodic checkups increase survival chances by 40 percent, according to current estimates.

Prostate Cancers

The prostate is a male gland adjacent to the urinary bladder. Examinations via the rectum can reveal prostate cancers as lumpy growths on the surface of the gland. In the last 10 years, scientists have developed a blood test for a substance that indicates the possible presence of a malignancy. It's called the PSA test. Although controversy has arisen about the blood test, many doctors prescribe the assay for men 40 or older with male relatives who've had this disease.

Prostate cancer killed 32,378 men in 1990. This disease—probably because it was found too late—killed the actor-director Bill Bixby at age 59 and the musician-composer Frank Zappa at 52. The American Urological Association urges yearly tests for prostate cancer for all men aged 50 and older: 80 percent of prostate cancers strike men over 65.

Note: Some doctors argue that an enlarged prostate gland that is not cancerous might benefit more from careful medical scrutiny than from drugs or surgery.

Cervical Cancer

The number of women this disease killed in the United States dropped from 8,487 in 1960 to 4,627 in 1990. A major cause was early detection with the help of Pap tests and treatment with surgery. There is controversy about the effectiveness of Pap tests, but deaths from cervical and uterine cancers have fallen more than 70 percent since the introduction of the tests in the 1950s, reports the College of American Pathologists. Sexually active women (especially those with more than one partner) would do well to have three successive yearly Pap tests. If each test result is negative, a test every three years is then advised.

Genital warts (papilloma) warn women to get a Pap test. The warts are caused by viruses that may also cause cervical cancer. Prompt removal of these warts is urged for men and women.

Ovarian Cancer

Can screenings detect ovarian cancer early enough to remove it? Dr. Eyre says researchers are trying to determine that answer: "We are testing the effectiveness of pelvic exams, a blood test for a substance called CA 125, as well as a sonar examination of the ovaries."

Breast Cancer
In 1990 in the United States, 43,391 women died of breast cancer. Tests for early signs of this disease also are controversial. If, as a woman, you have a family history of breast cancer, ask your doctor when, how, and how often you should be tested. Self-examination of the breasts and mammography have saved lives through early detection. But some doctors rate the tests as ineffective, saying much is missed in self-exams. Because of denser breast tissue in younger women, mammograms don't always reveal cancerous sites.

Dr. Eyre urges that initial mammograms be taken at age 40, then—depending on the study's results, the patient's risk factors, and family history—every 2 years until age 50, and yearly after that.

Some risk factors for breast cancer reportedly include alcohol consumption, a high-fat diet, and obesity. Researchers are testing a diet low in animal fats as a possible preventive. Detection is difficult: "Of women who get breast cancer," Dr. Eyre says, "seventy percent have no known or identifiable risk factor."

Lung Cancer
"In America, statistics show that smoking accounts for 90 percent of lung can-

cer in men and 85 percent in women," Dr. Eyre says.

The American Cancer Society projects that lung cancer will kill 94,000 men and 59,000 women this year, and it cites a terrifying mortality rate rise since 1960—up by 104 percent in men and 452 percent in women! And a jump in lung cancer for the young is almost certain: a new study by the University of Michigan showed a 2 percent rise in smoking among schoolchildren in the 8th, 10th and 12th grades.

Diabetes

A nine-year study of 1,441 diabetic patients shows that those who succeeded in keeping their blood-sugar levels near normal had far fewer complications of eyes, nerves, and kidneys than others. If you are a diabetic, you can reap the same benefits by regularly measuring your blood sugar, following your prescribed meal plan, and exercising. Engineers have developed small, accurate machines that test for sugar levels in the blood from a single drop.

Stomach Ulcers

In the last decade, several powerful compounds—including Tagamet, Pepcid, Axid, and Zantac—have reduced stomach acid for ulcer patients. Now, after 12 years of study, researchers say a specific bacterium in the stomach causes peptic ulcers and may be linked to cases of gastritis and gastric cancer. To kill it and prevent reinfection, antibiotics and bismuth are prescribed.

Influenza

Flu is especially deadly for the elderly or those harboring a chronic disease. If you are 60 or older, ask your doctor whether you should be vaccinated yearly against the flu. Influenza opens the door to pneumonia, which is even deadlier.

Pneumonia

A one-time-only lifetime pneumonia vaccine can halve your risk of this dangerous disease. It can protect against a score of different types of pneumonia-causing bacteria. Doctors recommend it for most individuals aged 60 and over.

Think about it: If you would use the medical knowledge available, you could add years to your life.

Is a Retirement Community for You?

PEOPLE DON'T LIKE TO TALK MUCH ABOUT THE problems of being old. But one day—when the kids are gone, or your finances or health aren't what they used to be—you may have to make up your mind about where you're going to spend your remaining years.

Most people stay put. Census data suggest 70 percent of people over 60 have lived in the same home for 5 years or more. They want to stay close to friends and family. Robert B. Maxwell, a former president of the American Association of Retired Persons, says, "The American dream of the young is to own your own home. The American dream of older folks is to remain in your own home."

Would you be different?

In the 1970s, there was a mass migration of elderly Americans seeking sun or fun or both. Between 1975 and 1980, 3 million folks 65 or over left their old homes for new housing—1.5 million of them moving to other states, mostly Florida, California, Arizona, and Texas. Today, a variety of options exist for those who want to retire "somewhere else."

I found Charlotte and La Grand Wilberg at Sunflower Resort, a trailer park in Surprise, Arizona. She's 59; he's 60. When La Grand's emphysema got worse in 1985, his doctors advised him to move to a lower altitude, down from the 5,500 feet of Price, Utah, where he lived. There was a series of visits to Arizona, and things began to change.

"From the moment we pulled into Sunflower in our motor home, we found the people here warm and helpful," Charlotte says. "In a few weeks, we felt as though we had lived here all our lives."

Sunflower Resort is not what most people imagine when they hear the words "trailer park." It's a new type of camp for adults at least 50 years old—inexpensive but rich with things to do. It features two swimming pools; tennis; billiard rooms; classes in art, languages, computers, sculpting—you name it. And no children are allowed.

The 1,100 recreational vehicles here are really factory-made homes with wheels. They run about $50,000 or less, with a completely furnished living room, bedroom, kitchen, and bathroom. At Sunflower, $1,668 a year pays for a site with water and sewage services and also gives you access to the leisure activities. Gas and electric are extra. A couple could live here for $15,000 a year.

Like the other residents, the Wilbergs picked out the activities they wanted; for La Grand, it was golf and making wicker furniture; for Charlotte, church work.

"The first time we saw the place," Charlotte says, "I thought, 'Everybody is so old. Get me out of here.' Now, I don't notice people's ages. They're not sitting around being sick."

When it gets really hot in the summer, the Wilbergs seek cooler climes, visiting their daughter on the East Coast or traveling abroad. They sold their house in Utah. That part of their lives was over.

Of course, you don't have to move out of your longtime home just to prove you're a go-go senior. Usually, you can find plenty to do right in your hometown. Rose Dobrof, executive director of the Brookdale Center on Aging of Hunter College in Manhattan, points out, "Seniors who don't migrate are not, as a group, less active than those who do move. Activity and zest for life are found everywhere."

In weighing whether to move or stay put after retirement, assess your needs and resources. Examine your income and expenses, the services you'll need, the distance from relatives and friends, personal safety, health care, work opportunities, and the chance to have fun.

David Savageau, a relocation counselor in Gloucester, Massachusetts, gathered data across the United States for his book *Retirement Places Rated*. When relocating, he says in the book, it is important to "develop a very strong psychic connection with the place where you are going to live before you actually move there." That means spending time at the place and getting to know the people, and renting before buying. Many people take years to decide.

There's a lot to choose from these days. Some places just evolve—unplanned communities where elderly people have congregated because they heard that a particular neighborhood or town fits an older person's needs. These are called *naturally occurring retirement communities*. Such places, however, may not have the leisure activities you want or the medical or home-care services you need. *Congregate housing* refers to places that offer meals, leisure activities, trips, vans to take residents shopping, and crime protection. An example is St. Margaret's House in Manhattan, a 20-story high-rise for the elderly underwritten by the Department of Housing and Urban Development (HUD), which also pays a portion of each resident's rent.

Charlotte Leyden, 88, pays $474 a month at St. Margaret's, which includes one meal a day. "Imagine," she said, "if I were alone in my last apartment, and I fell—as I did here. There, I had no one to call. I could have died. Here, I phoned the maintenance man, who came and got me."

For people who have some money, the choices for retirement open up. In communities built only for older persons, you can buy a home for as little as $50,000 or as much as $250,000.

Sun Cities, Arizona, begun in 1960, is a two-city complex northwest of Phoenix with 68,000 residents. The two communities share 11 golf courses, plus tennis courts, swimming pools, and recreation buildings where you can sculpt, paint, do pottery or woodwork, sing, play instruments, and learn languages. All that costs $100 a year. The one- to four-bedroom homes stand neat and clean in the Arizona sun. For a condominium, as little as $90 a month covers garden and building maintenance. There is no maintenance charge for a single-family house.

Most of the people I talked with in Sun City liked the way they've made tight friendships very quickly. They say they get emotional support from their peers more readily than they do from younger persons—often more so than from their own children. Formal studies of retirement centers uphold this observation.

Elderly people with disabilities or health problems—and enough money—are moving in increasing numbers to *continuing-care communities*. There you pay an entrance fee that ranges from $5,000 to $300,000, depending on the elegance and size of the place, and a monthly fee, from as little as $300 up to $2,700, to cover food, housekeeping, and other services. In some cases, up to 90 percent of the entrance fee is returned when you leave. (If you die, it's given to your family.) Some communities offer nothing back, so it's wise to go over the contract with a lawyer or financial adviser.

These villages guarantee continuing care in a nursing home attached to the community. In some, the monthly fee can go as high as $3,600 if you transfer to the nursing home—which, over time, could pauperize anyone except the very rich.

To overcome that problem, some villages offer a "life-care" program that promises nursing-home care for the rest of your life, if you need it. The financial arrangement varies with each organization. If Medicare or Medicaid approves of the nursing home, the costs will be covered.

Meadow Lakes, in Hightstown, New Jersey, looks like a fancy hotel—a series of low buildings connected by all-weather corridors sitting in a lush, well-kept garden. The 400 residents, whose average age is 85, live in one- or two-bedroom apartments. They receive one meal a day for their monthly fee, which ranges up to $4,730.

Louise Cook, 78, a retired telephone representative living at Meadow Lakes, spoke of being surrounded by people her own age all the time. Sometimes, she admits, she needs "a youth fix." Then, smiling slyly, she adds, "Of course, the need is over in a few hours of visiting, and, happily, it's time to go home."

If you want to be sure that no young people can move into your retirement village, check to see whether it meets HUD's new standard, which says 80 percent of a retirement community's residents must be older than 55. In 1988, Congress voted that unless they meet this rule, retirement communities must open up their housing to young families.

A strong warning comes from Dr. Charles F. Longino, Jr., professor of sociology at Wake Forest University in Winston-Salem, North Carolina, and an expert on migration during later years. "People tend to fantasize about places that are the opposite of where they are living," Longino says. "When you move to a place, it tends not to live up to your fantasy because, when you vacationed there, it was the best time of the year." The lesson: Get to know the place year-round before you move or plunk down a deposit to buy new housing.

If you're inclined to move for whatever reason, study the situation carefully. It may be your last migration. With care, you can make it a happy one.

For more information, write to the American Association of Retired Persons, Consumer Affairs, 601 E Street, N.W., Washington, D.C. 20049.

Should Death Be a Patient's Choice?

JUNE 1990: A RETIRED PATHOLOGIST FROM ROYAL Oak, Michigan, grants the use of his "suicide machine" to a woman who has sought his help to avoid the horrors of Alzheimer's disease. She pushes a button and dies. Despite the publicity and ensuing furor, two more women enlist Dr. Jack Kevorkian's help to commit suicide a year later. The 61-year-old retired pathologist gives one woman a canister of lethal carbon monoxide to breathe into her lungs.

March 1991: In Rochester, New York, a doctor reports that he has given a hopelessly ill leukemia victim a full prescription of sleeping pills. She takes the pills and dies.

August 1991: A book with recipes for suicide becomes a best-seller. The author's ex-wife, in what appears to be a fit of depression, kills herself.

November 1991: By a slim majority, voters in Washington State reject a referendum that would legalize suicides assisted by a physician; 46 percent of the voters approve the initiative.

December 29, 1990: A 94-year-old woman dies of bowel cancer after prolonged suffering. Her son, Dr. Fred Hechinger, a nationally known educator and writer, says he felt that his mother had been "tortured to death" by one medical machination after another. Cases like Lilly Hechinger's occur much more often than the news headlines might lead us to think.

"We took her to the hospital because she was bleeding internally," Fred Hechinger recalls with some bitterness. "It would have been better had we let her bleed to death. She would have just gone to sleep."

Instead, Mrs. Hechinger fell into a high-technology medical care trap. Her doctor performed an operation for bowel cancer. She survived the surgery but, once put on a breathing machine, could not be weaned from it.

"I could see in her eyes the horror," her son recalls. "She raised her arms as if to say, 'Why are you doing this to me?'" Finally, and mercifully, her kidneys shut down and her heart stopped.

Fred Hechinger wrote an article for the *New York Times* about his mother's tragedy. More than 200 readers sent him letters relating similar experiences. (Dr. Hechinger has since died.)

These are but a few of the events revealing that growing numbers of Americans want to avoid long, painful deaths at the hands of modern medicine. Many say that respirators, feeding tubes, and other gadgets can stretch out life beyond points that make it worth living. And, they add, the costs for such care can financially sicken the patients' families. Their concerns are grave, indeed.

Still, this move toward "death with dignity" worries many doctors, lawyers, and students of ethics. They contend that we are lurching rapidly toward a state of euthanasia on demand. If this situation actually is arrived at, they argue, it inevitably not only will lead to the killing of conscious terminally ill patients who want to end their suffering, but, they maintain, it also will affect others not so stricken.

For example, it will impact the comatose, who are unable to choose or refuse euthanasia (a Greek word meaning "easy death"). It also will imperil—from infancy through old age—those who are merely ailing or somehow socially dependent.

Yale Kamisar, a professor of law at the University of Michigan at Ann Arbor, reminds everyone, "Not all people are kind, understanding, and loving. Yet they will be making decisions about the elderly and the helpless. A lot of pressure may be placed on people to choose euthanasia when they don't really want it."

A *Parade* survey indicates that public opinion favors helping the terminally ill to avoid a needlessly long, painful, and costly death. We mailed questionnaires to 3,750 individuals aged 21 or older. We asked them to respond to various statements—including four concerning the right to choose death, which appear in this chapter. The first concerns terminally ill persons who are conscious and rational:

1. *If a person has a fatal illness, that person should have the right to have all life-sustaining devices removed, including feeding tubes.*

Of the 2,203 persons who responded, 79 percent said they agree with the statement; 12 percent disagreed; and the other 9 percent said they neither agreed nor disagreed or indicated no answer.

Susan M. Wolf, an associate for law at The Hastings Center, a think-tank for biomedical ethics in Briarcliff Manor, New York, said our courts long have given patients the right to turn down medical treatment of any kind, even if it leads to their deaths. But what if patients aren't conscious and can't choose for themselves? Consider these two cases:

• On April 15, 1975, Karen Ann Quinlan of Roxbury, New Jersey, sank into a coma at the age of 21 after ingesting alcohol and tranquilizers. The widening of criteria on a patient's suitability for euthanasia then began. A respirator kept Quinlan breathing; a feeding tube supplied nutrition. Most experts agreed she was in a "vegetative state," with no chance of a normal life. When healthy, however, she had not prepared a living will, and, in her coma, she certainly could not consent to the respirator's removal.

In March 1976, Quinlan's parents sued to have the respirator removed. After a New Jersey court consented, her machine was stopped. Quinlan lived 9 more years, never regaining consciousness. At that time, however, in states such as neighboring New York, the parents and other relatives of patients like Karen Ann Quinlan could not remove their life support systems, including feeding tubes, unless the comatose person previously had made a clear request to do so, preferably in writing.

• In June 1990, the U.S. Supreme Court rejected the request of the parents of Nancy Beth Cruzan, 32, to end her treatment at the Missouri Rehabilitation Center in Mount Vernon, Missouri. She had suffered severe brain damage in a car accident on January 11, 1983, and lay for 7 years in what doctors termed "a vegetative state." Given more evidence that Cruzan would "wish to terminate" her treatment, however, a Missouri court finally allowed the removal of her feeding tube on December 14, 1990. She died 12 days later.

Professor Kamisar says the euthanasia drive began in the 1950s to ease the "helpless pain and hopeless suffering" of a dying patient who had requested death. Now, he warns, the movement to bring easy death to anyone who wants it—and to some who do not want it—threatens to swell to tidal wave proportions.

The second question on the *Parade* magazine survey on dying:

2. If a person is in a coma that cannot be reversed, relatives should be allowed to tell doctors to remove all life-sustaining devices, including feeding tubes.

The Missouri probate court's decision in the Cruzan case reflects the views of 81 percent of those surveyed by *Parade,* who said they agreed with this statement. Only 11 percent said they disagreed, and 8 percent either had no answer or neither agreed nor disagreed.

In 1990, a federal law was passed requiring all hospitals and nursing homes receiving federal aid to inform patients of their rights—or lack of them—to refuse treatment under their state's law. Here are two legal aids, recognized by some states and rejected by others:

• **Living will.** This document tells your relatives what you want done (or do not want done) should you get so sick you cannot tell the doctors yourself. For example, you can say under what conditions you want life support systems to stay or go.

You can say in your living will whether you want chemotherapy, surgery, or radiation treatments for cancer, or nothing at all. You can instruct your future doctors via a living will whether you want doctors to get your heart started if it

stops. You can also order hospitals or your doctor not to revive you if you have a severe brain hemorrhage.

• **Proxy.** This is a person you choose to make health decisions for you, should you be unable to make them for yourself. Some states require you to sign a power of attorney to do so. If your state recognizes a living will, the will then guides your proxy.

David Smith is director of legal services for Choice in Dying, an organization headquartered in New York City and devoted to protecting a patient's rights to self-determination. Mr. Smith says that, in states which recognize living wills, doctors have an obligation either to honor the patient's wishes or to try to find another doctor who will honor them.

Arthur Caplan, director of the Center for Biomedical Ethics at the University of Minnesota in Minneapolis, says he thinks living wills and proxies are good ideas. He adds, however, "I'm just skeptical that most Americans will fill them out. I've done mine but cannot get my wife to do it. She's afraid the doctors won't treat her aggressively."

Dr. Marca L. Sipski is medical director of the Kessler Institute for Rehabilitation in West Orange, New Jersey. Dr. Sipsky treats patients who became paraplegics and quadriplegics as a result of accidents. (She was one of Christopher Reeve's physicians.) Dr. Sipski says she feels that many of her patients are emotionally unable to fill out living wills.

"In the first hours, days, and weeks," she observes, "they all want to die. If they fill out the living will forms when they're first admitted to the hospital, they will tell us not to resuscitate them if they get a lung clot, which often happens. Yet we know that, in a few months, when they see life is not only possible but often good, they change their minds."

The third *Parade* survey question:

3. *In case of fatal illness, a doctor should be allowed to help that person end his or her life.*

In our survey, 49 percent said they agreed with this statement, while 35 percent disagreed, and 16 percent neither agreed nor disagreed or chose no answer.

Like the Washington State referendum, this response indicates that many people want doctors to assist conscious, rational dying patients with their suicides. Fewer, however, would leave suicide solely up to the patient.

Many ethicists and physicians decry the euthanasia movement. Some reflect the view of Arthur Caplan of the Center for Biomedical Ethics, who fears that, with medical costs skyrocketing, there will be pressure to do away with the high-cost, low-benefit patients, mostly the old and the poor. "Doctors are trained to save lives," declares Mr. Caplan. "We shouldn't turn them into killers.

"In 12 years," he adds, "I've had the chance to talk with many mentally alert patients. I have not seen one case in which, had they wanted to kill themselves, they couldn't have done it alone."

In the Netherlands, physician-assisted suicide is allowed—not by statute. Instead of a law, the Dutch have a system that, if the guidelines are strictly followed, prosecutors will not indict doctors for giving the lethal injections.

A report in the September 14, 1991, issue of *The Lancet,* the British medical journal, reviewed nearly 10,000 deaths in the Netherlands. The researchers found that Dutch doctors had given lethal drugs at the patient's request in 1.8 percent of the cases studied. They provided the means of suicide in 0.3 percent of the cases and performed life-ending maneuvers without explicit request in 0.8 percent.

In 17.5 percent of the cases, doctors—unasked—gave their patients pain-killing drugs in amounts that could have shortened life. Equally, they withheld or withdrew treatment that might have prolonged life.

"It's impressive that there are so few problems," says Mr. Caplan. "I would not change the Dutch situation. They feel comfortable with it. They are not afraid the doctor will kill them because they lack insurance."

Dr. Leon Kass, a professor of social thought at the University of Chicago, disagrees with Mr. Caplan and says the Dutch have "started us on a decline that will take us all the way to eliminating everyone deemed unfit."

In his analysis in *Commentary* magazine (December 1991) of a Dutch government report on the issue of euthanasia, Dr. Kass calculated that 25,300 cases of euthanasia in some form occur in the Netherlands each year. He cites figures from the Dutch report showing that 60 percent of morphine-overdose euthanasia cases were done without the patients' knowledge or consent.

In 45 percent of the cases in which patients' lives were ended in a hospital, the physician acted not only without the patient's consent but also without telling the family.

Dr. Carlos F. Gomez, a medical resident at the University of Virginia Hospital, has made his own study of the Dutch practices. In his book *Regulating Death,* Dr. Gomez calls attempts to protect vulnerable patients "half-hearted and ineffective at best."

He says that his in-depth interviews with Dutch physicians and others involved in 26 euthanasia cases has led him to believe that doctors in the Netherlands do not routinely follow the accepted guidelines. Yet, he adds, when they do not, there are no repercussions. Dr. Gomez says physicians sometimes take lives without consent and without getting a second opinion.

Despite this alarming revelation, Americans seem to be moving ever closer to the Dutch approach to euthanasia. Physician-assisted suicide was defeated in Washington State, but similar initiatives are coming in Oregon and California.

The final question in the *Parade* survey:

4. If a person has been diagnosed as having a fatal illness, he or she should be allowed to take his or her own life.

Apparently, more Americans are opposed to euthanasia when the death is not physician assisted: only 39 percent agreed with the above statement; 45 percent disagreed; 16 percent neither agreed nor disagreed or indicated no answer.

Undeniably, two advocates of patient suicide, whether physician assisted or not, have captured the public's attention: Dr. Jack Kevorkian, with his "death machine," and the author Derek Humphry, whose book *Final Exit* is a compendium of suicide recipes.

Using Dr. Kevorkian's machine, 54-year-old Janet Adkins of Portland, Oregon, ended her life in a minivan in a park near Flint, Michigan. Dr. Kevorkian said Ms. Adkins told him she had been diagnosed as having Alzheimer's disease, which destroys memory and thinking, and that she did not want to face the future with this terrible disease. When she hit the switch on his machine, a sleeping potion flowed into her vein. In minutes, she was asleep. A timing device then released a second drug that paralyzed her heart. Minutes later, she was dead.

Dr. Kevorkian refused to be interviewed, but his attorney, Michael Alan

Schwartz, of Southfield, Michigan, answered some of our questions. Essentially, Mr. Schwartz said that Dr. Kevorkian was performing a "vital service"—one that other doctors were not brave enough to perform. He added that Dr. Kevorkian charged no fee for this service.

Although Janet Adkins was not in pain, Marjorie Wantz, 58, of Sodus, Michigan, complained of a severe pelvic pain that, Mr. Schwartz said, was not helped by traditional pain control methods. She became the second person to seek Dr. Kevorkian's help.

The third was Sherry Miller, 43, of Roseville, Michigan, paralyzed by multiple sclerosis. Dr. Kevorkian said he gave her a canister of carbon monoxide because her veins were too small to permit the injection of a lethal drug.

Only 20 states have clear-cut laws against assisting suicide. Because Michigan does not, a judge there dismissed a murder charge against Dr. Kevorkian. He later was forbidden to use his "death machine" again in the state.

Physicians have condemned Dr. Kevorkian's actions and his machine. Dr. Leon Kass wrote of Kevorkian, "I feel the deepest shame for my profession that he should be counted a member."

Derek Humphry, 61, is the founder of the Hemlock Society, based in Eugene, Oregon. He has professed to be devoted to helping the terminally ill end their lives if they wish. In his book, Mr. Humphry says that Dr. Kevorkian "performed a public service by forcing the medical profession to rethink its attitude about euthanasia." Once a journalist for U.S. and British papers, Mr. Humphry obviously struck a nerve with *Final Exit,* which sold 500,000 copies in 9 months.

"The public," he says, "is disillusioned with how medicine and the law handle the dying process. People are taking the law into their own hands."

Mr. Humphry says that the fear of pain drives many to ask for euthanasia. In his book, he reports that 10 percent of pain can't be controlled. He also says that he helped his first wife, Jean, a cancer patient, to commit suicide in 1975 at age 42. Headlines last October told of the death at age 49 of his second wife, Ann, who was diagnosed with cancer in 1989 and left by Mr. Humphry a month later. They subsequently were divorced. She killed herself after *Final Exit* was published, discussing her suicide and doubts about euthanasia in a note and a videotape. Mr. Humphry has asserted that his ex-wife's death had nothing to do with his book.

Dr. Kathleen Foley, a neurologist in charge of pain services at Memorial Sloan-Kettering Cancer Center in New York City, says, "For terminal illness, such as advanced cancer, a variety of approaches adequately control pain. For me to kill the patient because of pain is unconscionable."

In his *Commentary* article, Leon Kass calls *Final Exit* evil: "This is humanitarian evil, evil with a smile: well-meaning, gentle and rational, especially rational." He voices concern that depressed high school students will follow the book's prescriptions.

"Thanks to Derek Humphry's book," he writes, "our youth need no longer fail. Even if only one teenager is helped to suicide, Derek Humphry will have a lot to answer for."

To obtain a copy of your state's living will and medical power of attorney forms, write to Choice in Dying, 200 Varick Street, 10th floor, New York, NY 10014. Send a check for $3.50. To order by phone call (800) 989-WILL. You can download the forms free if you visit the website http://www.choices.org.

For Dying Children and Their Families, Hospices Provide Loving Care and Comfort

THIS IS A STORY ABOUT LIFE, NOT DEATH. IT IS about children who have only a few months or few years to live. Some can no longer speak or see or hear or think. But, in their last moments, they are surrounded by love.

Daniel Faith was born in 1988 with only part of a brain, a deformity of the skull, a single nostril, and a flat forehead. He was not expected to live for more than a few years. This tiny boy in overalls and a yellow shirt sits upright in a special chair. His eyes remain hooded, as if in a waking sleep. He moves his arms and hands but without purpose.

Angela Leale, a musician in her 20s, strums a guitar beside Danny's chair. She sings a bright little children's song. In a minute or two, a funny small smile lights

his sad face, like a rainbow springing up after a storm. Danny is cooing now.

When I visit St. Mary's Hospital for Children in Bayside, New York, and see these two human beings connect with one another, I fight back tears and force myself to ask, Why spend money and effort to keep such a child alive?

"We believe that such children need to make the most out of every moment of life remaining to them," replies Dr. Burton Grebin, executive director of the hospital. "We cannot let them die in pain and alone. And if a smile is all the child gets, that's enough."

Danny is one of 10 children in the Palliative Care Unit (PCU) at St. Mary's. *Palliative* refers to lessening the pain or discomfort of a disease without curing it.

Essentially, the PCU is a hospice—a place where a child can die in dignity and comfort. The 95-bed hospital, founded by Episcopalian nuns, serves other children with long-term medical problems, physical deformities, cancer, or victims of accidents who need rehabilitation. It has a full complement of doctors, nurses, teachers, nutritionists, social workers, and therapists (physical, speech, music, art). The PCU lessens the suffering of the dying child.

St. Mary's is just one of a growing number of institutions offering love and comfort to dying children. In response to their increase, in 1983 Ann Armstrong-Dailey founded Children's Hospice International in Washington, D.C. This group encourages the establishment of children's hospices and shows them how to care for sick and dying children. When she began, only four hospices for children existed in the nation. Today, 200 hospices include children, and, Mrs. Armstrong-Dailey says, 800 more institutions are thinking about providing places for children.

Ann Armstrong-Dailey's work developed out of deep frustration. "A doctor friend had asked me to meet with a family whose 8-year-old son was dying," she explains. "There were five hospices in Washington with adult programs only. None would take him. That made me angry."

She also tells the story of Timmy, 5, who suffered from severe kidney disease. As long as the doctors and nurses be-

lieved there was hope for his recovery, they rallied round him. When the treatments failed, they seemed to withdraw from him emotionally.

"No one would talk to Timmy about death, not even his parents," recalls Mrs. Armstrong-Dailey. "He felt so isolated."

Timmy's last act was to draw a yellow butterfly with 'I love you, Mom' written on it."

His parents were overcome by grief and guilt that they had not been at Timmy's side when he died. They later were divorced; his father became an alcoholic, his mother a pill taker. His sister, ignored at home, failed at school.

"None of this might have happened had there been hospice support," Mrs. Armstrong-Dailey declares. "Mother Teresa says that the greatest pain on Earth is not the pain of poverty and hunger but the feeling of isolation."

Many hospices have home-care programs. St. Mary's has one that sends nurses, therapists, and sometimes doctors to the home of a dying child. Edmarc Hospice for Children in Portsmouth, Virginia, only provides in-home care. Formed 10 years ago by a Presbyterian minister, Edward Page, who had cancer, and a young couple, Allen and Joan Hogge, whose son Marcus was dying of a rare brain disease (Edmarc combines their names), the hospice has since served more than 200 children, more than half of whom have died.

"We can't cure the dying child," says Julie Simpson, Edmarc's executive director. "But we can help heal the family. And we can promise them that they won't go through this alone."

At the Children's Hospital of Wisconsin, in Milwaukee, most of the patients die at home. "We try to have parents be the focus of the care," says Patricia Quinn-Casper, a nurse-coordinator. "They know their children best. We are supportive visitors who come into the home. We work as advocates to help them get through this."

Dan Marks, who is vice president of finance of the San Diego Hospice Children and Adults, took a job there. He had experienced the hospice staff's help for him and his son, Jacob, who died at home 9 weeks after a diagnosis of cancer.

"I don't know what my family would have done without the hospice," he says. "Your life shatters at the diagnosis. They gave us hope that we could take care of our son. He died in his mom's arms. He was smiling. You can't put a price on that."

Marks adds that the San Diego hospice loses money—72 cents on the dollar—in its effort to provide care for those children who need it even if their families can't pay for it.

Even a brief contact with a hospice provides deep comfort for the parents of a dying child. Debbie, 23, and Ken Fuqua, 22, of San Diego became the parents of Stephanie. During her pregnancy, Debbie's doctors learned through a sonogram of the fetus in the womb that the baby had water on the brain. After birth,

surgery failed to correct the resultant brain impairment.

"They didn't think she'd live past a year," Debbie says. "They gave her 60 days. She didn't move much. She could hear a little, and she was blind."

The Fuquas turned to the San Diego hospice. Staff members there gave Stephanie care at home and counseled her young parents on how to cope with a terminally ill child. A nurse and a social worker visited them once a week.

"They comforted me," says Debbie. "I don't know what I would have done without them. It's like living on the edge. A lot of stress. Oh, but it's worth it. She was my daughter, and I loved her."

Later that year, the Fuquas moved to Chicago, where Ken enrolled in college. The couple had learned enough to provide routine care for Stephanie on their own. They tried their best to make her days as comfortable as possible. But a month later, the baby suffered a seizure and had to be taken for emergency treatment to Rush-Presbyterian Hospital.

"I told the hospital, 'No heroic measures,'" Debbie says. "I told them, 'Don't put Stephanie on a machine. If she stops breathing, it is time for her to go.' We felt she'd go when she was ready."

In New York, Ann Armstrong-Dailey calls St. Mary's "the gold standard of hospices for children." It has everything. Its low brick building stands on a knoll overlooking Long Island Sound. In spring, clumps of flowering trees dot the green lawns. You can see them from the

PCU on the fourth floor. As you step off the elevator, bright sunlight showers down from the skylight. Although each child shares a room with one or two others, the children gather every day on the bright green carpet of the large and cheerful anteroom.

On a couch lies Danielle de Jong, 5, wearing a white dress with blue dots, blue knee socks, white shoes, and a little gold ring on her left hand. Blue bows keep her long, blond hair neat. Her mother, Ellen, makes many of Danielle's clothes.

Danielle was born with a brain stem but no brain. Her head is the size of a basketball, and it is constantly filling with an overabundance of spinal fluid that must be drained regularly. Her face looks like a small mask.

"To me she is a vision of loveliness," Ellen de Jong says. "We have surrounded her with beautiful things. We have dressed her like a little princess. These are a few little things we can do for her. I get a lot of joy from that."

Despite her doctors' efforts, the pressure created by the spinal fluid in Danielle's skull was so bad that she could no longer see. Seizures gripped her body from time to time. And she had trouble breathing. When I last saw her, doctors gave her a year or so to live.

"She knew her mother," says Mrs. de Jong, "She had her own way of seeing and feeling me. She knew when she was in Mommy's lap."

The de Jongs lived miles away. But they visited Danielle at least twice a week.

"I've never felt she would be better off if she were gone," Mrs. de Jong says, remembering those days.

"She has given us a lot. We've been able to love her. She has a life worth living. It will be devastating to me when she goes. I want happy moments to remember when she is gone."

"We regard the patient as part of the family," says Dr. Burton Grebin, the hospice's director. The PCU has overnight accommodations for parents. Most important, there is a staff upon whom the parents can lean for emotional support.

"This place is filled with love," says Mrs. Lillian Baumann of Athens, New York. Her son, Carter, 21, had been hospitalized at St. Mary's for 11 years. He had been in the PCU since it opened in 1984.

Carter was a healthy, bright boy who loved sports and music. But in his 9th year, he began to lose his hearing. Medical diagnosis found a neurological disease that destroys a part of the brain. Month by month, Carter's faculties declined. First, walking became slow, then difficult, then impossible. Later, his sight declined. His speech and thinking abilities suffered next. For a while he watched baseball on TV, which he loved. But, bedridden and blind, he could only smile when someone sang "Take Me Out to the Ball Game."

"His smile and laughter could light up a room," says his mother. "Seeing the good care he got here, I could go back to a normal life. This is one of the greatest, most important elements—not just the care they give your child but the trust you feel. It allows you to relax."

Dr. Grebin, himself the father of two healthy sons, says he chose to take care of dying children because he met such a child in a large hospital during his medical training, a child with cystic fibrosis. She was 14 and alone in her room.

Dr. Grebin recalls, "She called to me and said, 'I know I am dying, and I don't want to die alone this way.' I told her I would come back. She started crying out, 'Please don't let me die this way.' I heard her voice trailing off. She had no family member present. I should have stayed at her bedside. I could have been the warmth of human presence. I came back—too late. She died alone. It made me sad."

This often happens to children in hospitals. In their last days, people in gowns and masks poke them, take blood, examine them, shoot them full of powerful chemicals. Few people (if any) spend time talking or singing to them or holding them.

Besides being more humane, the PCU costs only $325 a day for each child, compared with $700 a day or more in a general hospital in the New York area.

Before the age of 5, few children have any conception of what death is. So, the dying youngsters are content with talking, singing, and holding. As they get older, their views become more realistic, and they become frightened by death.

Dr. Grebin speaks of a 6-year-old girl with leukemia who told him, "I know I am dying. I know what it means. They dig a big hole. They throw you in the hole. They cover you up with dirt, and they walk all over you. Now get out of my room."

A couple of days later, he brought her some brightly colored pens and started to draw. Soon the little girl was drawing, too. In the days that followed, the subject of death did not arise again. She had somehow made peace with her thoughts.

Music also helps. Angela Leale, St. Mary's music therapist, sings to each child for up to 45 minutes twice a week. Danny Faith responds with his radiant smile. Danielle de Jong sighs deeply at the end of the song. For Carter Baumann, the music helps him fall asleep. "I use the rhythm of their breathing to pace the music," Ms. Leale says. "Sometimes they can follow along and sing along in their own way."

Because these children have hopeless conditions, at St. Mary's no cure is attempted. To get a child admitted, parents must sign an agreement that if the patient's heart or breathing stops, the doctors and nurses will not use high-tech medicine to bring back the heart and lungs. Medication for pain is provided, and pneumonia and other infections are treated; the hospital also tries to improve the child's ability to function.

Sandra Jackson, director of rehabilitation, works to improve the quality of life. "I gave Danny Faith an upright seat so that he can have toys in front of him," she says. She worked hard to stretch the muscles of a 3-year-old stricken with an incurable disease that usually kills by age 3. "He now has an infant walker," she says. "He can propel himself around the room."

Dr. Grebin and his staff provide the same kind of services to dying children who can be treated at home. Home care lowers the cost and, more important, keeps the child with caring parents and siblings.

But many children cannot go home. Anthony Donatich and his wife, Noreen, say they never could have managed Patrick at home. He was born with an underdeveloped brain and a defect in the skull. "St. Mary's was a miracle for us," says Anthony. "Patrick needed dressing changes every 3 to 4 hours. The way they cared for Patrick! It was so gentle. We felt comfortable going home, and the hardest thing is to leave."

In his 2nd year, Patrick died. But St. Mary's continued to work with the Donatiches, helping them cope with their loss. Paul Alexander Klincewicz, the hospital's bereavement specialist, brings together the parents of children who died. "Parents feel guilty about not being there when the child dies," he says. "Each person finds his own solution to the devastating feelings. Talking it out with other parents in the same situation helps the grieving process."

"We have moved from curing to caring," Dr. Grebin reflects, "When you can't cure, what else do you have to offer people? The children are alive."

For more information, write to Children's Hospice International, 1101 King Street, Suite 131, Alexandria, Virginia 22314.

INDEX